Personalized Medicine for Parkinson's Disease: New Concepts and Future of Individualized Management

Personalized Medicine for Parkinson's Disease: New Concepts and Future of Individualized Management

Editors

Nataliya Titova
K. Ray Chaudhuri

MDPI • Basel • Beijing • Wuhan • Barcelona • Belgrade • Manchester • Tokyo • Cluj • Tianjin

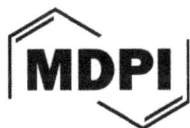

Editors

Nataliya Titova
Department of Neurology,
Neurosurgery and Medical
Genetics
N.I. Pirogov Russian National
Research Medical University,
The Ministry of Health of the
Russian Federation
Moscow
Russia

K. Ray Chaudhuri
Department of Basic &
Clinical Neuroscience
King's College London
London
United Kingdom

Editorial Office
MDPI
St. Alban-Anlage 66
4052 Basel, Switzerland

This is a reprint of articles from the Special Issue published online in the open access journal *Journal of Personalized Medicine* (ISSN 2075-4426) (available at: www.mdpi.com/journal/jpm/special_issues/new_concepts).

For citation purposes, cite each article independently as indicated on the article page online and as indicated below:

LastName, A.A.; LastName, B.B.; LastName, C.C. Article Title. *Journal Name* **Year**, *Volume Number*, Page Range.

ISBN 978-3-0365-6212-4 (Hbk)
ISBN 978-3-0365-6211-7 (PDF)

© 2023 by the authors. Articles in this book are Open Access and distributed under the Creative Commons Attribution (CC BY) license, which allows users to download, copy and build upon published articles, as long as the author and publisher are properly credited, which ensures maximum dissemination and a wider impact of our publications.

The book as a whole is distributed by MDPI under the terms and conditions of the Creative Commons license CC BY-NC-ND.

Contents

About the Editors vii

Kallol Ray Chaudhuri, Nataliya Titova, Mubasher A. Qamar, Iulia Murășan and Cristian Falup-Pecurariu
The Dashboard Vitals of Parkinson's: Not to Be Missed Yet an Unmet Need
Reprinted from: *J. Pers. Med.* **2022**, 12, 1994, doi:10.3390/jpm12121994 1

Vinod Metta, Huzaifa Ibrahim, Tom Loney, Hani T. S. Benamer, Ali Alhawai and Dananir Almuhairi et al.
First Two-Year Observational Exploratory Real Life Clinical Phenotyping, and Societal Impact Study of Parkinson's Disease in Emiratis and Expatriate Population of United Arab Emirates 2019–2021: The EmPark Study
Reprinted from: *J. Pers. Med.* **2022**, 12, 1300, doi:10.3390/jpm12081300 9

Ștefania Diaconu and Cristian Falup-Pecurariu
Personalized Assessment of Insomnia and Sleep Quality in Patients with Parkinson's Disease
Reprinted from: *J. Pers. Med.* **2022**, 12, 322, doi:10.3390/jpm12020322 23

Anna Fedosova, Nataliya Titova, Zarema Kokaeva, Natalia Shipilova, Elena Katunina and Eugene Klimov
Genetic Markers as Risk Factors for the Development of Impulsive-Compulsive Behaviors in Patients with Parkinson's Disease Receiving Dopaminergic Therapy
Reprinted from: *J. Pers. Med.* **2021**, 11, 1321, doi:10.3390/jpm11121321 39

Thomas F. Tropea and Alice Chen-Plotkin
Are Parkinson's Disease Patients the Ideal Preclinical Population for Alzheimer's Disease Therapeutics?
Reprinted from: *J. Pers. Med.* **2021**, 11, 834, doi:10.3390/jpm11090834 57

Valentina Leta, Haidar S. Dafsari, Anna Sauerbier, Vinod Metta, Nataliya Titova and Lars Timmermann et al.
Personalised Advanced Therapies in Parkinson's Disease: The Role of Non-Motor Symptoms Profile
Reprinted from: *J. Pers. Med.* **2021**, 11, 773, doi:10.3390/jpm11080773 65

Valentina Varalta, Paola Poiese, Serena Recchia, Barbara Montagnana, Cristina Fonte and Mirko Filippetti et al.
Physiotherapy versus Consecutive Physiotherapy and Cognitive Treatment in People with Parkinson's Disease: A Pilot Randomized Cross-Over Study
Reprinted from: *J. Pers. Med.* **2021**, 11, 687, doi:10.3390/jpm11080687 77

Vinod Metta, Lucia Batzu, Valentina Leta, Dhaval Trivedi, Aleksandra Powdleska and Kandadai Rukmini Mridula et al.
Parkinson's Disease: Personalized Pathway of Care for Device-Aided Therapies (DAT) and the Role of Continuous Objective Monitoring (COM) Using Wearable Sensors
Reprinted from: *J. Pers. Med.* **2021**, 11, 680, doi:10.3390/jpm11070680 89

Takayasu Mishima, Shinsuke Fujioka, Takashi Morishita, Tooru Inoue and Yoshio Tsuboi
Personalized Medicine in Parkinson's Disease: New Options for Advanced Treatments
Reprinted from: *J. Pers. Med.* **2021**, 11, 650, doi:10.3390/jpm11070650 109

Itsasne Sanchez-Luengos, Yolanda Balboa-Bandeira, Olaia Lucas-Jiménez, Natalia Ojeda, Javier Peña and Naroa Ibarretxe-Bilbao
Effectiveness of Cognitive Rehabilitation in Parkinson's Disease: A Systematic Review and Meta-Analysis
Reprinted from: *J. Pers. Med.* **2021**, *11*, 429, doi:10.3390/jpm11050429 125

Xylena Reed, Artur Schumacher-Schuh, Jing Hu and Sara Bandres-Ciga
Advancing Personalized Medicine in Common Forms of Parkinson's Disease through Genetics: Current Therapeutics and the Future of Individualized Management
Reprinted from: *J. Pers. Med.* **2021**, *11*, 169, doi:10.3390/jpm11030169 145

Nupur Nag, Xin Lin, Maggie Yu, Steve Simpson-Yap, George A. Jelinek and Sandra L. Neate et al.
Assessing Lifestyle Behaviours of People Living with Neurological Conditions: A Panoramic View of Community Dwelling Australians from 2007–2018
Reprinted from: *J. Pers. Med.* **2021**, *11*, 144, doi:10.3390/jpm11020144 157

Piyush Varma, Lakshanaa Narayan, Jane Alty, Virginia Painter and Chandrasekhara Padmakumar
An Innovative Personalised Management Program for Older Adults with Parkinson's Disease: New Concepts and Future Directions
Reprinted from: *J. Pers. Med.* **2021**, *11*, 43, doi:10.3390/jpm11010043 169

Federica Piras, Daniela Vecchio, Francesca Assogna, Clelia Pellicano, Valentina Ciullo and Nerisa Banaj et al.
Cerebellar GABA Levels and Cognitive Interference in Parkinson's Disease and Healthy Comparators
Reprinted from: *J. Pers. Med.* **2020**, *11*, 16, doi:10.3390/jpm11010016 177

João Botelho, Patrícia Lyra, Luís Proença, Catarina Godinho, José João Mendes and Vanessa Machado
Relationship between Blood and Standard Biochemistry Levels with Periodontitis in Parkinson's Disease Patients: Data from the NHANES 2011–2012
Reprinted from: *J. Pers. Med.* **2020**, *10*, 69, doi:10.3390/jpm10030069 193

About the Editors

Nataliya Titova

Dr. Nataliya Titova is currently an Associate Professor and consulting Neurologist in the Department of Neurology, Neurosurgery and Medical Genetics at the Federal State Budgetary Educational Institution of Higher Education .I. Pirogov Russian National Research Medical Universityof the Ministry of Healthcare of the Russian Federation in Moscow. She graduated from Pirogov Russian National Research Medical University in Moscow and obtained her Ph.D. with a thesis on controlled cross-sectional and prospective study on clinical and neurophysiological evaluation of patients with de novo Parkinson's disease (PD). She, thereafter, trained to become a specialist in movement disorders and a parkinsonologist. Dr. Titova is also part of the overseas research faculty at the Parkinson Foundation International Parkinson Centre of Excellence at Kings College Hospital in London. She is an active teacher and researcher in the field of PD and related conditions and has a special interest in PD non-motor pathophysiology, genetics, and biomarker-driven assessment of natural history and endophenotypes. She is leading an international programme on developing strategies for personalised medicine in PD.

K. Ray Chaudhuri

Professor K. Ray Chaudhuri is Professor of Neurology/Movement Disorders at King's College Hospital and King's College London and the Medical Director of the Parkinson Foundation International Centre of Excellence at King's College.

He is internationally known for pioneering modern care for people with Parkinson's particularly advanced therapies in addition to care for restless legs syndrome. He is the founding Chairman of the International Movement Disorders Society Non-motor Study Group and member MDS-ES Education and palliative care committee and ex Chair of the MDS Membership and Public Relations committee as well as member MDS congress scientific programme committee (2013–2017).

He is the founding and consulting editor and ex editor-in-chief of the Nature group *Nature Parkinson's* journal (2020 Impact Factor 8.8), as well as Guest Editor for Special Issues of Frontiers in Neurology, *Journal of Personalised Medicine* (Impact Factor 4.8), Movement Disorders in Older Adults (Geriatrics) and Journal of Parkinson's Disease, reviewer for all mainstream Movement Disorders journals as well as JAMA, Neurology, Annals of Neurology, BMJ, Brain, Lancet and JNNP.

He won the Andrew Wilson Prize for services to RLS patients by RLS:UK, William Koller Memorial Fund Award by MDS, the 2018 Van Andel award in the USA for outstanding nonmotor research contribution in the field of nonmotor Parkinson, as well as NIHR/Royal College of Physicians London award for outstanding research leadership in 2017.

In 2020, he was elected as lead for Equality Diversity charter for NIHR London South Applied Research Collaboration (ARC) and was elected as a Honorary Member for the Movement Disorders Society in 2021. In 2022, he was awarded UK NHS Gold merit clinical impact award and is currently ranked 6th in the world and top from the UK for publications related to Parkinson's (Expertscape-Parkinson's disease).

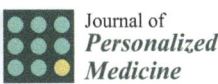

Editorial

The Dashboard Vitals of Parkinson's: Not to Be Missed Yet an Unmet Need

Kallol Ray Chaudhuri [1,2,*], Nataliya Titova [3,4], Mubasher A. Qamar [1,2], Iulia Murășan [5] and Cristian Falup-Pecurariu [5,6]

1. Institute of Psychiatry, Psychology & Neuroscience, Department of Basic & Clinical Neuroscience, Division of Neuroscience, King's College London, London SE5 9RT, UK
2. Parkinson Foundation Centre of Excellence in Care and Research, King's College Hospital NHS Foundation Trust, London SE5 9RS, UK
3. Department of Neurology, Neurosurgery and Medical Genetics, Federal State Autonomous Educational Institution of Higher Education, N.I. Pirogov Russian National Research Medical University, The Ministry of Health of the Russian Federation, 117997 Moscow, Russia
4. Department of Neurodegenerative Diseases, Federal State Budgetary Institution, Federal Center of Brain Research and Neurotechnologies, The Federal Medical Biological Agency, 117997 Moscow, Russia
5. Faculty of Medicine, Transilvania University of Brașov, 500036 Brașov, Romania
6. Department of Neurology, County Clinic Hospital, 500365 Brașov, Romania
* Correspondence: ray.chaudhuri@kcl.ac.uk; Tel.: +44-20-299-7154

1. Commentary

The vitals of Parkinson's disease (PD) address the often-ignored symptoms, which are considered either peripheral to the central core of motor symptoms of PD or secondary symptoms, which, nevertheless, have a key role in the quality of life (QoL) and wellness of people with Parkinson's (PwP) [1]. Unmet needs in PwP have recently been discussed, with many being related to motor symptoms and, specifically, non-motor symptoms (NMSs), which continue to pose a major challenge to PwP and their clinicians [2]. In addition, several other factors related to enablers of PD expression, progression, as well as co-morbidities and co-medication issues compound the wellness of PwP and we proposed all PwP to have a dashboard, whereby clinical assessment for these symptoms must be noted and managed as bespoke to the individual person, a key element in modern personalized medicine for PD [3,4].

The key elements of the vitals to form a dashboard for PwP are shown in Figure 1. These include the essential motor assessment, which is completed in almost all clinics as the initial evaluation in consultations. Motor function can be graded by clinical examination and assigning the Hoehn and Yahr (H&Y) staging [5], which, despite its clinimetric drawbacks, continues to be the most widely used clinical assessment for tangible and real-life motor assessment of PD and has stood the test of time. If time permits and there is capacity, then detailed motor examinations are possible using the Scales for Outcomes in PD (SCOPA)-motor [6], Movement Disorder Society Unified PD Rating scale (MDS-UPDRS) [7], or even the older UPDRS parts 3 and 4 [8]. In the future, PD-validated wearable monitoring scores with sensors, such as Parkinson kinetograph (PKG), could be added [9,10].

Then, there is the burden of NMS assessments, which can be carried out and graded using either the validated NMS Questionnaire (NMS Quest) or, if time permits, utilizing the PD-NMS scale (NMSS) [11–14]. NMS burden (NMSB) should be performed for every patient and graded, alongside the patients and their caregivers, rating their top named bothersome NMS. NMSB is contributed to by a range of NMS, from cognitive issues, neuropsychiatric problems, such as depression, apathy, and anxiety, to sleep dysfunction, hyposmia, bladder, bowel, and upper gastrointestinal dysfunction, such as the dribbling of saliva. NMSB has a direct correlation with QoL and a guide to using the NMS Quest in the clinic has also been published. NMSB score should be integral to the dashboard and ideally measured on a yearly basis [15].

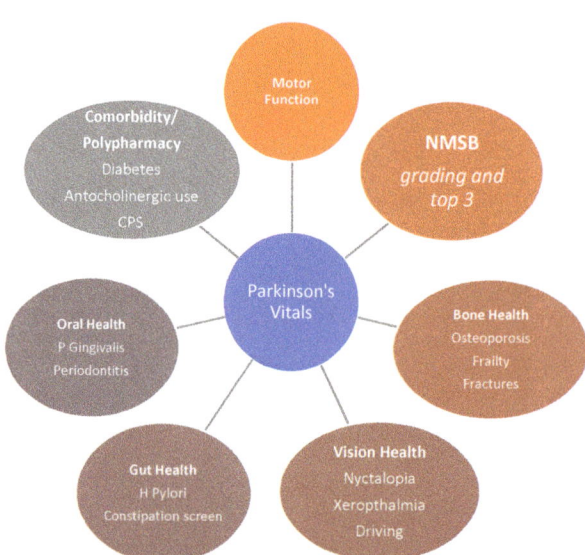

Figure 1. A diagram of the essential "vitals" to be considered in Parkinson's disease which should form a dashboard of symptoms to be considered and managed in every person with Parkinson's. NMSB non-motor symptom burden; H Pylori Helicobacter pylori; P Gingivalis porphyromonas gingivalis; CPS comorbidity polypharmacy score.

Vision is a critical aspect of living with PD and is rarely formally addressed in a PD clinic. A range of visual problems can occur in PD and these have been explored in several studies [16–20]. Vision assessment is important for PwP who continue to drive and, in this respect, night blindness (nyctalopia) and convergence insufficiency are important. Subsequently, a patient may have significant discomfort related to dry eyes (xeropthalmia), which is treatable with eye drops as well as glaucoma. The NMS Quest also allows for declaration of diplopia, which is common in PD and may be related to dyskinesias or convergence insufficiency. Nyctalopia may be related to vitamin A deficiency and may require night-time bedroom lighting to prevent falls at night-time should the patient need to get out of bed, for instance, to go to the toilet. Significant issues need a referral to an ophthalmologist [21].

Bone health is an integral aspect of Parkinson's wellness and relates to a very high incidence of osteoporosis or osteopenia in PD and related risk of fractures with falls and frailty as well as subsequent risk of hospitalization. A global longitudinal study of osteoporosis in women, the GLOW study, reported PD to be the strongest and most robust contributor to risk of fractures compared with other studied factors [22]. Motor dysfunction, frailty, gait impairment and freezing, postural instability, diphasic or troublesome dyskinesias and falls, polypharmacy, and reduced bone density contribute towards the increased risk of fracture in PD [23–26]. Vitamin D deficiency along with disease duration and severity, age, and low body mass index (BMI) with secondary hyperparathyroidism may also contribute to low bone density and need to be evaluated in all PwP periodically and added to the dashboard [22].

When assessing PwP holistically, the issue of weight is often ignored in clinical consultations, although blood pressure, height, and weight are often routinely collected in the clinic. Low body weight poses a specific challenge in PD and a low body weight phenotype in PD, the Park-weight phenotype, has been proposed to have a high risk of dyskinesias, as well as possible links with cognitive dysfunction and hyposmia [27–29]. Weight and BMI, therefore, need to be noted at baseline in all PD cases and routinely charted for monitoring. Unexplained weight loss is a question asked in the NMS Quest and, in addition, may be a problem with some medications, such as intrajejunal levodopa infusion, as well as those with severe dyskinesias. Unexplained weight loss coupled with rising frailty has also been linked to future cognitive dysfunction and, therefore, also may have prognostic consequences [30,31].

Gut and oral health is another important enabler of wellness and health in PD and constitutes the important "vital" aspect for the dashboard. Gut dysfunction in PD is well documented and ranges from upper gastrointestinal dysfunction, such as dysphagia and delayed gastric emptying, to constipation [32].

While many of these symptoms are flagged up in the NMS Quest and constitute part of the NMSB, some need key and focused attention as they are often ignored in clinics. These include:

1. Specific attention and query about oral health, gum, and gingivitis and an examination by a dentist in all cases. Infection with porphyromonas gingivalis, a Gram-negative anaerobic bacterium, can cause chronic periodontitis and possibly systemic inflammation, together with gingipains, and may have an overall effect on worsening of the Parkinsonian state and even pathogenesis [33]. A recent study suggested that high serum C-reactive protein (CRP) level may be a good indicator of periodontitis and should trigger a referral to a dentist and needs to feature in the dashboard [34].
2. Delayed oral drug absorption as well as clinical phenomena of "delayed on" or "no on" or even dyskinesias-related erratic absorption may relate to delayed gastric emptying and "gastric blocks". Helicobacter pylori (H Pylori) infection, a Gram-negative bacteria, in the stomach is common in PD and several case-control studies report that prevalence of H Pylori infection is five-times higher in older PD patients, specifically those over 80 years of age, and up to three-times higher in PD patients compared to healthy individuals [35].
3. Eradication of H Pylori infection using combined antibiotic therapies can improve bioavailability and pharmacokinetics of levodopa and drug bioavailability by increasing its absorption by 21 to 54%, despite one single-centre negative study. The latter study, however, did not address blood levels of levodopa and instead focused on quality of life and motor scores [36]. Any patient with delayed time to 'ON' after oral levodopa absorption, as well as upper gastrointestinal symptoms of heartburn, bloating, and reflux, must have H Pylori infection tested and, if positive, be treated [37].
4. Severe constipation may arise from chronic dehydration and impacted faeces. This also interferes with oral drug absorption and a simple abdominal X-ray may show dilated bowel loops and impacted faeces [38,39]. Treatment with regular laxatives and even an enema may then be warranted, as part of the vitals, in relevant cases.

Finally, there is the issue of comorbidity- and medication-related enablers of health, such as impulse control disorders (ICD) as well as medication management. Diabetes mellitus has been proposed to be a risk factor of PD and comorbid diabetes can affect PD [40–42]. Consequently, blood glucose is often listed, along with urate, as associates in the revised MDS criteria for PD, while antidiabetic drugs are being examined for possible neuroprotection in PD [43]. Diabetes is a risk factor for worsening neurodegeneration, delayed gastric emptying as well as cognitive dysfunction and, hence, should be actively listed in the dashboard [44]. Other important co-morbidities, which have been proposed as risk factors for PD, also include REM Sleep behaviour disorder (RBD), with 80% of RBD patients developing neurodegenerative diseases, such as PD [45,46]. Development of PD Dementia (PDD) has been proposed to be greater in those with higher UPDRS scores, male gender, have hypertension, and, most commonly, have a history of neuropsychiatric disorders [47]. As such, greater emphasis should be on managing cognitive and psychological disorders in PwP given the risk of significant progression in PD that can occur in these cohorts; as such, the dashboard includes MoCa and MDS NMS, both of which aid in the surveillance of the emergence and presence of psychiatric and other neurological comorbidities.

Polypharmacy is common in PD related to comorbidities and risks side effects, which includes ICD with dopaminergic drugs, specifically dopamine agonists. Withdrawal of dopaminergic drugs, specifically dopamine agonists, also needs to follow a graded pattern to avoid dopamine agonist withdrawal syndrome [48,49]. The use of dopaminergic drugs carries with it side effects, which must be reviewed in each consultation with PwP, to ensure adequate support and holistic care are provided. Side effects include ICD, which can range from hypersexuality, gambling, binge eating, or impulsively, and other side effects, including neuropsychiatric (hallucinations, delusions) and dyskinesias [50,51]. The dashboard includes assessment of these concurrently during consultation (see Figure 2). Furthermore, specific attention needs to be given to anticholinergic drugs and a reference to the anticholinergic index of all drugs being given to PwP, as these drugs should not be used in the cholinergic subtype of PD and generally can worsen cognition and gait in PD. In this respect, a comorbidity polypharmacy score (CPS), which is defined as the sum of baseline medication and all known comorbidities, may be useful, and the severity of CPS has been traditionally stratified as mild (CPS 0–7), moderate (8–14), severe (15–21), and morbid ($\geq$22 points). Pill burden, comorbidity, and swallowing all come into play in this respect [52,53].

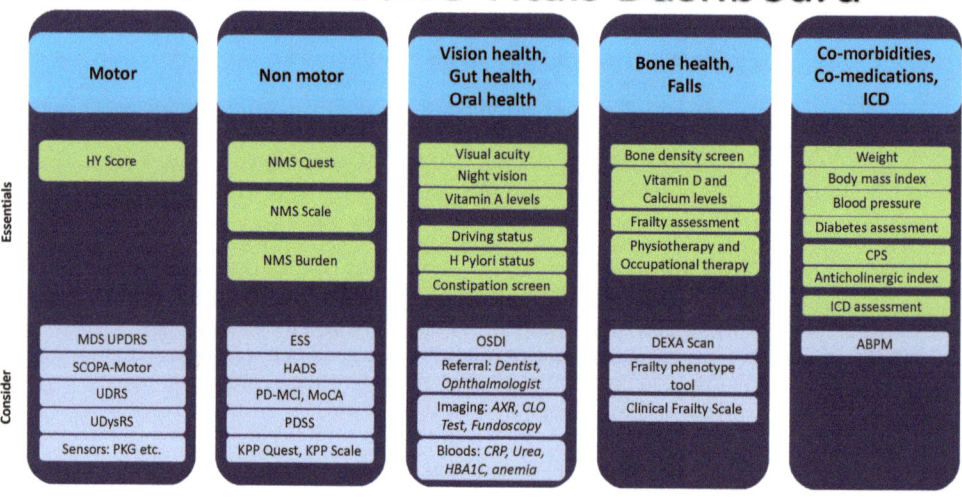

Figure 2. A proposed "Parkinson's vitals dashboard" comprising the vitals and some specific measures that should be undertaken. Divided into the *essentials* which should be performed annually at review and *consider* some optional investigations and assessments if time permits. ABPM ambulatory blood pressure monitoring; AXR abdominal X-ray; CLO campylobacter-like organism test; CPS co-morbidities polypharmacy score; CRP C-reactive protein; DEXA dual energy X-ray absorptiometry scan; ESS Epworth Sleepiness Scale; HADS Hospital anxiety and depression scale; HY Hoehn and Yahr, H Pylori helicobacter pylori; ICD impulse control disorder; KPP King's Parkinson's Pain; MCI mild cognitive impairment; MDS-UPDRS Movement disorder society unified Parkinson's disease rating scale; MoCA Montreal Cognitive Assessment; NMS nonmotor symptoms; NMS Quest NMS questionnaire; OSDI Ocular Surface Disease Index; PDSS PD Sleep Scale; PKG Parkinson's kinetograph; SCOPA-motor Scales for outcomes in Parkinson's disease motor function; UDRS unified dystonia rating scale; UDysRS unified dyskinesia rating scale.

2. Conclusions

A dashboard of the vital symptoms, which are enablers of wellness in PD, needs to be considered in every patient with PD, regardless of stage and setting, see Figure 2. The process is simple and needs to be preferably recorded on an annual basis, as part of their regular review. Attention to these vitals would ensure continuing good care for PwP and function as the cornerstone of a holistic personalised modern symptom-driven management strategy.

Author Contributions: Conceptualization, K.R.C., N.T., M.A.Q.; methodology, K.R.C., N.T., M.A.Q.; validation, K.R.C., N.T., M.A.Q., I.M., C.F.-P.; formal analysis, N.T., M.A.Q.; investigation, K.R.C., N.T., M.A.Q., I.M., C.F.-P.; data curation K.R.C., N.T., M.A.Q., I.M., C.F.-P.; writing—original draft preparation, K.R.C., N.T., M.A.Q.; writing—review and editing, K.R.C., N.T., M.A.Q., I.M., C.F.-P.; visualization, K.R.C., N.T., M.A.Q., I.M., C.F.-P.; supervision, K.R.C., N.T., M.A.Q., I.M., C.F.-P.; project administration, K.R.C., N.T., M.A.Q. All authors have read and agreed to the published version of the manuscript.

Funding: This research received no external funding.

Conflicts of Interest: The authors declare no conflict of interest.

References

1. Subramanian, I.; Brindle, S.; Perepezko, K.; Chaudhuri, K.R. Wellness, sexual health, and nonmotor Parkinson's. *Int. Rev. Neurobiol.* **2022**, *162*, 171–184. [CrossRef] [PubMed]
2. LeWitt, P.A.; Chaudhuri, K.R. Unmet needs in Parkinson disease: Motor and non-motor. *Park. Relat. Disord.* **2020**, *80*, S7–S12. [CrossRef] [PubMed]
3. Titova, N.; Chaudhuri, K.R. Personalized Medicine and Nonmotor Symptoms in Parkinson's Disease. *Int. Rev. Neurobiol.* **2017**, *134*, 1257–1281. [CrossRef]
4. Titova, N.; Chaudhuri, K.R. Personalized medicine in Parkinson's disease: Time to be precise. *Mov. Disord.* **2017**, *32*, 1147–1154. [CrossRef] [PubMed]
5. Hoehn, M.M.; Yahr, M.D. Parkinsonism: Onset, progression and mortality. *Neurology* **1967**, *17*, 427–442. [CrossRef]
6. Martínez-Martín, P.; Benito-León, J.; Burguera, J.A.; Castro, A.; Linazasoro, G.; Martínez-Castrillo, J.C.; Valldeoriola, F.; Vázquez, A.; Vivancos, F.; del Val, J.; et al. The SCOPA-Motor Scale for assessment of Parkinson's disease is a consistent and valid measure. *J. Clin. Epidemiol.* **2005**, *58*, 674–679. [CrossRef]
7. Goetz, C.G.; Tilley, B.C.; Shaftman, S.R.; Stebbins, G.T.; Fahn, S.; Martinez-Martin, P.; Poewe, W.; Sampaio, C.; Stern, M.B.; Dodel, R.; et al. Movement Disorder Society-sponsored revision of the Unified Parkinson's Disease Rating Scale (MDS-UPDRS): Scale presentation and clinimetric testing results. *Mov. Disord.* **2008**, *23*, 2129–2170. [CrossRef]
8. Disease, M.D.S.T.F.o.R.S.f.P.s. The Unified Parkinson's Disease Rating Scale (UPDRS): Status and recommendations. *Mov. Disord.* **2003**, *18*, 738–750. [CrossRef]
9. Joshi, R.; Bronstein, J.M.; Keener, A.; Alcazar, J.; Yang, D.D.; Joshi, M.; Hermanowicz, N. PKG Movement Recording System Use Shows Promise in Routine Clinical Care of Patients With Parkinson's Disease. *Front. Neurol.* **2019**, *10*, 1027. [CrossRef]
10. Pahwa, R.; Bergquist, F.; Horne, M.; Minshall, M.E. Objective measurement in Parkinson's disease: A descriptive analysis of Parkinson's symptom scores from a large population of patients across the world using the Personal KinetiGraph®. *J. Clin. Mov. Disord.* **2020**, *7*, 5. [CrossRef]
11. Romenets, S.R.; Wolfson, C.; Galatas, C.; Pelletier, A.; Altman, R.; Wadup, L.; Postuma, R.B. Validation of the non-motor symptoms questionnaire (NMS-Quest). *Park. Relat. Disord.* **2012**, *18*, 54–58. [CrossRef] [PubMed]
12. Martinez-Martin, P.; Ray Chaudhuri, K. Comprehensive grading of Parkinson's disease using motor and non-motor assessments: Addressing a key unmet need. *Expert Rev. Neurother.* **2018**, *18*, 41–50. [CrossRef] [PubMed]
13. Sauerbier, A.; Qamar, M.A.; Rajah, T.; Chaudhuri, K.R. New concepts in the pathogenesis and presentation of Parkinson's disease. *Clin. Med.* **2016**, *16*, 365–370. [CrossRef]
14. Chaudhuri, K.R.; Sauerbier, A.; Rojo, J.M.; Sethi, K.; Schapira, A.H.; Brown, R.G.; Antonini, A.; Stocchi, F.; Odin, P.; Bhattacharya, K.; et al. The burden of non-motor symptoms in Parkinson's disease using a self-completed non-motor questionnaire: A simple grading system. *Park. Relat. Disord.* **2015**, *21*, 287–291. [CrossRef] [PubMed]
15. Todorova, A.; Martin, A.; Chaudhuri, K.R. How Do I Examine Nonmotor Aspects of Parkinson's Disease? What Not to Miss and What to Ignore? *Mov. Disord. Clin. Pract.* **2014**, *1*, 274. [CrossRef]
16. Ekker, M.S.; Janssen, S.; Seppi, K.; Poewe, W.; de Vries, N.M.; Theelen, T.; Nonnekes, J.; Bloem, B.R. Ocular and visual disorders in Parkinson's disease: Common but frequently overlooked. *Park. Relat. Disord.* **2017**, *40*, 1–10. [CrossRef]
17. Armstrong, R.A. Visual Dysfunction in Parkinson's Disease. *Int. Rev. Neurobiol.* **2017**, *134*, 921–946. [CrossRef]
18. Armstrong, R.A. Oculo-Visual Dysfunction in Parkinson's Disease. *J. Parkinsons. Dis.* **2015**, *5*, 715–726. [CrossRef]

19. Borm, C.; Werkmann, M.; Visser, F.; Peball, M.; Putz, D.; Seppi, K.; Poewe, W.; Notting, I.C.; Vlaar, A.; Theelen, T.; et al. Towards seeing the visual impairments in Parkinson's disease: Protocol for a multicentre observational, cross-sectional study. *BMC Neurol.* **2019**, *19*, 141. [CrossRef]
20. Meppelink, A.M.; de Jong, B.M.; Renken, R.; Leenders, K.L.; Cornelissen, F.W.; van Laar, T. Impaired visual processing preceding image recognition in Parkinson's disease patients with visual hallucinations. *Brain* **2009**, *132*, 2980–2993. [CrossRef]
21. Sauerbier, A.; Ray Chaudhuri, K. Parkinson's disease and vision. *Basal Ganglia* **2013**, *3*, 159–163. [CrossRef]
22. Dennison, E.M.; Compston, J.E.; Flahive, J.; Siris, E.S.; Gehlbach, S.H.; Adachi, J.D.; Boonen, S.; Chapurlat, R.; Díez-Pérez, A.; Anderson, F.A., Jr.; et al. Effect of co-morbidities on fracture risk: Findings from the Global Longitudinal Study of Osteoporosis in Women (GLOW). *Bone* **2012**, *50*, 1288–1293. [CrossRef] [PubMed]
23. Bezza, A.; Ouzzif, Z.; Naji, H.; Achemlal, L.; Mounach, A.; Nouijai, M.; Bourazza, A.; Mossadeq, R.; El Maghraoui, A. Prevalence and risk factors of osteoporosis in patients with Parkinson's disease. *Rheumatol. Int.* **2008**, *28*, 1205–1209. [CrossRef] [PubMed]
24. Abou-Raya, S.; Helmii, M.; Abou-Raya, A. Bone and mineral metabolism in older adults with Parkinson's disease. *Age Ageing* **2009**, *38*, 675–680. [CrossRef]
25. Wood, B.; Walker, R. Osteoporosis in Parkinson's disease. *Mov. Disord.* **2005**, *20*, 1636–1640. [CrossRef]
26. Can, N.U.; Alagöz, A.N. The Relationship Among Bone Mineral Density, Bone Biomarkers and Vitamin D Levels in Patients with Parkinson's Disease. *Clin. Lab.* **2020**, *66*, 8. [CrossRef]
27. Sharma, J.C.; Lewis, A. Weight in Parkinson's Disease: Phenotypical Significance. *Int. Rev. Neurobiol.* **2017**, *134*, 891–919. [CrossRef]
28. Sharma, J.C.; Vassallo, M. Prognostic significance of weight changes in Parkinson's disease: The Park-weight phenotype. *Neurodegener. Dis. Manag.* **2014**, *4*, 309–316. [CrossRef]
29. Lorefält, B.; Ganowiak, W.; Pålhagen, S.; Toss, G.; Unosson, M.; Granérus, A.K. Factors of importance for weight loss in elderly patients with Parkinson's disease. *Acta Neurol. Scand.* **2004**, *110*, 180–187. [CrossRef]
30. Urso, D.; van Wamelen, D.J.; Batzu, L.; Leta, V.; Staunton, J.; Pineda-Pardo, J.A.; Logroscino, G.; Sharma, J.; Ray Chaudhuri, K. Clinical trajectories and biomarkers for weight variability in early Parkinson's disease. *NPJ Parkinsons Dis.* **2022**, *8*, 95. [CrossRef]
31. Borda, M.G.; Pérez-Zepeda, M.U.; Jaramillo-Jimenez, A.; Chaudhuri, K.R.; Tovar-Rios, D.A.; Wallace, L.; Batzu, L.; Rockwood, K.; Tysnes, O.B.; Aarsland, D.; et al. Frailty in Parkinson's disease and its association with early dementia: A longitudinal study. *Park. Relat. Disord.* **2022**, *99*, 51–57. [CrossRef] [PubMed]
32. Metta, V.; Leta, V.; Mrudula, K.R.; Prashanth, L.K.; Goyal, V.; Borgohain, R.; Chung-Faye, G.; Chaudhuri, K.R. Gastrointestinal dysfunction in Parkinson's disease: Molecular pathology and implications of gut microbiome, probiotics, and fecal microbiota transplantation. *J. Neurol.* **2022**, *269*, 1154–1163. [CrossRef] [PubMed]
33. Auffret, M.; Meuric, V.; Boyer, E.; Bonnaure-Mallet, M.; Vérin, M. Oral Health Disorders in Parkinson's Disease: More than Meets the Eye. *J. Parkinsons Dis.* **2021**, *11*, 1507–1535. [CrossRef] [PubMed]
34. Lyra, P.; Botelho, J.; Machado, V.; Rota, S.; Walker, R.; Staunton, J.; Proença, L.; Chaudhuri, K.R.; Mendes, J.J. Self-reported periodontitis and C-reactive protein in Parkinson's disease: A cross-sectional study of two American cohorts. *NPJ Parkinsons Dis.* **2022**, *8*, 40. [CrossRef] [PubMed]
35. Çamcı, G.; Oğuz, S. Association between Parkinson's Disease and Helicobacter Pylori. *J. Clin. Neurol.* **2016**, *12*, 147–150. [CrossRef] [PubMed]
36. Tan, A.H.; Mahadeva, S.; Marras, C.; Thalha, A.M.; Kiew, C.K.; Yeat, C.M.; Ng, S.W.; Ang, S.P.; Chow, S.K.; Loke, M.F.; et al. Helicobacter pylori infection is associated with worse severity of Parkinson's disease. *Park. Relat. Disord.* **2015**, *21*, 221–225. [CrossRef]
37. Nyholm, D.; Hellström, P.M. Effects of Helicobacter pylori on Levodopa Pharmacokinetics. *J. Parkinsons Dis.* **2021**, *11*, 61–69. [CrossRef]
38. Frazzitta, G.; Ferrazzoli, D.; Folini, A.; Palamara, G.; Maestri, R. Severe Constipation in Parkinson's Disease and in Parkinsonisms: Prevalence and Affecting Factors. *Front. Neurol.* **2019**, *10*, 628. [CrossRef]
39. van Kessel, S.P.; de Jong, H.R.; Winkel, S.L.; van Leeuwen, S.S.; Nelemans, S.A.; Permentier, H.; Keshavarzian, A.; El Aidy, S. Gut bacterial deamination of residual levodopa medication for Parkinson's disease. *BMC Biol.* **2020**, *18*, 137. [CrossRef]
40. Chohan, H.; Senkevich, K.; Patel, R.K.; Bestwick, J.P.; Jacobs, B.M.; Bandres Ciga, S.; Gan-Or, Z.; Noyce, A.J. Type 2 Diabetes as a Determinant of Parkinson's Disease Risk and Progression. *Mov. Disord.* **2021**, *36*, 1420–1429. [CrossRef]
41. Brauer, R.; Wei, L.; Ma, T.; Athauda, D.; Girges, C.; Vijiaratnam, N.; Auld, G.; Whittlesea, C.; Wong, I.; Foltynie, T. Diabetes medications and risk of Parkinson's disease: A cohort study of patients with diabetes. *Brain* **2020**, *143*, 3067–3076. [CrossRef]
42. Xu, Q.; Park, Y.; Huang, X.; Hollenbeck, A.; Blair, A.; Schatzkin, A.; Chen, H. Diabetes and risk of Parkinson's disease. *Diabetes Care* **2011**, *34*, 910–915. [CrossRef] [PubMed]
43. Sportelli, C.; Urso, D.; Jenner, P.; Chaudhuri, K.R. Metformin as a Potential Neuroprotective Agent in Prodromal Parkinson's Disease-Viewpoint. *Front. Neurol.* **2020**, *11*, 556. [CrossRef] [PubMed]
44. Cereda, E.; Barichella, M.; Pedrolli, C.; Klersy, C.; Cassani, E.; Caccialanza, R.; Pezzoli, G. Diabetes and risk of Parkinson's disease: A systematic review and meta-analysis. *Diabetes Care* **2011**, *34*, 2614–2623. [CrossRef] [PubMed]
45. Postuma, R.B.; Gagnon, J.F.; Bertrand, J.A.; Génier Marchand, D.; Montplaisir, J.Y. Parkinson risk in idiopathic REM sleep behavior disorder: Preparing for neuroprotective trials. *Neurology* **2015**, *84*, 1104–1113. [CrossRef]

46. Schenck, C.H.; Montplaisir, J.Y.; Frauscher, B.; Hogl, B.; Gagnon, J.F.; Postuma, R.; Sonka, K.; Jennum, P.; Partinen, M.; Arnulf, I.; et al. Rapid eye movement sleep behavior disorder: Devising controlled active treatment studies for symptomatic and neuroprotective therapy–a consensus statement from the International Rapid Eye Movement Sleep Behavior Disorder Study Group. *Sleep Med.* **2013**, *14*, 795–806. [CrossRef]
47. Xu, Y.; Yang, J.; Shang, H. Meta-analysis of risk factors for Parkinson's disease dementia. *Transl. Neurodegener.* **2016**, *5*, 11. [CrossRef]
48. Pondal, M.; Marras, C.; Miyasaki, J.; Moro, E.; Armstrong, M.J.; Strafella, A.P.; Shah, B.B.; Fox, S.; Prashanth, L.K.; Phielipp, N.; et al. Clinical features of dopamine agonist withdrawal syndrome in a movement disorders clinic. *J. Neurol. Neurosurg. Psychiatry* **2013**, *84*, 130–135. [CrossRef]
49. Nirenberg, M.J. Dopamine agonist withdrawal syndrome: Implications for patient care. *Drugs Aging* **2013**, *30*, 587–592. [CrossRef]
50. Weintraub, D.; Claassen, D.O. Impulse Control and Related Disorders in Parkinson's Disease. *Int. Rev. Neurobiol.* **2017**, *133*, 679–717. [CrossRef]
51. Ceravolo, R.; Rossi, C.; Del Prete, E.; Bonuccelli, U. A review of adverse events linked to dopamine agonists in the treatment of Parkinson's disease. *Expert Opin. Drug Saf.* **2016**, *15*, 181–198. [CrossRef] [PubMed]
52. Fackrell, R.; Carroll, C.B.; Grosset, D.G.; Mohamed, B.; Reddy, P.; Parry, M.; Chaudhuri, K.R.; Foltynie, T. Noninvasive options for 'wearing-off' in Parkinson's disease: A clinical consensus from a panel of UK Parkinson's disease specialists. *Neurodegener. Dis. Manag.* **2018**, *8*, 349–360. [CrossRef] [PubMed]
53. Stawicki, S.P.; Kalra, S.; Jones, C.; Justiniano, C.F.; Papadimos, T.J.; Galwankar, S.C.; Pappada, S.M.; Feeney, J.J.; Evans, D.C. Comorbidity polypharmacy score and its clinical utility: A pragmatic practitioner's perspective. *J. Emerg. Trauma Shock* **2015**, *8*, 224–231. [CrossRef] [PubMed]

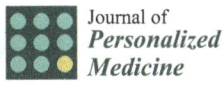

Article

First Two-Year Observational Exploratory Real Life Clinical Phenotyping, and Societal Impact Study of Parkinson's Disease in Emiratis and Expatriate Population of United Arab Emirates 2019–2021: The EmPark Study

Vinod Metta [1,2,3,*], Huzaifa Ibrahim [4], Tom Loney [5], Hani T. S. Benamer [5], Ali Alhawai [6], Dananir Almuhairi [4], Abdulla Al Shamsi [4], Sneha Mohan [3], Kislyn Rodriguez [3], Judith Mohan [3], Margaret O'Sullivan [3], Neha Muralidharan [3], Sheikha Al Mazrooei [7], Khadeeja Dar Mousa [8,9], Guy Chung-Faye [1,2,3], Rukmini Mrudula [10], Cristian Falup-Pecurariu [11], Carmen Rodriguez Bilazquez [12], Maryam Matar [13], Rupam Borgohain [10] and K. Ray Chaudhuri [1,2,3]

1 Psychology & Neuroscience, Department of Neurosciences, Institute of Psychiatry, King's College London, London, UK
2 Parkinson's Foundation Centre of Excellence, King's College Hospital, London, UK
3 Kings College Hospital London, Dubai, United Arab Emirates
4 Parkinson's Association, Dubai, United Arab Emirates
5 College of Medicine, Mohammed Bin Rashid University of Medicine and Health Sciences, Dubai, United Arab Emirates
6 Higher Colleges of Technology, Dubai, United Arab Emirates
7 Stem Cell Association, Dubai, United Arab Emirates
8 Dubai Statistics Centre, Dubai, United Arab Emirates
9 People of Determination Council (POD) Council of Dubai Police, Dubai, United Arab Emirates
10 Nizams Institute of Medical Sciences, Hyderabad, Telangana, India
11 Department of Neurology, Transilvania University of Brasov, Brasov, Romania
12 Institute of Salud Carlos 111, Madrid, Spain
13 Genetic Disease Association, Dubai, United Arab Emirates
* Correspondence: vinod.metta@nhs.net

Abstract: Background: Phenotypic differences in Parkinson's Disease (PD) among locals (Emiratis) and Expatriates (Expats) living in United Arab Emirates have not been described and could be important to unravel local aspects of clinical heterogeneity of PD pointing towards genetic and epigenetic variations. Objective: To investigate the range and nature of motor and nonmotor clinical presentations of PD and its impact on time to diagnosis, local service provisions, and quality of life in Emiratis and Expats in UAE, as well as address the presence of current unmet needs on relation to care and etiopathogenesis of PD related to possible genetic and epigenetic factors. Methods: a cross-sectional one point in time prospective, observational real-life study of 171 patients recruited from PD and Neurology clinics across United Arab Emirates from 2019–2021. Primary outcomes were sociodemographic data, motor and nonmotor symptoms (NMS), including cognition and sleep, and quality of life (QOL) assessments, Results: A total of 171 PD patients (52 Emiratis 119 Expats) were included with mean age (Emiratis 48.5 (13.1) Expats 64.15 (13.1)) and mean disease duration (Emiratis 4.8 (3.2) Expats 6.1 (2.9)). In the Emiratis, there was a significant mean delay in initiating treatment after diagnosis (Emiratis 1.2 (0.9) Expats 1.6 (1.1)), while from a clinical phenotyping aspect, there is a high percentage of akinesia 25 (48.1) or tremor dominant (22 (42.3)) phenotypes as opposed to mixed subtype 67 (56.3) in Expat cohorts; double tremor dominant, especially Emirati females (25%), had a predominant lower limb onset PD. Both Emirati (27.9 (24.0)) and Expat 29.4 (15.6) showed moderate NMS burden and the NMS profile is dominated by Sleep, Fatigue, Mood, Emotional well-being 3.0 (1.1) and Social Stigma 3.5 (0.9) aspects of PDQ8 SI measurements are predicted worse QOL in Emiratis, while lack of social support 2.3 (1.3) impaired QOL in Expat population. Awareness for advanced therapies was low and only 25% of Emiratis were aware of deep brain surgery (DBS), compared to 69% Expats. Only 2% of Emiratis, compared to 32% of Expats, heard of Apomorphine infusion (CSAI), and no (0%) Emiratis were aware of intrajejunal levodopa

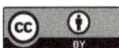

infusion (IJLI), compared to 13% of expats. Conclusion: Our pilot data suggest clinical phenotypic differences in presentation of PD in Emiratis population of UAE compared to expats. Worryingly, the data also show delayed treatment initiation, as well as widespread lack of knowledge of advanced therapies in the Emirati population.

Keywords: young onset Parkinson's (YOPD); Emiratis; expatriate; genetic; epigenetics; societal impact; device aided therapies; quality of life; non motor symptoms

1. Background

Parkinson's disease (PD) is the second most common neurodegenerative disorder, with an increasing prevalence with age; according to a recent study by Post et al. [1], 1 in 10 people aged 45 to 100 are at risk of developing PD and 4 out of every 100 people are diagnosed with PD before the age of 50 (young onset PD) YOPD [1]. Whether or not the frequency of PD varies by race/ethnicity or gender, it is now the leading cause of disability worldwide. Unlike in European and United Kingdom Parkinson's cohorts, Arab families have a high rate of consanguineous marriages [2] which may increase the risk of genetic phenotypes (YOPD) albeit Familial PD accounts for less than 10% of all cases of PD [3]. Some studies show low prevalence of PD in some Arab communities, especially in the Al Thuqbah region of Saudi Arabia (27 per 100,000) [4], in contrast to relatively high prevalence in north African Arabs [5] (31.4–557.4 per 100,000), whereas varied genetically heterogenous patterns were reported in Tunisian study by Gouider-Khouja N [6].

A pilot study conducted by the Movement Disorders International task force [7] identified unmet needs in the Middle East, North Africa, South Asia (MENASA) region and recommended requirement and need for multidisciplinary care, increased movement disorders specialists, educational programs, accurate epidemiologic/genetic data, awareness and availability of more advanced therapies, and suitable infrastructure to provide care to the people with PD. However, no tangible developments in relation to the aforementioned unmet needs are currently obvious, and our study aimed to address the awareness and range and nature of PD in a granular manner in a local UAE population here a comparison with settled expat communities. There are also genetic aspects that have to be considered. For instance, the LRRK2, G2019S, autosomal dominant PD with inadequate penetrance and autosomal recessive inheritance patterns were discovered in a genomic analysis of familial PD in Tunisia [8] and are now known to be prevalent in North African Arabs in Gulf cooperation council countries (GCC) with Arabic population [8–10]. This could be due to ancestry disparities between Arabs from the Gulf Cooperation Council and Arabs from North Africa, with the latter being considerably more closely linked to Berber ancestry [11]. As an example, Al-Mubarak et al. [11] reported no LRRK2 G2019S mutations in the Saudi population they studied.

Furthermore, epidemiologic evidence suggests that ethnicity/race may play a significant impact on genetic, epigenetic, environmental, cultural, and socioeconomic factors, which may affect the pathophysiology and symptomatic expression in PD [12–14]. Given its multi- ethnic population, the United Arab Emirates (UAE), particularly the Dubai area, allows our study and comparison of endophenotypic variations in carefully selected locals and expats. The results may aid in the establishment of a biobanking share initiative with the local setup, specifically to study genetic and epigenetic aspects of diseases. Aside from a few anecdotal studies, as discussed above, no obvious robust prevalence or any endophenotypic studies have been reported or been described among UAE patient cohorts to date. Ours is possibly the first UAE real-life study seeking to understand any specific clinical phenotypic (motor and nonmotor, predictors of QOL) differences in the local Emirati population compared to a wider Expat group in addition to differences in perception of treatment and delivery of care.

2. Methods

Study Design

This was a cross-sectional one-point-in-time prospective, observational real-life study of 171 patients recruited from PD and Neurology clinics across United Arab Emirates from 2019 to 2021. Primary outcomes were sociodemographic data, motor and nonmotor symptoms (NMS), including cognition and sleep, and quality of life (QOL) assessments.

This study was carried out in accordance with local ethical committee guidelines. Prior to participating in the study, all patients provided written consent and all data were stored in an anonymized fashion in accordance with the ongoing UK portfolio adopted NILS longitudinal cohort study at the National Parkinson's Centre of Excellence at Kings College Hospital in London, Dubai, in accordance with the General Data Protection Regulation (GDPR UAE). The NILS (UK) study has been authorized by local ethics committees (NRES South-East London REC3, 10,084, 10/H0808/141).

3. Informed Consent

Informed consent was obtained from patients/carers/all participants involved in this study.

3.1. Patient Selection

Patients with a confirmed diagnosis of Parkinson's disease (PD) who met the UK PD Brain Bank criteria were recruited. Referrals to national Parkinson's Centre of Excellence Kings College Hospital, Dubai, from all around the UAE (mainly from Dubai, Abu Dhabi Sharjah, Al Ain, Ras Al Khaimah, and others) and self-referrals were included.

Separation of Emirati and Expat groups were carried out following established local methodology. Emirates were UAE nationals and Expats were carefully selected to provide for a comparator group and only included subjects from outside Asia and settled in UAE.

3.2. Assessments

During the consultation, as a part of good clinical practice, standardized assessment protocols such as the demographics of (Emirati vs. Expat), age, gender, disease duration, were used, Levodopa Equivalent Daily Dose Calculation (LEDD) [15]. other scales like Hoehn and Yahr Staging (H&Y) [16], and Non-Motor Symptoms Scale (NMSS) [17], Parkinson's Disease Questionnaire-8 (PDQ-8) [18], Kings Parkinson's Pain Scale (KPPS) [19], PDSS (Parkinson's Disease Sleep Scale) [20], MMSE (Mini-Mental State Examination) [21], PFS 16 (Parkinson's Fatigue Scale) [22], and the Hospital Anxiety Depression Scale (HADS) [23] were applied. Details of these validated scales have been published elsewhere and the assessments were performed in line with the NILS assessment; a national study by the National Institute of Health Research in the UK (UKCRN No: 10,084) currently containing data for over 1600 PD patients.

4. Statistical Methods

Data did not fit normal distribution; thus, non-parametric statistics were applied. Descriptive statistics (frequencies and percentages, mean, standard deviation—SD-, median, and inter-quartile range—IQR) were calculated for socio-demographic and clinical variables and scale scores. Differences in scores between Emiratis and Expats were explored using Mann–Whitney and chi-square tests (significance, $p < 0.05$).

5. Results

In total, 171 patients of all ages and HY stages of Parkinson's disease from across the UAE (primarily from Dubai, Abu Dhabi Sharjah, Ain, Abu Dhabi, Ras Al Khaimah, etc.) were recruited during the period 2019–2021. A total of 171 PD patients (52 Emiratis 119 Expats) were included, with mean age (Emiratis 48.5 (13.1), Expats 64.15 (13.1)) and mean disease duration (Emiratis 4.8 (3.2), Expats 6.1 (2.9)), respectively, regardless of their origin, similar to other European and Caucasian cohorts. Male preponderance (73.1%) compared to females (26.9%) is observed in both Emiratis and Expat patients, whereas disease duration in Expats cohorts 6.1 (2.9) was longer than Emiratis 4.8 (3.2) in years (Table 1).

Table 1. Demographic and clinical variables by origin of the patients.

	Total Sample	Emiratis	Expats	p
Age	59.4 (14.9)	48.5 (13.1)	64.15 (13.1)	<0.001 *
Disease Duration (years)	5.7 (3.05)	4.8 (3.2)	6.1 (2.9)	<0.001 *
H&Y	2.5 (0.5) [a]	2.5 (0.5) [a]	3 (0.5) [a]	<0.001 **
LED	752.1 (457.8)	473.08 (473.7)	874.03 (394.06)	<0.001 *
Delay in treatment (years)	1.5 (1.06)	1.2 (0.9)	1.6 (1.1)	0.03
Number of neurologists seen	2.9 (1.1)	3.6 (1.1)	2.5 (0.9)	<0.001 *
PD subtypes				
Akinetic	51 (29.8) [b]	25 (48.1) [b]	26 (21.8)	
Tremor	48 (28.1) [b]	22 (42.3) [b]	26 (21.8)	<0.001 **
Mixed	72 (42.1) [b]	5 (9.6) [b]	67 (56.3)	

All values are expressed as mean (standard deviation), except [a] median (inter-quartile range) and [b] frequency (percentage). * Mann-Whitney test; ** chi-square test.

There was a 1.5 (1.06) delay in starting PD treatment after formal diagnosis with an average delay of 1.2 (0.9) years in Emiratis and 1.6 (1.1) years in Expats, and, interestingly, we discovered at least three neurologists 3.6 (1.1) were seen by Emiratis compared to expats 2.5 (0.9) consulted after onset of symptoms, before diagnosis and initiation of PD treatment (Table 1). Surprisingly, 37% of Emirati patients were not on any treatment even after 2–5 years of diagnosis.

Emiratis appeared to have a higher rate of young onset Parkinson's disease (PD onset below 50 years) (YOPD) and while from a clinical phenotyping aspect, there is a high percentage of akinesia 25 (48.1) or tremor dominant 22 (42.3) phenotypes as opposed to mixed subtype 67 (56.3), in Expat cohorts, double tremor dominant especially Emirati females (25%) had a predominant lower limb onset PD (Table 1).

In Table 2, the differences in the applied rating scales between Emiratis and Expats are displayed.

Table 2. Scales scores and differences by origin of the patients.

Variables	Total Sample (N = 171)	Emiratis (N = 52)	Expats (N = 119)	p *
NMSS Total	29.0 (18.5)	27.9 (24.0)	29.4 (15.6)	0.030
Cardiovascular	2.0 (1.5)	1.4 (1.5)	2.3 (1.5)	<0.001
Sleep/fatigue	4.0 (2.7)	5.2 (3.6)	3.5 (2.1)	0.006
Mood/Apathy	2.7 (3.0)	3.2 (4.9)	2.4 (1.6)	0.028
Perceptual problems/Hallucinations	2.1 (1.6)	1.5 (1.4)	2.4 (1.6)	<0.001
Attention/memory	2.4 (2.4)	1.6 (1.8)	2.7 (2.6)	<0.001
Gastrointestinal	3.0 (2.0)	2.6 (2.4)	3.1 (1.7)	0.013
Urinary	3.0 (2.0)	2.2 (3.4)	3.3 (4.6)	<0.001
Sexual function	7.5 (5.4)	8.0 (6.5)	7.2 (4.8)	0.954
Miscellaneous	2.2 (1.8)	2.0 (2.3)	2.3 (1.5)	0.012
PDQ-8 SI	61.6 (21.2)	54.6 (18.3)	64.6 (21.6)	0.002
Bodily Discomfort	2.4 (1.2)	2.3 (1.2)	2.4 (1.2)	0.645
Communication	2.0 (1.3)	1.6 (1.2)	2.1 (1.3)	0.038
Cognition	2.0 (1.3)	1.4 (1.0)	2.2 (1.3)	<0.001
Social Support	2.0 (1.3)	1.5 (1.2)	2.3 (1.3)	<0.001
Stigma	3.4 (1.0)	3.5 (0.9)	3.3 (1.1)	0.266
Emotional well-being	3.2 (1.1)	3.0 (1.1)	3.1 (1.1)	0.625
Activities of daily living	2.5 (1.3)	2.0 (1.1)	2.7 (1.3)	0.003
Mobility	2.2 (1.3)	1.7 (1.2)	2.4 (1.3)	0.007

Table 2. Cont.

Variables	Total Sample (N = 171)	Emiratis (N = 52)	Expats (N = 119)	p *
KPPS Total	16.1 (8.0)	13.3 (7.2)	17.3 (8.1)	0.002
Musculoskeletal pain	2.1 (1.2)	1.7 (1.1)	2.2 (1.2)	0.002
Chronic pain	2.1 (1.2)	1.6 (0.9)	2.3 (1.2)	<0.001
Fluctuation-related pain	2.1 (1.2)	1.6 (0.8)	2.3 (1.2)	<0.001
Nocturnal pain	3.1 (1.8)	2.7 (1.7)	3.3 (1.8)	0.018
Orofacial pain	2.4 (2.4)	2.3 (3.9)	2.4 (1.4)	<0.001
Discoloration/oedema	2.2 (1.3)	1.7 (1.0)	2.4 (1.5)	0.002
Radicular Pain	2.1 (1.3)	1.6 (1.0)	2.3 (1.3)	<0.001
PFS-16	10.5 (2.8)	11.1 (2.7)	10.2 (2.8)	0.089
MMSE	28.1 (2.9)	29.2 (2.1)	27.6 (3.0)	<0.001
PDSS	70.7 (19.6)	77.3 (17.2)	67.8 (19.9)	0.003
HADS-Anxiety	9.4 (2.2)	9.9 (2.2)	9.2 (2.2)	0.079
HADS-Depression	8.2 (2.8)	7.5 (2.8)	8.5 (2.7)	0.023

* Mann-Whitney test.

Based on NMSS score and staging, both Emirati (27.9) (24.0) and Expats 29.4 (15.6) had moderate NMS burden. NMS profile is dominated by Sleep, Fatigue, Mood, Emotional well-being 3.0 (1.1), and Social Stigma 3.5 (0.9) aspects of PDQ8 measurements are predicted worse QOL in Emiratis, while lack of social support 2.3 (1.3) impaired QOL in Expat population. Nocturnal pain 2.7 (1.7) dominates in Emiratis, whereas both nocturnal and radicular pain, 3.3 (1.8) and 2.3 (1.3), respectively, dominates in Expat population.

6. Discussion

Our study reports some key findings highlighting differences in PD presentation and delivery of Parkinson's care among local Emirati population versus a comparator Expat PD population in UAE.

These are: Emirati PD patients tended to have young onset Parkinson's (YOPD) 48.5 (13.1) which is lower than a global average, Khalil et al. [7]. This may underpin a genetic causation or predisposition possibly contributed to by consanguinity in Arab population, although this was not specifically studied and is certainly worthy of further larger suitable powered clinical genetic cohort studies. Moreover, 93.8% of Emiratis presented to our clinics were YOPD within 1–5 years' duration. It is also considered that the general age of the Emirate population tends to be lower and as such there may be a bias to this observation.

The occurrence of higher proportion of Lower limb tremor (LLT) in emirate female PD is of interest. LLT has been specifically described to occur in some genetic variants of PD such as in Parkin mutation [24], as well as in those with LRRK2 [25] and the data, therefore, need more specific observation, and genetic and biomarker analysis, as well as clinical follow up of this specific cohort. There was a higher representation of nocturnal, fluctuation, and radicular pain in the LLT group. This is a preliminary finding and needs to be investigated in more granular detail. Lower back pain and shoulder pain (variants of musculoskeletal and radicular pain) have been reported in PINK1 and GBA mutation related PD cases [26]. Fluctuation is often seen at a greater level in YOPD and parkin positive cases. These factors, therefore, need exploring as Emirati patients, who were either on low levodopa doses or those who were eligible or unaware of advanced device aided therapies (DAT), respond very well either to escalating dopaminergic regime or DAT therapies.

When data on the Emirate PD are examined in a more granular fashion, it emerges that the Emirate PD, in spite of lower disease duration, have similar HY stage compared to the expat group and similar burden of overall NMS scores. Moreover, 29.0 (18.5) was seen in both Emiratis and Expats and NMS profile is dominated by Sleep, Fatigue, Mood. On the whole the overall NMS burden were similar cross both groups, and given that the emirate PD group had a significantly lower disease duration, this may mean that the clinical PD phenotype in this group may have a greater representation of the recently described

NMS endophenotypes [27]. Greater understanding and clarity around this pattern of endophenotype would be important to assign sub type specific treatment and delivery of personalized medicine [28] in this group. A faster disease progression in this group, therefore, could be proposed on the basis of this observation although lower LED intake in the Emirate group could be a confounder.

Another striking feature of our study we would like to highlight is Emotional well-being and Social Stigma aspects of PDQ8 SI measurements, which were predicted worse QOL in Emiratis, while lack of social support impaired QOL in Expat population Pain in Parkinson's is independent of disease severity so is with disease duration. Nocturnal pain Predominates in Emiratis, whereas both nocturnal and radicular pain dominate in Expat population (Figure 1).

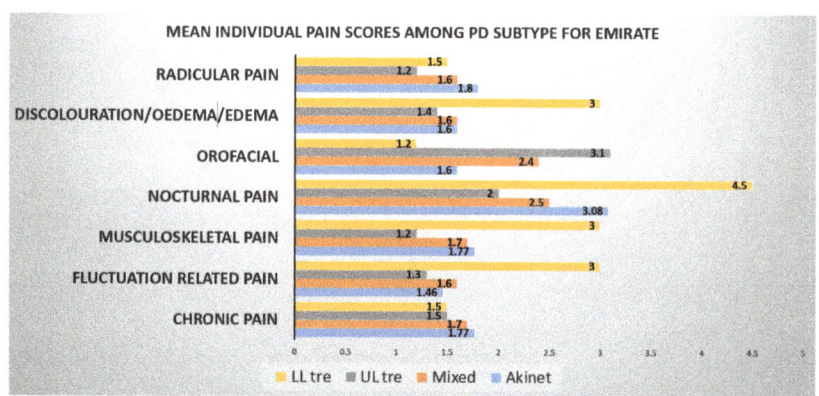

Figure 1. Graphical representation of PD subtype vs. pain domains (KPPS) in Emiratis. In this graph it can be seen that Nocturnal pain (NP) is found to be higher in all the PD Subtypes where as Radicular pain scores high in Tremor Dominant Subtype.

Finally, we consider vignettes of care delivery of PD across both groups. The Emirates saw more neurologists, and, in spite of seeing at least three neurologists, there was a significant delay in initiation of treatment, even after diagnosis in general UAE PD patients (both Emiratis and Expats). Surprisingly, 33% Emiratis were not on any treatment, even after 2–5 years of diagnosis, and this observation is in conflict with the wider consensus that treatment in PD ought to be started at diagnosis as patients otherwise report progressive deterioration in QoL [29].

Delivery of care in PD is also underpinned by successful provision of advanced infusion (apo IJLI) and surgical treatments. Here, awareness of patient about these treatments is paramount and our data suggest (Figure 2) that only 25% of Emiratis are aware of the deep brain stimulation surgery (DBS), compared to 69% of Expats. Interestingly only 2% of Emiratis are aware of Apomorphine infusion treatment (CSAI), compared with 32% of Expats. Surprisingly, no (0%) Emiratis, compared to 13% of expats, were aware of intrajejunal levodopa infusion (IJLI). Out of 171 (our study sample), only 8% were treated with device aided therapies, despite the fact that nearly 50% were eligible based on Delphi 5-2-1 criteria [30]. This may be due to lack of awareness, or specialist skills or experience or advanced device aided therapy (DAT) treatment guidelines to implement these therapies. Some of the Arabic patients and care givers struggled with clinical scales/questionnaires being in English; perhaps Arabic translated ones would be beneficial.

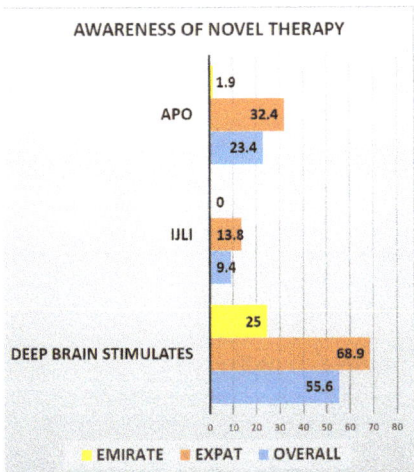

Figure 2. Graphical representation of the awareness of novel therapies in PD treatment among the Emiratis and Expats. This graph shows only 25% of Emirates are aware of deep brain stimulation test compared to 69% Expats and 2% of Emirates are aware of Apomorphine pump treatment compared to 32% of Expats. Whereas Not even a single (0%) Emirati is aware of Ileo-jejunal levodopa infusion compared to 13% of expats.

The findings consolidate several key unmet needs related to MENASA countries as articulated in the 2020 paper by Khalil et al. [7]. In the Emirate PD, well controlled longitudinal cohort studies need to be undertaken seeking genotype phenotype correlations from a care perspective; awareness for advanced therapies needs to be improved and this needs to be a multilevel educational exercise related to both patients and health care professionals. Such access to therapies can be improved by implementation of a culturally bespoke local clinical guideline for pharmacological as well as non-pharmacological therapies for PD.

6.1. Why Early Diagnosis and Treatment Important in PD?

Parkinson's disease is a progressive neurodegenerative condition attributed to progressive loss of dopaminergic neurons emerging evidence supports early intervention may help preserving the functioning of neurons helps in slowing disease progression and improving overall quality of life [31]. Early treatment depends and relies on early diagnosis; a UK autopsy study of 100 subjects who had been diagnosed with PD found a misdiagnosis rate of 24% [32], while another study [33] showed nearly 47% of PD diagnosis are incorrect when performed in primary care setting and by non-movement disorder specialists. It is necessary that the required skill set and resources are refined as early detection and treatment have potential to improve the experience and quality of life [34].

6.2. Clinical Benefits of Early Diagnosis and Treatment in PD?

Several studies demonstrated clinical benefit of early treatment. A multicenter controlled clinical trial of Selegiline for 24 months' follow-up on 800 patients in 1987 demonstrated a delayed onset of disability and reduction in motor function (UPDRS) and requirement of Ldopa [35]. Early Parkinson's disease can be managed successfully for up to five years with the use of Ropinirole alone and supplementing it with levodopa if necessary. This result is observed in a 5-year follow up study comparing the role of Ropinirole vs. L-DOPA and Benserazide [36]. In another study, Rasagiline treatment demonstrated significant improvement in motor (UPDRS) and no change in onset/frequency of adverse events in a 26-week follow-up study comparing Rasagiline vs. Placebo [37]. A 46-month SPECT study of individuals treated with Pramipexole and Carbidopa Levodopa revealed that the Pramipexole-treated group had less dopaminergic neuron degeneration than the Carbidopa-treated group, with identical UPDRS scores in both groups [38]. After a 24-month follow-up, in a PET study of patients treated with Ropinirole and Carbidopa Levodopa, the Ropinirole-treated group showed decreased dopaminergic neuron degeneration, with equivalent UPDRS ratings in both groups [39]. A 42-week follow-up study of varied multiple doses of carbidopa levodopa revealed a dose-related improvement in motor UPDRS scores [40]. With Pramipexole, there was a reduction in dyskinesia and wear-off, but the L-dopa group had a better overall score and motor score, as well as fewer side effects (freezing, somnolence, and edema) [41]. In a meta-analysis of 5247 individuals treated with dopamine agonists and levodopa, patients treated with dopamine agonists had fewer motor problems (dyskinesias or dystonia) than patients treated with levodopa [42]. Individuals treated with MAO B inhibitors had improvements in both motor scores and activities of daily living in a meta-analysis study of 3525 patients treated with MAO B inhibitors and levodopa [43]. Rasagiline 1 mg and 2 mg were compared to placebo in a 72-week follow-up study. With Rasagiline 1 mg, but not with 2 mg dosage, the early-start group had better UPDRS scores than the delayed-start group [44]. The 6.5-year extension of the TEMPO research confirmed that the early treated group had less UPDRS score degradation than the delayed onset group [45]. The intervention group experienced a slow onset of dyskinesia and had a higher frequency of dyskinesia [46]. L-dopa improves mobility and gives higher quality of life than dopamine agonists (DA) and monoamine oxidase type B inhibitors, according to a 36-month follow-up study of 1620 patients comparing levodopa and dopamine agonists and MAOB inhibitors [47] all these studies (randomized clinical trials and meta-analysis) summarized in (Table 3) supports treatment should be initiated at the time of diagnosis, delaying the treatment has worst prognostic implications (Table 3).

Table 3. Studies showing clinical benefits of early diagnosis of Parkinson's disease.

Year	Study	Outcome
1993	DATATOP	Selegiline compared with placebo, 24-month follow up of 800 patients showed Selegiline delayed the onset of disability and reduction in motor (UPDRS) and requirement of L-dopa
2000	RASCOL et al.	A 5-year follow up study comparing Ropinirole vs. L-dopa and Benserazide, patients treated with Ropinirole had longer time to dyskinesia's and no significant difference or change in motor scores or quality of between two groups
2002	TEMPO	A 26-week follow up study comparing Rasagiline vs. Placebo, Rasagiline treated group showed significant improvement in motor (UPDRS) and no difference in onset/frequency of adverse events.
2002	CALM-PD-CIT	A 46-month follow up SPECT study of patients treated with Pramipexole and carbidopa Levodopa showed less dopaminergic neuron degeneration in Pramipexole treated group with similar UPDRS scores in both groups.
2003	REAL-PET	A 24-month follow-up PET study of patients treated with Ropinirole and Carbidopa Levodopa showed less dopaminergic neuron degeneration in Pramipexole treated group with similar UPDRS scores in both groups.
2004	ELLDOPA	A 42-week follow up study of various multiple doses of carbidopa levodopa showed significant improvement in motor UPDRS scores in a dose related fashion.
2008	STOOWE et al.	A meta-analysis study 5247 patients treated with dopamine agonists and Levodopa; patients treated with dopamine agonists has less motor complications (dyskinesia's, dystonia)

Table 3. Cont.

Year	Study	Outcome
2008	Ives et al.	A meta-analysis study 3525 patients treated with MAO B inhibitors and Levodopa; patients treated with MAO B inhibitors have improvements in both motor scores and activities of daily living.
2009	ADAGIO	A 72-week follow up study comparing Rasagiline 1 mg and 2 mg compared with placebo showed Improved UPDRS scores in the early-start group compared to delayed-start group, with Rasagiline 1 mg but not with 2 mg dosage
2009	Hauser et al.	A 6.5-year extension of TEMPO study indeed showed early treated group has less worsening of UPDRS scores compared to delayed onset
2014	PD MED TRIAL	A 36-month follow up study of 1620 patients comparing levodopa and dopamine agonists and MAOB inhibitors showed L-dopa improves mobility and provides better quality of life compared to dopamine agonists (DA) and monoamine oxidase type B inhibitors (MAOBI)

6.3. Economical Benefits of Early Diagnosis and Treatment in PD?

Early intervention is likely to have a significant impact on healthcare costs, as well as societal impact; several studies showed the impact of social healthcare burden and economic costs and quality of life is severe in the later stages of the disease, when symptoms are at their most severe, necessitating more healthcare services or caregiver support [34,35,48,49]. Motor difficulties (motor fluctuations, dyskinesias, and dystonia, which manifests as uncontrollable and sometimes painful muscular spasms) have been recognized as variables contributing to the rise in PD-related expenditures. Social, healthcare burden, and economic costs impact quality of life in patients with advanced Parkinson's disease (APD) [48–50].

Patients with Parkinson's disease (PwP) experience more unpredictable and troublesome motor and non-motor fluctuations as they progress through advanced stages, with the emergence of severe motor (progressive disability) and non-motor symptoms, such as mood, cognitive, and behavioral problems, causing a severe impact on QoL and necessitating more healthcare services or caregivers [48–50].

According to a study by Schrag et al. [48], the overall burden of Parkinson's disease and healthcare resource consumption expenses grew dramatically as the disease progressed with advanced Parkinson's disease (APD). Annual costs for early Parkinson's disease were €2110, but for advanced Parkinson's disease, they were about twenty times higher (€38,625), and majority of patients with advanced disease not on any device aided therapies (DAT) elderly over 70 years old [48]. A Spanish study by Zecchinelli et al. [51] revealed roughly 30% of Parkinson's patients are in advanced stages, and the cost of illness rose sharply, primarily due to costs linked with in-patient treatment and nursing homes because advanced-stage patients are bedridden, wheelchair-bound, or hospitalized [52,53]. The primary drivers and determinants of the socio-economic burden of PD were hospitalization, nursing care, drug costs, indirect costs (loss of work, etc.), predictors of quality of life, societal socio-economic impact healthcare burden, and QOL in PwP [54–56] (Figure 3).

A study by Popov et al. [57] looked at costs of PD illness and societal burden in a cohort of 100 patients showed over all annual burden of 1 billion euros with direct costs accounting to 67% and indirect costs accounting 33% and main drivers of the burden being informal care and drugs [58]. Another UK study by McCrone [59] et al. showed the informal care compared to formal (80% vs. 20%) impact on societal burden and the main predictors being male gender, level of disability and non-motor symptoms like depression [59], as well as adherence to oral medications, especially in elderly patients with advanced disease where they have to take several pills multiple times

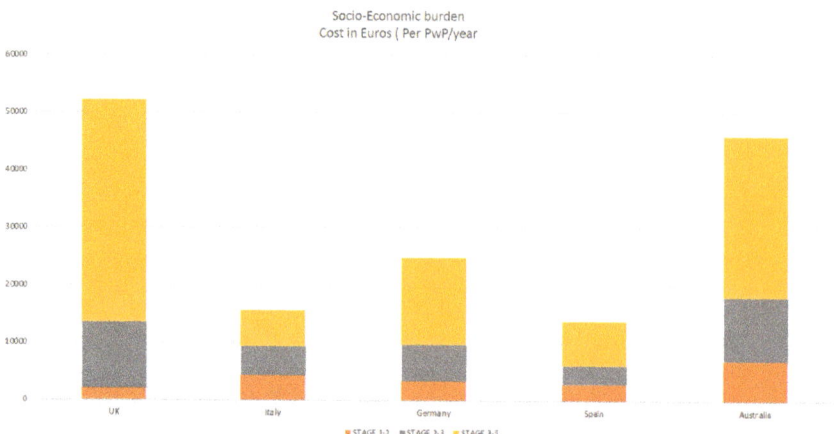

Figure 3. highlighting socio-economic burden increases as disease progress (yellow).

Strong predictors of socio-economic burden 61% of PD patients were non-adherent to oral therapy and medical costs were significantly higher among non-adherent versus adherent ($15,826 vs. $9228) [60]. A multicenter (France, Germany, and UK) observational study by Pechevis et al. [61] showed dyskinesia (motor complications measured using UPDRS scale) was associated with significant socio-economic and societal burden and increasing total healthcare costs with each unit increase in dyskinesia score led to 562 euros additional costs per patient over a 6-month period [61].

The economic and clinical evidence gathered in the literature shows and confirms that early diagnosis and initiation of treatment is crucial, halts risk of disease progression, and reduces the effects on QOL. This can potentially reduce treatment costs if possible non-oral therapeutic device aided therapies are offered to patients as they progress to an advanced stage before significant deterioration has occurred. Patients' QOL and well-being are improved when the Multidisciplinary care approach and timely referrals to a movement disorders specialist with expertise in PD, as selection of patients for advanced device aided therapies (IJLI, CSAI, DBS) are likely to be most effective and patients are likely to be more complaint with these therapies.

7. Conclusions

Our study highlights heterogenetic and endophenotype variations of Parkinson's disease in UAE population comparing local Emirati and Expat populations. Our study identifies the importance of early diagnosis, prompt treatment initiation, which has huge societal socio-economic impact, and healthcare burden. Moreover, timely implementation of advanced therapies help delay PD disease progression. A bio banking share initiative with the local setup specifically to study genetic and epigenetic aspects focusing on: GBA, LRRK2, Parkin gene mutation. Screening of Emirati patients with young onset Lower limb tremor dependent Parkinson's disease would be beneficial, identifying these endophenotypes is paramount as these patients will respond very well to dopaminergic dose escalation or to advanced device aided therapies and also helps to formulate gene-targeted therapies. Setting up a local expert committee panel, implementation of national treatment protocols involving patients and care giver groups (expert patient panel) will help empower patients and caregivers.

Author Contributions: V.M., H.I., T.L., H.T.S.B., A.A., D.A., A.A.S., S.M., K.R., J.M., M.O., N.M., S.A.M., K.D.M., G.C.-F., R.M., C.F.-P., C.R.B., M.M., R.B. and K.R.C. contributed to the designing, drafting, and revision of the manuscript for intellectual content; V.M. and K.R.C. oversaw the entire writing and editing process. All authors have read and agreed to the published version of the manuscript.

Funding: This research received no external funding.

Institutional Review Board Statement: This study was carried out in accordance with local ethical committee guidelines. Prior to participating in the study, all patients provided written consent and all data were stored in an anonymized fashion in accordance with the ongoing UK portfolio adopted NILS longitudinal cohort study at the National Parkinson's Centre of Excellence at Kings College Hospital in London, Dubai, in accordance with the General Data Protection Regulation (GDPR UAE). The NILS (UK) study has been authorized by local ethics committees (NRES South-East London REC3, 10,084, 10/H0808/141).

Informed Consent Statement: Informed consent was obtained from patients/carers/all participants involved in this study.

Data Availability Statement: Raw data were generated at Kings College hospital London, Dubai. Derived data supporting the findings of this study are available from the corresponding author VM on request.

Conflicts of Interest: The authors declare no conflict of interest.

References

1. Post, B.; van den Heuvel, L.; van Prooije, T.; van Ruissen, X.; van de Warrenburg, B.; Nonnekes, J. Young onset Parkinson's disease: A modern and tailored approach. *J. Park. Dis.* **2020**, *10*, S29–S36. [CrossRef] [PubMed]
2. Tadmouri, G.O.; Nair, P.; Obeid, T.; Al Ali, M.T.; Al Khaja, N.; Hamamy, H.A. Consanguinity and reproductive health among Arabs. *Reprod. Healh* **2009**, *6*, 17. [CrossRef] [PubMed]
3. McInerney-Leo, A.; Hadley, D.W.; Gwinn-Hardy, K.; Hardy, J. Genetic testing in Parkinson's disease. *Mov. Disord. Off. J. Mov. Disord. Soc.* **2005**, *20*, 1–10. [CrossRef]
4. Al Rajeh, S.; Bademosi, O.; Ismail, H.; Awada, A.; Dawodu, A.; Al-Freihi, H.; Assuhaimi, S.; Borollosi, M.; Al-Shammasi, S. A community survey of neurological disorders in Saudi Arabia: The Thuqbah study. *Neuroepidemiology* **1993**, *12*, 164–178. [CrossRef] [PubMed]
5. Benamer, H.T.; De Silva, R. LRRK2 G2019S in the North African population: A review. *Eur. Neurol.* **2010**, *63*, 321–325. [CrossRef] [PubMed]
6. Gouider-Khouja, N.; Belal, S.; Hamida, M.B.; Hentati, F. Clinical and genetic study of familial Parkinson's disease in Tunisia. *Neurology* **2000**, *54*, 1603–1609. [CrossRef]
7. Khalil, H.; Chahine, L.; Siddiqui, J.; Aldajani, Z.; Bajwa, J.A. Parkinson's disease in the MENASA countries. *Lancet Neurol.* **2020**, *19*, 293–294. [CrossRef]
8. Belarbi, S.; Hecham, N.; Lesage, S.; Kediha, M.I.; Smail, N.; Benhassine, T.; Ysmail-Dahlouk, F.; Lohman, E.; Benhabyles, B.; Hamadouche, T.; et al. LRRK2 G2019S mutation in Parkinson's disease: A neuropsychological and neuropsychiatric study in a large Algerian cohort. *Parkinsonism Relat. Disord.* **2010**, *16*, 676–679. [CrossRef]
9. Jasinska-Myga, B.; Kachergus, J.; Vilariño-Güell, C.; Wider, C.; Soto-Ortolaza, A.I.; Kefi, M.; Middleton, L.T.; Ishihara-Paul, L.; Gibson, R.A.; Amouri, R.; et al. Comprehensive sequencing of the LRRK2 gene in patients with familial Parkinson's disease from North Africa. *Mov. Disord.* **2010**, *25*, 2052–2058. [CrossRef]
10. Alrefai, A.; Habahbih, M.; Alkhawajah, M.; Darwish, M.; Batayha, W.; Khader, Y.; El-Salem, K. Prevalence of Parkinson's disease in Northern Jordan. *Clin. Neurol. Neurosurg.* **2009**, *111*, 812–815. [CrossRef] [PubMed]
11. Al-Mubarak, B.R.; Bohlega, S.A.; Alkhairallah, T.S.; Magrashi, A.I.; AlTurki, M.I.; Khalil, D.S.; AlAbdulaziz, B.S.; Abou Al-Shaar, H.; Mustafa, A.E.; Alyemni, E.A.; et al. Parkinson's disease in Saudi patients: A genetic study. *PLoS ONE* **2015**, *10*, e0135950. [CrossRef]
12. Hu, M.; Richards, M.; Agapito, C.; Brooks, D.; Clough, C.; Ray Chaudhuri, K. Parkinsonism in immigrant Afro-Caribbean and Indian subjects living in the United Kingdom. *J. Neurol. Neurosurg. Psychiatry* **1999**, *66*, 258–259.
13. Chaudhuri, K.R.; Hu, M.; Brooks, D. Atypical parkinsonism in Afro-Caribbean and Indian origin immigrants to the UK. *Mov. Disord. Off. J. Mov. Disord. Soc.* **2000**, *15*, 18–23. [CrossRef]
14. Dorsey, E.R.; Bloem, B.R. The Parkinson pandemic—A call to action. *JAMA Neurol.* **2018**, *75*, 9–10. [CrossRef] [PubMed]
15. Tomlinson, C.L.; Stowe, R.; Patel, S.; Rick, C.; Gray, R.; Clarke, C.E. Systematic review of levodopa dose equivalency reporting in Parkinson's disease. *Mov. Disord.* **2010**, *25*, 2649–2653. [CrossRef] [PubMed]
16. Hoehn, M.M.; Yahr, M.D. Parkinsonism: Onset, progression, and mortality. *Neurology* **1998**, *50*, 318. [CrossRef] [PubMed]
17. Ray Chaudhuri, K.; Rojo, J.M.; Schapira, A.H.; Brooks, D.J.; Stocchi, F.; Odin, P.; Antonini, A.; Brown, R.J.; Martinez-Martin, P. A proposal for a comprehensive grading of Parkinson's disease severity combining motor and non-motor assessments: Meeting an unmet need. *PLoS ONE* **2013**, *8*, e57221. [CrossRef]

18. Jenkinson, C.; Fitzpatrick, R.; Peto, V.; Greenhall, R.; Hyman, N. The PDQ-8: Development and validation of a short-form Parkinson's disease questionnaire. *Psychol. Health* **1997**, *12*, 805–814. [CrossRef]
19. Chaudhuri, K.R.; Rizos, A.; Trenkwalder, C.; Rascol, O.; Pal, S.; Martino, D.; Carroll, C.; Paviour, D.; Falup-Pecurariu, C.; Kessel, B.; et al. King's Parkinson's disease pain scale, the first scale for pain in PD: An international validation. *Mov. Disord.* **2015**, *30*, 1623–1631. [CrossRef] [PubMed]
20. Chaudhuri, K.R.; Pal, S.; DiMarco, A.; Whately-Smith, C.; Bridgman, K.; Mathew, R.; Pezzela, F.R.; Forbes, A.; Högl, B.; Trenkwalder, C. The Parkinson's disease sleep scale: A new instrument for assessing sleep and nocturnal disability in Parkinson's disease. *J. Neurol. Neurosurg. Psychiatry* **2002**, *73*, 629–635. [CrossRef]
21. Folstein, M.F.; Folstein, S.E.; McHugh, P.R. Mini-mental state: A practical method for grading the cognitive state of patients for the clinician. *J. Psychiatr. Res.* **1975**, *12*, 189–198. [CrossRef]
22. Brown, R.; Dittner, A.; Findley, L.; Wessely, S. The Parkinson fatigue scale. *Parkinsonism Relat. Disord.* **2005**, *11*, 49–55. [CrossRef]
23. Zigmond, A.S.; Snaith, R.P. The hospital anxiety and depression scale. *Acta Psychiatr. Scand.* **1983**, *67*, 361–370. [CrossRef]
24. Camargos, S.T.; Dornas, L.O.; Momeni, P.; Lees, A.; Hardy, J.; Singleton, A.; Cardoso, F. Familial Parkinsonism and early onset Parkinson's disease in a Brazilian movement disorders clinic: Phenotypic characterization and frequency of SNCA, PRKN, PINK1, and LRRK2 mutations. *Mov. Disord. Off. J. Mov. Disord. Soc.* **2009**, *24*, 662–666. [CrossRef] [PubMed]
25. Clark, L.; Wang, Y.; Karlins, E.; Saito, L.; Mejia-Santana, H.; Harris, J.; Louis, E.D.; Cote, L.J.; Andrews, H.; Fahn, S.; et al. Frequency of LRRK2 mutations in early-and late-onset Parkinson disease. *Neurology* **2006**, *67*, 1786–1791. [CrossRef] [PubMed]
26. Criscuolo, C.; Volpe, G.; De Rosa, A.; Varrone, A.; Marongiu, R.; Mancini, P.; Salvatore, E.; Dallapiccola, B.; Filla, A.; Valente, E.M.; et al. PINK1 homozygous W437X mutation in a patient with apparent dominant transmission of parkinsonism. *Mov. Disord. Off. J. Mov. Disord. Soc.* **2006**, *21*, 1265–1267. [CrossRef]
27. Sauerbier, A.; Qamar, M.A.; Rajah, T.; Chaudhuri, K.R. New concepts in the pathogenesis and presentation of Parkinson's disease. *Clin. Med.* **2016**, *16*, 365. [CrossRef]
28. Titova, N.; Chaudhuri, K.R. Personalized medicine in Parkinson's disease: Time to be precise. *Mov. Disord.* **2017**, *32*, 1147–1154. [CrossRef] [PubMed]
29. Grosset, D.; Taurah, L.; Burn, D.J.; MacMahon, D.; Forbes, A.; Turner, K.; Bowron, A.; Walker, R.; Findley, L.; Foster, O.; et al. A multicentre longitudinal observational study of changes in self-reported health status in people with Parkinson's disease left untreated at diagnosis. *J. Neurol. Neurosurg. Psychiatry* **2007**, *78*, 465–469. [CrossRef] [PubMed]
30. Antonini, A.; Stoessl, A.J.; Kleinman, L.S.; Skalicky, A.M.; Marshall, T.S.; Sail, K.R.; Onuk, K.; Odin, P.L.A. Developing consensus among movement disorder specialists on clinical indicators for identification and management of advanced Parkinson's disease: A multi-country Delphi-panel approach. *Curr. Med. Res. Opin.* **2018**, *34*, 2063–2073. [CrossRef]
31. Vlaar, A.M.; van Kroonenburgh, M.J.; Kessels, A.G.; Weber, W.E. Meta-analysis of the literature on diagnostic accuracy of SPECT in parkinsonian syndromes. *BMC Neurol.* **2007**, *7*, 1–13. [CrossRef]
32. Hughes, A.J.; Daniel, S.E.; Kilford, L.; Lees, A.J. Accuracy of clinical diagnosis of idiopathic Parkinson's disease: A clinico-pathological study of 100 cases. *J. Neurol. Neurosurg. Psychiatry* **1992**, *55*, 181–184. [CrossRef]
33. Conditions, N.C.C.f.C. CRoyal College of Physicians.
34. Gage, H.; Hendricks, A.; Zhang, S.; Kazis, L. The relative health related quality of life of veterans with Parkinson's disease. *J. Neurol. Neurosurg. Psychiatry* **2003**, *74*, 163–169. [CrossRef]
35. Group, P.S. Effects of tocopherol and deprenyl on the progression of disability in early Parkinson's disease. *N. Engl. J. Med.* **1993**, *328*, 176–183.
36. Rascol, O.; Brooks, D.J.; Korczyn, A.D.; De Deyn, P.P.; Clarke, C.E.; Lang, A.E. A five-year study of the incidence of dyskinesia in patients with early Parkinson's disease who were treated with Ropinirole or levodopa. *N. Engl. J. Med.* **2000**, *342*, 1484–1491. [CrossRef] [PubMed]
37. Group, P.S. A controlled trial of Rasagiline in early Parkinson disease: The TEMPO Study. *Arch. Neurol.* **2002**, *59*, 1937–1943.
38. Parkinson Study Group; Parkinson Study Group. Dopamine transporter brain imaging to assess the effects of Pramipexole vs levodopa on Parkinson disease progression. *JAMA* **2002**, *287*, 1653–1661. [CrossRef]
39. Whone, A.L.; Watts, R.L.; Stoessl, A.J.; Davis, M.; Reske, S.; Nahmias, C.; Lang, A.E.; Rascol, O.; Ribeiro, M.J.; Remy, P.; et al. Slower progression of Parkinson's disease with Ropinirole versus levodopa: The REAL-PET study. *Ann. Neurol.* **2003**, *54*, 93–101. [CrossRef] [PubMed]
40. Group, P.S. Levodopa and the progression of Parkinson's disease. *N. Engl. J. Med.* **2004**, *351*, 2498–2508.
41. Group, P.S. Pramipexole vs levodopa as initial treatment for Parkinson disease: A randomized controlled trial. *JAMA* **2000**, *284*, 1931–1938. [CrossRef] [PubMed]
42. Stowe, R.; Ives, N.; Clarke, C.E.; Ferreira, J.; Hawker, R.J.; Shah, L.; Wheatley, K.; Gray, R. Dopamine agonist therapy in early Parkinson's disease. *Cochrane Database Syst. Rev.* **2008**, CD006564. [CrossRef]
43. Ives, N.J.; Stowe, R.L.; Marro, J.; Counsell, C.; Macleod, A.; Clarke, C.E.; Gray, R.; Wheatley, K. Monoamine oxidase type B inhibitors in early Parkinson's disease: Meta-analysis of 17 randomized trials involving 3525 patients. *BMJ* **2004**, *329*, 593. [CrossRef] [PubMed]
44. Olanow, C.W.; Rascol, O.; Hauser, R.; Feigin, P.D.; Jankovic, J.; Lang, A.; Langston, W.; Melamed, E.; Poewe, W.; Stocchi, F.; et al. A double-blind, delayed-start trial of Rasagiline in Parkinson's disease. *N. Engl. J. Med.* **2009**, *361*, 1268–1278. [CrossRef] [PubMed]

45. Hauser, R.A.; Lew, M.F.; Hurtig, H.I.; Ondo, W.G.; Wojcieszek, J.; Fitzer-Attas, C.J.; TEMPO Open-Label Study Group. Long-term outcome of early versus delayed Rasagiline treatment in early Parkinson's disease. *Mov. Disord.* **2009**, *24*, 564–573. [CrossRef] [PubMed]
46. Stocchi, F.; Rascol, O.; Kieburtz, K.; Poewe, W.; Jankovic, J.; Tolosa, E.; Barone, P.; Lang, A.E.; Olanow, C.W. Initiating levodopa/carbidopa therapy with and without entacapone in early Parkinson disease: The STRIDE-PD study. *Ann. Neurol.* **2010**, *68*, 18–27. [CrossRef]
47. Group, P.M.C. Long-term effectiveness of dopamine agonists and monoamine oxidase B inhibitors compared with levodopa as initial treatment for Parkinson's disease (PD MED): A large, open-label, pragmatic randomized trial. *Lancet* **2014**, *384*, 1196–1205. [CrossRef]
48. Schrag, A.; Jahanshahi, M.; Quinn, N. What contributes to quality of life in patients with Parkinson's disease? *J. Neurol. Neurosurg. Psychiatry* **2000**, *69*, 308–312. [CrossRef] [PubMed]
49. Kuopio, A.M.; Marttila, R.J.; Helenius, H.; Toivonen, M.; Rinne, U.K. The quality of life in Parkinson's disease. *Mov. Disord. Off. J. Mov. Disord. Soc.* **2000**, *15*, 216–223. [CrossRef]
50. Duncan, G.W.; Khoo, T.K.; Yarnall, A.J.; O'Brien, J.T.; Coleman, S.Y.; Brooks, D.J.; Barker, R.A.; Burn, D.J. Health-related quality of life in early Parkinson's disease: The impact of nonmotor symptoms. *Mov. Disord.* **2014**, *29*, 195–202. [CrossRef] [PubMed]
51. Zecchinelli, A.; Caprari, F.; Ponzi, P.; Bonetti, A.; Pezzoli, G. PNL5 Social Costs of Parkinson Disease in Italy. *Value Health* **2004**, *6*, 788. [CrossRef]
52. Weir, S.; Samnaliev, M.; Kuo, T.C.; Tierney, T.S.; Walleser Autiero, S.; Taylor, R.S.; Schrag, A. Short-and long-term cost and utilization of health care resources in Parkinson's disease in the UK. *Mov. Disord.* **2018**, *33*, 974–981. [CrossRef] [PubMed]
53. Keränen, T.; Kaakkola, S.; Sotaniemi, K.; Laulumaa, V.; Haapaniemi, T.; Jolma, T.; Kola, H.; Ylikoski, A.; Satomaa, O.; Kovanen, J.; et al. Economic burden and quality of life impairment increase with severity of PD. *Parkinsonism Relat. Disord.* **2003**, *9*, 163–168. [CrossRef]
54. Winter, Y.; Balzer-Geldsetzer, M.; von Campenhausen, S.; Spottke, A.; Eggert, K.; Oertel, W.H.; Dodel, R. Trends in resource utilization for Parkinson's disease in Germany. *J. Neurol. Sci.* **2010**, *294*, 18–22. [CrossRef]
55. Richard Dodel, J.-P.R.M.B.a.W.H.O. The Economic Burden of Parkinson's Disease. *Rep. Touch Brief.* 2008.
56. Martinez-Martin, P.; Rodriguez-Blazquez, C.; Paz, S.; Forjaz, M.J.; Frades-Payo, B.; Cubo, E.; de Pedro-Cuesta, J.; Lizán, L.; ELEP Group. Parkinson symptoms and health related quality of life as predictors of costs: A longitudinal observational study with linear mixed model analysis. *PLoS ONE* **2015**, *10*, e0145310. [CrossRef]
57. Popova, V.; Pishtiyski, I. Isolation of cyclodextrin glucanotransferase preparations of different purities. *Eur. Food Res. Technol.* **2001**, *213*, 67–71. [CrossRef]
58. Winter, Y.; von Campenhausen, S.; Popov, G.; Reese, J.P.; Balzer-Geldsetzer, M.; Kukshina, A.; Zhukova, T.V.; Bertschi, N.; Bötzel, K.; Gusev, E.; et al. Social and clinical determinants of quality of life in Parkinson's disease in a Russian cohort study. *Parkinsonism Relat. Disord.* **2010**, *16*, 243–248. [CrossRef] [PubMed]
59. McCrone, P.; Allcock, L.M.; Burn, D.J. Predicting the cost of Parkinson's disease. *Mov. Disord.* **2007**, *22*, 804–812. [CrossRef]
60. Davis, K.L.; Edin, H.M.; Allen, J.K. Prevalence and cost of medication nonadherence in Parkinson's disease: Evidence from administrative claims data. *Mov. Disord.* **2010**, *25*, 474–480. [CrossRef]
61. Pechevis, M.; Clarke, C.E.; Vieregge, P.; Khoshnood, B.; Deschaseaux-Voinet, C.; Berdeaux, G.; Ziegler, M.; Trial Study Group. Effects of dyskinesias in Parkinson's disease on quality of life and health-related costs: A prospective European study. *Eur. J. Neurol.* **2005**, *12*, 956–963. [CrossRef]

Review

Personalized Assessment of Insomnia and Sleep Quality in Patients with Parkinson's Disease

Ștefania Diaconu [1] and Cristian Falup-Pecurariu [1,2,*]

[1] Department of Medical and Surgical Specialties, Faculty of Medicine, Transilvania University, 500036 Brașov, Romania; stefi_diaconu@yahoo.com
[2] Department of Neurology, County Emergency Clinic Hospital, 500365 Brașov, Romania
* Correspondence: crisfp100@yahoo.co.uk

Abstract: Sleep disturbances are more common in patients with Parkinson's disease (PD) than in the general population and are considered one of the most troublesome symptoms by these patients. Insomnia represents one of the most common sleep disturbances in PD, and it correlates significantly with poor quality of life. There are several known causes of insomnia in the general population, but the complex manifestations that might be associated with PD may also induce insomnia and impact the quality of sleep. The treatment of insomnia and the strategies needed to improve sleep quality may therefore represent a challenge for the neurologist. A personalized approach to the PD patient with insomnia may help the clinician to identify the factors and comorbidities that should also be considered in order to establish a better individualized therapeutic plan. This review will focus on the main characteristics and correlations of insomnia, the most common risk factors, and the main subjective and objective methods indicated for the assessment of insomnia and sleep quality in order to offer a concise guide containing the main steps needed to approach the PD patient with chronic insomnia in a personalized manner.

Keywords: Parkinson's disease; insomnia; sleep quality; assessment; personalized medicine

1. Introduction

Several non-motor symptoms are known to affect the quality of life in patients with Parkinson's disease (PD), both in the early and advanced stages. Sleep disorders are found in all stages of PD, including in the pre-motor ones. Neurodegenerative processes that affect the normal functioning of neurotransmitters and the various effects of antiparkinsonian drugs could be involved in the pathogenesis of sleep disorders in PD [1]. Insomnia is reported by almost half of PD patients, and it is significantly related to motor fluctuations and other non-motor features [2].

The diagnosis of insomnia is based on the definition criteria established by the International Classification of Sleep Disorders, 3rd edition: difficulties to initiate and/or to maintain sleep and/or early morning awakenings [3]. For chronic insomnia, the above symptoms should be experienced by the patient at least 3 times a week for a minimum of 3 months. The association of daytime symptoms as consequences of insomnia is usually mandatory to establish the diagnosis [3]. Insomnia is commonly reported by PD patients, regardless of the severity of the disease, with a reported prevalence of 37–83% [4,5]. Polysomnographic studies revealed that PD patients have a shorter total sleep time and lower sleep efficiency compared to controls [6]. A polysomnographic analysis of 50 PD patients showed prolonged sleep latencies in almost half of the patients (mean duration: approximate 22 min) and a mean total sleep time of approximately 5 h/night [7]. Regarding the duration of sleep during the daytime, a study that objectively measured napping using wrist actigraphy in 85 PD patients showed a mean nap time of 39.2 ± 35.2 min/day [8]. All subtypes of insomnia (derived from the main definition) can be identified in PD, with variations across PD stages [9]. According to the results of a study performed on 689 PD patients, sleep maintenance insomnia due to disrupted sleep was the most commonly encountered (81.54%), followed by early morning awakenings (40.4%) [10]. Sleep disturbances, especially insomnia and reduced sleep quality, affect the quality of life [11]. Moreover, worsening of sleep disturbances and other neuropsychiatric complaints may contribute to the progression of other non-motor symptoms [12]. Some of the motor and non-motor symptoms are interrelated; for instance, gastrointestinal dysfunction may lead to poor absorption of antiparkinsonian drugs and to worsening motor symptoms [13]. Certain sleep disturbances might influence disease-related disability as well [14]. A proper and careful assessment of insomnia and other comorbidities is therefore mandatory in order to choose the right therapeutic intervention for each patient. Depending on the main causes of insomnia, the therapeutic options may vary from recommending sleep hygiene or cognitive behavioral therapy to pharmacological options such as benzodiazepine and nonbenzodiazepine hypnotics [15].

2. Assessment

2.1. Clinical Interview

A thorough history taking is essential when evaluating a patient with complaints suggestive of insomnia. The anamnesis should be obtained from the patient but also from the bed partner or caregiver. It is important to highlight the most important subjective symptoms, the time of the night when these complaints occur (first part of the night or after the patient falls asleep) and information regarding sleep patterns and habits. Regarding this aspect, the physician should be interested in the consistency or not of a sleep schedule, naps during the day, the consumption of alcohol, caffeine or other energizing products, as well as the type of physical activity performed by the patient. The patient's medication should be reviewed in search of insomnia as a side effect. Even if dopaminergic medication is known to induce daytime sleepiness, it can also be associated with insomnia [16]. According to a meta-analysis, levodopa, dopamine agonists, acetyl-cholinesterase inhibitors, and certain antidepressants may cause insomnia as an adverse effect [17]. Therefore, the medication regimen of the patient and the effects of polypharmacy should be carefully evaluated. Additionally, the medication and personal strategies used to alleviate insomnia should be assessed.

The clinician should search for the associated non-motor symptoms that can impair sleep quality and might sustain insomnia (an easy method in this regard is to use the Non-Motor Symptoms Questionnaire [18], which is described below) and also for the motor features that might interfere with satisfactory nighttime sleep (tremor, rigidity, dystonia). It is also essential to assess the consequences of insomnia that are experienced by the patient (e.g., headache, fatigue, daytime sleepiness, depression, anxiety) and the effects of insomnia on daily life activities. As daytime sleepiness frequently occurs in PD patients and is associated with episodes of sudden onset of sleep that might potentially be dangerous [19], it is important to ask PD patients with chronic insomnia if they feel sleepy during the day. A quick evaluation method of this symptom is to use the Epworth Sleepiness Scale (ESS) [20], which is one of the most commonly used scales for the evaluation of daytime sleepiness in the general population and also in PD. The Movement Disorders Society (MDS) Task Force considers the ESS a "recommended" instrument to screen for daytime sleepiness in the PD population [21]. Cognitive decline might also be considered as a negative consequence of sleep disorders, including insomnia [22]. For further assessment of cognitive function, the Mini-Mental State Examination (MMSE) and the Montreal Cognitive Assessment (MoCA) [23] are among the tools most commonly used in the general population. The MoCA has been shown to be more sensitive than the MMSE in detecting cognitive impairment in patients with PD [24] and other neurodegenerative disorders, such as progressive supranuclear palsy or multiple system atrophy [25]. The MDS Task Force recommends the following scales for cognitive screening in PD: MoCA, Mattis Dementia Rating Scale 2nd Edition (DRS-2) [26] and Parkinson's Disease-Cognitive Rating Scale (PD-CRS) [27].

A sleep diary is an easy method of assessing patients' sleep patterns that is used in the general population [28] and in PD patients for clinical evaluation [29], for comparison with other evaluation methods or for monitoring therapeutic effects [30]. There are several designs of sleep logs, but generally, the following information should be recorded by the patient: the bedtime hour, the estimated time of sleep onset, total sleep duration, wake-up time and awakenings overnight, sleep quality and the presence of naps/physical exercises/medication/alcohol or caffeine intake during daytime [28]. The sleep diary could also be used in association with other objective measurements.

2.2. The Assessment of Specific Risk Factors for Insomnia Associated with PD

Risk factors that lead to insomnia or are known to aggravate insomnia in the general population (e.g., age, stress, mood, maladaptive lifestyle, behavioral and environmental factors [31]) may also be found in PD. According to recent studies, overall sleep disturbances in PD were associated with napping during the day, watching the clock repeatedly and staying in bed when not able to fall asleep [32], or other inadequate sleep habits [33]. In addition to these factors, there are some specific symptoms in PD patients that contribute to insomnia and should be carefully assessed by the clinician.

2.2.1. Motor Symptoms

Motor features that are persistent or worsen during the night are associated with frequent awakenings and therefore, with sleep-maintenance insomnia. Nocturnal hypokinesia and rigidity might impair mobility and turning in bed and, therefore, might lead to sleep disturbances such as insomnia and reduced sleep quality and efficiency [34,35]. The persistence of tremors or dyskinesia during nighttime may also contribute to sleep fragmentation and poor sleep quality [36]. Motor symptoms may interfere with sleep maintenance even in the early stages; nocturnal dystonia, cramps and tremor were the motor features most commonly associated with sleep dysfunction in drug-naïve PD patients [37]. These motor symptoms, increased muscular tension, sleep apnea, age and disease duration may contribute to the concept of sleep fragmentation [38]. According to recent polysomnographic research, sleep fragmentation has a high rate in PD patients and might be considered a promising marker of PD progression [39].

2.2.2. Non-Motor Symptoms

Urinary dysfunction, especially nocturia, is a common symptom in the general elderly population and is a major factor that contributes to sleep disturbances [40]. Nocturia is a commonly encountered dysautonomic feature in PD patients, and it may correlate with subjective insomnia [41], frequent awakenings and insufficient total sleep time [2].

Another non-motor symptom that is significantly associated with sleep disturbances is pain. This symptom was found in almost half of PD patients, and the most reported type of pain was musculoskeletal pain [42]. Martinez-Martin et al. reported that any type of pain, but mostly the musculoskeletal subtype, was significantly correlated with overall sleep disorders [43]. Polysomnographic (PSG) studies demonstrated sleep fragmentation and modifications of sleep architecture in patients with PD and pain, characteristics which were less prominent in PD patients without pain [42]. An easy and robust method to assess pain is to use the King's Parkinson's Disease Pain Scale, which was demonstrated to be reliable and valid for the evaluation of this complex symptom in PD patients [44].

Among psychiatric non-motor symptoms, depression and anxiety were the most associated with sleep disturbances and reduced sleep quality. The severity of insomnia is correlated with the severity of depression in PD patients [45]. Moreover, an interconnection between depression, anxiety and pain may be found in conjunction with sleep disturbances and poor sleep quality in PD patients [46,47].

2.2.3. Other Associated Sleep Disorders

Restless legs syndrome (RLS), defined as discomfort in lower limbs that induces the need for movement and occurs during the night and during periods of immobility, is found in higher rates among PD patients compared to the general population [48]. RLS in association with periodic limb movements may induce arousal and disrupt normal sleep continuity, contributing to chronic insomnia [48,49]. The clinical diagnosis of RLS is based on the International Restless Legs Syndrome Study Group (IRLSSG) criteria [50]. There are various screening scales that can help the clinician to better assess these symptoms [51].

Sleep-disordered breathing (SDB) and mainly obstructive sleep apnea (OSA) may contribute to a reduced quality of sleep. Difficulties maintaining sleep are more common in patients with OSA than in healthy controls [52], and there is evidence that more than half of OSA patients without treatment have chronic insomnia [53]. In PD patients, the prevalence of OSA is approximately 62% [54]. Sobreira-Neto et al. found that PD patients with OSA may present lower rates of chronic insomnia (probably due to their reduced insight of sleep onset latency caused by sleep deprivation), but they also show reduced time spent in the N3 sleep stage and higher numbers of arousals compared to PD patients without OSA [55].

REM sleep behavior disorder (RBD), a parasomnia with "dream enacting", expressed by abnormal movements instead of muscular atonia during the REM sleep stage, is commonly associated with PD and with other neurodegenerative disorders. Longitudinal studies, including patients with idiopathic RBD, show significant correlations with neurodegenerative disorders and even high rates of phenoconversion [56]. RBD in PD patients causes reduced quality of sleep and also induces other consequences, such as cognitive impairment and autonomic dysfunctions [57,58]. RBD is associated with disrupted sleep architecture, explained by lower percentages of N2 and N3 sleep and a high periodic limb movement index [59].

2.3. Rating Scales and Objective Assessment of Insomnia and Quality of Sleep in PD Patients

2.3.1. Multidomain Scales or Questionnaires Designed to Evaluate Non-Motor Symptoms in PD, including Insomnia

Many of these scales contain items for screening and/or assessment of the severity of sleep disturbances.

The Movement Disorders Society Unified Parkinson Disease Rating Scale (MDS-UPDRS) is one of the most commonly used scales for the complex evaluation of various features of PD. It contains four parts, and part I is designed for the assessment of non-motor complaints. There is one question regarding insomnia and one question about daytime sleepiness. For all the items in this first part of the scale, the answers can be chosen between "0 = normal" and "4 = severe" [60].

The Non-Motor Symptoms Questionnaire (NMSQ) [18] has proven its efficiency in screening non-motor features of patients with PD. It contains 30 questions with simple answer choices ("yes"/"not"), and five of them are dedicated to the assessment of sleep: the difficulty of staying awake in certain circumstances, the difficulty of falling asleep and maintaining sleep, vivid dreams or nightmares, speaking or having abnormal movements during sleep and unpleasant sensations in the lower limbs during nighttime or rest associated with the need to move. This questionnaire is very easy for the patient to complete. It offers an accurate overview of the main symptoms, but it does not offer any information regarding the severity or the frequency of these symptoms. There are no items addressing SDB.

The Non-Motor Symptoms Scale (NMSS) [61] was created to complete and deepen the information obtained with the NMSQ. It is completed by the examiner. It takes a longer time for scoring than the NMSQ, but it provides data regarding symptom frequency and severity. For all the 30 items, the severity of the symptoms is evaluated from "0 = none" to "3 = severe", and the frequency is scored from "1 = rarely" to "4 = very frequent". The total score for each item is obtained by multiplying its severity by its frequency. The sleep/fatigue domain is comprised of items about insomnia, daytime sleepiness, RLS and fatigue.

The International Parkinson and Movement Disorder Society Non-Motor Rating Scale (MDS-NMSS) [62] is a reviewed version of the NMSS. It is administered by the examiner; it contains 52 items about non-motor symptoms, and the scoring process is similar to the NMSS: the frequency of the symptom is rated from "0 = never" to "4 = majority of time" and the severity is chosen between "0 = never" to "4 = severe". The product (frequency × severity) is calculated for each question. The "sleep and wakefulness" domain contains six questions about insomnia, RBD, excessive daytime sleepiness (EDS), restlessness, periodic limb movements and SDB.

2.3.2. Specific Scales or Questionnaires Designed to Evaluate Insomnia and Sleep Quality

The Parkinson's Disease Sleep Scale (PDSS) [63] is a self-assessment rating scale encompassing 15 questions which assess general aspects of sleep/daytime symptoms within one (previous) week: items related to insomnia, restlessness, hallucinations, bladder dysfunctions, tremor, dystonia, overall quality of sleep, and EDS. It was designed to assess sleep disturbances in the PD population, with each item being evaluated based on a visual analogue scale (VAS) ranging from 0 (never/excellent) to 10 (always/awful). A cutoff of 82/83 is considered suggestive for sleep disturbances, and the maximum score is 150 points, representing the worse clinical picture [64].

Regarding the psychometric properties of the PDSS, in the original study, the PDSS was applied on 280 adults (143 PD patients in different stages of severity and 137 healthy controls). Test-retest reliability was very high; good internal consistency (Cronbach's alpha, 0.77) and high repeatability were also observed [63]. Floor and ceiling responses were low (1%) [58,60]. High scores on the PDSS regarding EDS correlated with low scores on the ESS, which is the main scale used to assess EDS [63]. The PDSS showed a good correlation with SCOPA-S scores as well [64].

Regarding the strengths of the PDSS, it was developed as a brief, easy-to-use, reliable bedside instrument to screen for sleep symptoms in PD patients. Based on the results, the clinician may have insights regarding the severity of the sleep complaints. The items addressing insomnia might help discriminate between the types of insomnia or the possible causes (e.g., nocturia, tremor). The MDS Task Force classified the PDSS as a "recommended" tool to assess the existence and the severity of sleep disorders in PD [21]. It was shown that the PDSS could discriminate between PD and controls and also within PD severity levels and duration [64].

The PDSS is in the public domain and has been validated in several languages (Spanish, Japanese, Portuguese), with good clinimetric properties [65–67]. It was also widely used in several clinical trials in the PD population—e.g., evaluating the effectiveness of rotigotine [68]).

Regarding the weaknesses of the PDSS, even if the VAS is considered a simple method of assessing the level of severity of symptoms, it may be necessary to first inform the patient or caregiver how to apply this scoring system correctly.

The scale has only one question regarding EDS; therefore, it does not represent a proper tool to assess daytime symptoms. There are no questions related to other sleep disturbances, like sleep apnea or RBD; regarding RLS, there is only one question about "restlessness" of the arms or legs that might be related to RLS symptoms, but the mandatory criteria for RLS diagnosis are not fulfilled. The proposed timeframe is the previous week.

Based on the experience gathered from the administration of the PDSS, a revised version, the *Parkinson's Disease Sleep Scale (PDSS-2)*, was designed with the intention of exploring several aspects of sleep in the PD population that were not evaluated in the first version. It was also intended to be a useful tool to assess the effects of treatment on sleep disturbances [69].

The PDSS-2 includes 15 questions for the self-evaluation of sleep symptoms, addressing sleep quality, insomnia, restlessness, nightmares/hallucinations, bladder problems, motor features like rigidity or tremor, pain and breathing difficulties. The VAS scoring system was replaced with a grading system of symptom severity from 0 (never) to 4 (very frequent), with a maximum score of 60, indicating severe nocturnal sleep disturbances [69]. A score of 15 or above was considered the cutoff for poor sleepers [69,70].

Regarding the psychometric properties of the PDSS-2, the total score was evaluated, as were the scores for the three subscales (motor problems at night; PD symptoms at night; sleep specific disturbances) in order to establish the clinimetric characteristics. The PDSS-2 was validated in order to investigate nighttime impairments for the PD population, with findings demonstrating satisfactory reliability (Cronbach's alpha coefficient of 0.73 for the total score and few variations for the sub-scores), good internal consistency for most of the items (>0.30), and high test-retest reliability within 1–3 days (ICC of 0.80 for the total score) [69]. The test-retest reliability for a longer timeframe (1 month) was evaluated in another study, and it was considered acceptable (ICC of 0.799 for the total score) [71].

Regarding the strengths of the PDSS-2, it was shown that the PDSS-2 is a brief, easy-to-use and easy-to-administer self-rating scale useful for both screening the existence of sleep symptoms and grading their severity. Compared to the previous version, it is easier for patients with PD to understand and complete the PDSS-2 scale due to its Likert scoring system. It has good discriminative power between the grades of disease severity as evaluated with the Hoehn and Yahr scale. PDSS-2 is an assessment tool belonging to the public domain, which was validated and translated into several languages (German [69], Spanish [72], Italian [73], and Chinese [74]). It has been widely used in prevalence studies to assess sleep symptoms and their associations with several other symptoms or objective investigations (e.g., the presence of sleep disturbances and their correlations with brain MRI morphometry [75]), and it was used in clinical trials to evaluate the efficiency of medication on sleep [76].

Regarding the weaknesses of the PDSS-2, it focuses on the existence and severity of nighttime symptoms and therefore is not a proper tool to investigate their diurnal consequences, such as EDS. Unlike the previous version, the PDSS-2 has more clear questions related to RLS, and it also assesses the existence of breathing disturbances, but these items are not precise enough to diagnose RLS or OSA. A caregiver might improve the accuracy of the answers for some of the items, like for those related to awakenings during the night or difficulties turning in bed (as the patient might underestimate the existence/severity of these issues). The proposed timeframe is the previous week.

The Scales for Outcomes in Parkinson's Disease—Sleep (SCOPA—Sleep) is a 12-item self-rating scale designed to specifically evaluate nighttime sleep and daytime consequences in PD patients [77]. The questionnaire is structured in three parts. The first part consists of five items representing nighttime-specific (NS) disturbances that the patient might have experienced in the previous month (most of them concerning different types of insomnia). To answer these 5 questions, the patient chooses the answer which fits best from 0 (not at all) to 3 (a lot). The maximum score for this part is 15, indicating severe nighttime impairments (cutoff: 6/7) [64,77]. The second part is composed of only one question regarding the quality of sleep during the night; there are seven response options, ranging from "very well" to "very badly". There is no numeric scoring for this part. The last part contains six items to evaluate the daytime symptoms (DS) in the previous month, including EDS and the existence of sudden onset of sleep. The scoring for each item varies from 0 "not at all" to 3 "very much", with a maximum of 18 and a cutoff of 4/5 indicating daytime disturbances [77].

Regarding the psychometric properties of SCOPA-sleep, it shows high internal consistency for both the NS and DS subscales (Cronbach's alpha: 0.88 and 0.91, respectively) and good test-retest reliability (ICC: 0.94 for the NS subscale and 0.89 for the DS subscale). There were robust correlations between the DS subscore and ESS; the subscores of the NS part correlated with the PDSS and PSQI [77]. The floor and ceiling effects are absent [64].

Regarding the strengths, this scale is a brief, easy-to-administer rating tool with good internal consistency and reproducibility which can be used for screening and quantifying nighttime and daytime symptoms (like sudden onset of sleep) in PD patients. The MDS task force indicated SCOPA-sleep as a "recommended" scale for the aforementioned purposes [16]. The scale has been translated into several languages, taking part of the public domain. Like other scales designed to assess sleep in PD, SCOPA-sleep was useful to analyze the effect of various therapeutic options on sleep [78], and it was also used for monitoring symptoms in longitudinal studies [2].

Regarding weaknesses, even if the scale is designed to screen for possible nighttime symptoms, SCOPA-sleep lacks questions addressing nocturia, RBD, RLS or OSA. There are no questions addressed to the caregiver.

The Pittsburgh Sleep Quality Index (PSQI) [79] represents a self-rating tool designed to assess sleep in the general population, with the timeframe being the previous month. The first four items are dedicated to sleep habits (like usual bedtime, the perceived sleep latency, and number of hours of sleep per night). This is followed by questions related to possible causes of sleep disturbances (e.g., insomnia, breathing difficulties, pain) and questions about sleep quality, use of sleep medication, difficulties staying awake during daytime activities, and difficulties maintaining enthusiasm in daily activities. The PSQI has an additional five informative questions for the bed partner, which do not accumulate to the final score. For each item, the answers can be scored from 0 to 3 (no impairment/severe impairment). Based on the type of sleep problem addressed, the results can be grouped into seven compounds. The total score reaches a maximum of 21 points (indicating severe sleep disturbances), and a score of more than 5 points (for the total items) was considered an indicator for "bad" sleepers [79]. For PD patients, a more appropriate cutoff was considered 8/9 [77].

Regarding the psychometric properties of the PSQI, in the original study published in 1989, it was demonstrated to have high internal consistency and homogeneity (Cronbach's alpha: 0.83) [79]. Test-retest reliability was high for a short interval (2 days apart), and it remained high for a longer timeframe considering the majority of the subscores and the total score (overall test-retest correlation coefficient: 0.87) [80]. The PSQI showed correlations with PSG only regarding sleep latency, but it has strong correlations with the SCOPA-Sleep scale [81].

Regarding its strengths, the PSQI is in the public domain, and it is used to assess sleep in the general population and in PD patients [54,82]. Even if not specifically validated for PD, the PSQI is considered by the MDS Task Force to be a "recommended" tool to investigate sleep in the PD population [21]. Furthermore, it is a commonly used scale to evaluate the occurrence of sleep disturbances in primary insomnia, dementia and other movement disorders [81]. It has been largely translated into several languages, and it is also useful for monitoring the impact of various interventional strategies on sleep parameters [83,84].

Regarding its weaknesses, even if it covers a large spectrum of sleep disturbances that might occur, the PSQI has limited power to assess some conditions, such as OSA or RBD, and has no items designed to evaluate RLS. The questions addressed to the bed partner can help the investigator to complete the picture of the patient's overall sleep disturbances, but the data is not included in the total score; consequently, the global severity may be underestimated. The scoring system is complex, and some additional time should be considered for this aspect; the investigator has a guide with instructions for scoring.

A summary of the main scales used to assess insomnia and sleep quality in PD patients is presented in Table 1.

Table 1. Main characteristics of the most commonly used scales for the assessment of insomnia and sleep quality.

Scale Name	Designed For	Nr. Items	Approximate Completion Time	Short Description	Time Frame	Cutoff	Advantages	Disadvantages
PDSS	• General sleep assessment in PD patients • EDS	15	10 min	• Self-assessment • Items regarding insomnia, restlessness, various symptoms during nighttime, EDS • Evaluation based on VAS (0–10) • Maximum: 150 points = no sleep problems	Previous week	82/83	• Brief, easy to administer • bet used to screen/assess the severity of nocturnal/diurnal sleep disturbances	• VAS scoring requires instruction to complete • No items addressing RBD, RLS, or breathing disturbances
PDSS-2	• General sleep assessment in PD patients • PD symptoms during sleep	15	10 min	• Self-assessment • Items regarding insomnia, restlessness, various symptoms during nighttime, including motor features and breathing difficulties • Evaluation based on Likert scale (0–4) • Maximum: 60 points = severe sleep disturbances	Previous week	≥15	• Brief, reliable, precise • Used to screen/assess the severity of nighttime complains	• No daytime symptoms assessment • The insight of a caregiver may be necessary for some items
SCOPA—sleep	• Nighttime symptoms, quality of life and daytime symptoms in PD patients	12	5–10 min	• Self-assessment • One part for assessing nighttime symptoms (mainly insomnia) • One question regarding sleep quality • One part for assessing daytime symptoms (EDS, sudden onset of sleep)	Previous month	6/7 for night symptoms 4/5 for day symptoms	• Brief, easy to administer • Useful for screening and grading nighttime + daytime symptoms	• No questions for SDB, RLS, RBD nocturia
PSQI	• General sleep assessment • EDS	19	5–10 min for completing 5 min for scoring	• Self-assessment • Sleep habits evaluation; insomnia, various causes for sleep disturbances; EDS • Scoring from 0 (no difficulties) to 3 (severe) based on a guide for investigator • Maximum: 21 points = severe sleep disturbances	Previous month	>5 in the general population; >8 in PD patients	• Good insight into quality of sleep, sleep habits and causes of sleep disturbances	• Questions related to SDB, RBD—ambiguous • No questions for RLS • Information from bed partner not accounted for in the total score • Additional time for scoring (which is complex)

EDS, excessive daytime sleepiness; PD, Parkinson's disease; PDSS, Parkinson Disease Sleep Scale; PSQI, Pittsburg Sleep Quality Index; RBD, REM sleep behavior disorder; RLS, restless legs syndrome; SCOPA, Scales for outcomes in PD; SDB, sleep-disordered breathing; VAS, Visual Analogue Scale.

2.4. Objective Methods to Assess Insomnia

Actigraphy is a non-invasive method that is able to investigate several sleep parameters based on recording limb activity via accelerometers [85]. The device is worn on the non-dominant hand for a minimum of one week, and the results are interpreted together with a sleep log. Actigraphy is a useful method for the assessment of insomnia in the general population, as patients have the tendency to overestimate their sleep onset latency and to have a lower perception regarding the total sleep time [86]. On the other hand, some studies have demonstrated that PD patients might actually have a more accurate perception of their sleep problems [87]. Actigraphy was validated in patients with insomnia in the general population [88–91] and also demonstrated accurate results in evaluating sleep quality in PD patients compared to other subjective measures [29]. Actigraphy has several limits, though, as it cannot offer information about sleep stages, and it may overestimate the total sleep time if the patient remains still in bed without moving, as the recorder misinterprets immobility as sleep [91]. Therefore, actigraphy is best indicated for characterizing sleep disruptions and not to certify sleep initiation insomnia [85].

The Parkinson's KinetiGraph (PKG) is a device using wearable sensors (accelerometers) to record movements in order to offer data regarding several motor parameters in PD. It can also provide relative information regarding sleep parameters, as a period of immobility detected for at least 14 min is considered as an episode of sleep. The presence of interruptions of immobility during the night might be interpreted as awakenings or abnormal movements caused by sleep disturbances (RLS, RBD, etc.) [92]. Klingelhoefer et al. reported that the immobility and mobility states recorded by the PKG might correspond to sleep/awakening periods during nighttime, and the recorded sleep parameters correlate with other subjective measures of sleep [92]. The information obtained with the PKG changed the therapeutic decision in almost one-third of PD patients and improved communication with the neurologist in the majority of cases [93]. Comparative studies with polysomnography indicated that the periods of immobility that were identified with PKG during daytime correspond in approximately 85% with sleep periods confirmed with PSG [94]. Considering this, PKG might be a useful tool to investigate sleep onset and maintenance insomnia [92] and to integrate the information with the concomitant objective measures of the motor symptoms (bradykinesia, tremor, dyskinesia and fluctuations) [95,96]. PKG might also provide information regarding sleep quantity and quality, with significant correlations with subjective measures, but it cannot establish the sleep stages only based on the immobility data recorded [92], nor can it establish other events such as OSA or periodic limb movements [97]. It is a reliable tool that should be used together with a thorough history and clinical examination [93].

Polysomnography (PSG) is considered the 'gold standard' assessment tool for sleep disorders, as it can evaluate in an objective manner the sleep stages, sleep architecture and the normal and abnormal events during sleep. Several studies have been conducted in order to evaluate the sleep differences between PD patients and healthy controls. In PD patients, most of the PSG studies revealed more awakenings in PD patients, but no differences in sleep stages 1, 2 and the slow-wave sleep stage were observed in comparison to controls [98]. Most of the PSG studies did not demonstrate an increased rate of periodic limb movements during sleep in PD patients, nor a certain association with obstructive sleep apnea [98]. The contribution of nocturia to disrupted sleep and poor sleep quality was also demonstrated objectively by PSG evaluation [99]. Regarding the suspicion of RBD in PD patients, the clinical interview of the patient and PD partner might underestimate the occurrence of the abnormal motor behavior during sleep; therefore, PSG is necessary for the correct diagnosis of RBD [100]. However, PSG does not take part in the routine assessment of insomnia, as it has several limits—it is laborious and it requires trained clinicians and special conditions for the assessment (sleep lab). It is neither useful nor recommended to diagnose insomnia, but it can be necessary to rule out other conditions that might induce and perpetuate insomnia, such as SDB, RBD, and periodic limb movements [101].

3. Personalized Medicine and the Assessment of the PD Patient with Insomnia and Impaired Quality of Sleep

The concept of personalized (precision) medicine emphasizes the need for multi-dimensional approaches to the PD patient considering the complexity of this disorder. Several factors should be reviewed in order to establish tailored management strategies: genomics, pharmacogenetics, personality, lifestyle, comorbidities, etc. [102]. For instance, the comorbidity of respiratory disorders/sleep apnea, which is related to excessive daytime sleepiness, sleep fragmentation, anxiety and memory difficulties, represents one of the interrelated clinical situations addressed by personalized medicine [103]. In that case, the proper assessment of sleep-maintenance insomnia could reveal an underlying respiratory problem and consultation with a pulmonologist would be necessary. Taking into account the various factors known to be associated with insomnia and the particularities of the sleep disturbances in PD, an individualized approach is therefore mandatory in order to better characterize sleep in PD and to develop adequate management strategies. We propose an algorithm for the personalized assessment of PD patients with insomnia and impaired sleep quality, which is shown in Figure 1. In this regard, the clinician should always approach the patient with sleep disturbances by asking for more details about the main complaints (the information obtained from a caregiver could be valuable). A full general and neurological exam should be performed; a proper examination of the motor symptoms should include assessment using the UPDRS part III & IV. As the non-motor symptoms have strong connections with insomnia and poor sleep quality, the NMSQ can be used as a screening tool that is brief and easy to apply. To better understand the patient's pre-sleep habits and symptoms, several aspects should be asked (for instance, sleep patterns during day and night, the intake of coffee or alcohol, if the patient leads a sedentary lifestyle, etc.). A sleep diary may bring valuable information in this regard, and the patient should be informed regarding how to overcome his or her bad sleep habits. The side effects of medications should be reviewed and changed accordingly. Once the clinician identifies certain symptoms that occur before sleep onset (for instance, RLS), the next step is to evaluate the severity of these symptoms and start a treatment (in this case, IRLS might be a useful tool for severity grading and monitoring). If the patient complains about poor sleep quality, frequent awakenings during nighttime and difficulties falling back asleep, the neurologist should try to identify and treat the cause(s), considering the common association with motor symptoms (nocturnal cramps, tremor, dyskinesia, etc.), non-motor symptoms (e.g., pain, nocturia) and other comorbidities (RLS/ PLMS, SDB, RBD). In the context of a busy medical practice, we strongly recommend the use of standardized scales for non-motor evaluation (NMSQ) and for overall sleep assessment (considering their main indications, advantages, and disadvantages—see Table 1). Daytime consequences of insomnia and poor quality of sleep should be asked about in order to appreciate the magnitude of the sleep complaints. For instance, if the patient or the clinician suspects that poor quality of sleep may be associated with memory and attention problems, a cognitive screening test such as the MMSE or MoCA can offer supplementary information. In some cases, when the causes or the consequences of insomnia and poor sleep quality are difficult to identify or are resistant to the recommended treatment, further objective assessment should be indicated. Wearable devices might be more convenient for the patient. They are useful for obtaining objective measurements of sleep parameters and motor function and can record information for a longer time (at least 1 week). PSG, on the other hand, should be indicated only in particular circumstances, for instance, when the diagnosis is uncertain or when other associated conditions such as SBD or RBD are suspected. Considering the many interconnected aspects of sleep disorders in PD patients, we suggest that a comprehensive assessment of sleep parameters and associated factors may be the key to personalized and successful management of these disturbances.

Main complaint and clinical evaluation	Pre-sleep habits and symptoms	Symptoms during sleep	Daytime consequences	Further objective assessments
• sleep initiation difficulties • sleep maintenance difficulties • early-morning awakenings ❖ Motor assessment • tremor; rigidity; dyskinesia (use UPDRS part III & IV) • RLS ❖ Non-motor assessment (e.g., use NMSQ for screening) • depression • anxiety • pain (e.g., use King's PD pain scale for grading)	• regular sleep pattern • caffeine or alcohol intake • physical exercises • medication (antiparkinsonian, for sleep) • anxiety • personal insomnia coping "strategies" • RLS (e.g. use IRLS) ❖ Sleep diary	❖ Motor symptoms • nocturnal cramps • tremor • rigidity • dystonia • dyskinesia ❖ Non-motor symptoms • pain • nocturia ❖ Other comorbid sleep disorders • RLS/PLMS • SDB • RBD ❖ Scales • PDSS • PDSS-2 • SCOPA-Sleep • PSQI	• excessive daytime sleepiness (e.g., use ESS) • fatigue • depression • irritability • headache • cognitive impairments (e.g., use MMSE, MOCA)	❖ Actigraphy • use for at least 1 week + sleep diary • objective estimates of sleep parameters ❖ PKG • useful for assessment of sleep parameters, assessment of motor function ❖ PSG • uncertainty of the diagnosis • suspected associated conditions (SDB, RLS, RBD) • treatment resistance

Figure 1. Proposed clinical interview components and subjective and objective methods for the personalized assessment of insomnia and sleep quality in PD patients. ESS, Epworth Sleepiness Scale; IRLS, International Restless Legs Syndrome Study Group rating scale; MMSE, Mini-Mental State Examination; MOCA, Montreal Cognitive Assessment; NMSQ, Non-Motor Symptoms Questionnaire; PD, Parkinson's disease; PDSS, Parkinson Disease Sleep Scale; PKG, Parkinson's KinetiGraph; PLMS, periodic limb movements of sleep; PSG, polysomnography; PSQI, Pittsburg Sleep Quality Index; RBD, REM sleep behavior disorder; RLS, restless legs syndrome; SCOPA, Scales for outcomes in PD; SDB, sleep-disordered breathing; UPDRS, Unified Parkinson Disease Rating Scale.

4. Conclusions

There are several aspects of sleep that should be carefully examined when investigating the PD patient with insomnia. Many behavioral factors, as well as the associated motor and non-motor symptoms, are interconnected with sleep disturbances and poor quality of life. An easy and methodical approach is to start from the main complaint and then assess the habits and symptoms before sleep, then the symptoms during sleep and the consequences during the day. There are several useful scales and questionnaires designed to help the clinician identify the main complaints and to grade their severity. When in doubt, further objective assessment methods should be recommended, such as actigraphy, the Parkinson KinetiGraph or polysomnography. A personalized approach to the PD patient with sleep disturbances would be therefore much effective in establishing the proper therapeutic strategies that can help improve the quality of life of these patients.

Author Contributions: Conceptualization, Ş.D. and C.F.-P.; methodology, Ş.D. and C.F.-P.; writing—original draft preparation, Ş.D.; writing—review and editing, Ş.D. and C.F.-P. All authors have read and agreed to the published version of the manuscript.

Funding: This research received no external funding.

Institutional Review Board Statement: Not applicable.

Informed Consent Statement: Not applicable.

Data Availability Statement: Not applicable.

Conflicts of Interest: The authors declare no conflict of interest.

References

1. Falup-Pecurariu, C.; Diaconu, Ş.; Țînț, D.; Falup-Pecurariu, O. Neurobiology of sleep (Review). *Exp. Ther. Med.* **2021**, *21*, 272. [CrossRef] [PubMed]
2. Zhu, K.; van Hilten, J.J.; Marinus, J. The course of insomnia in Parkinson's disease. *Parkinsonism Relat. Disord.* **2016**, *33*, 51–57. [CrossRef] [PubMed]
3. Darien, I. *The International Classification of Sleep Disorders (ICSD-3)*; American Academy of Sleep Medicine: Darien, IL, USA, 2014.
4. Barone, P.; Antonini, A.; Colosimo, C.; Marconi, R.; Morgante, L.; Avarello, T.P.; Bottacchi, E.; Cannas, A.; Ceravolo, G.; Ceravolo, R.; et al. The PRIAMO study: A multicenter assessment of nonmotor symptoms and their impact on quality of life in Parkinson's disease. *Mov. Disord.* **2009**, *24*, 1641-9. [CrossRef] [PubMed]
5. Gjerstad, M.D.; Wentzel-Larsen, T.; Aarsland, D.; Larsen, J.P. Insomnia in Parkinson's disease: Frequency and progression over time. *J. Neurol. Neurosurg. Psychiatry* **2007**, *78*, 476–479. [CrossRef]
6. Yong, M.H.; Fook-Chong, S.; Pavanni, R.; Lim, L.L.; Tan, E.K. Case control polysomnographic studies of sleep disorders in Parkinson's disease. *PLoS ONE* **2011**, *6*, e22511. [CrossRef]
7. Selvaraj, V.K.; Keshavamurthy, B. Sleep dysfunction in Parkinson's disease. *J. Clin. Diagn. Res.* **2016**, *10*, OC09–OC12. [CrossRef]
8. Bolitho, S.J.; Naismith, S.L.; Salahuddin, P.; Terpening, Z.; Grunstein, R.R.; Lewis, S.J.G. Objective measurement of daytime napping, cognitive dysfunction and subjective sleepiness in Parkinson's disease. *PLoS ONE* **2013**, *8*, e81233. [CrossRef]
9. Tholfsen, L.K.; Larsen, J.P.; Schulz, J.; Tysnes, O.B.; Gjerstad, M.D. Changes in insomnia subtypes in early Parkinson disease. *Neurology* **2017**, *88*, 352–358. [CrossRef]
10. Ylikoski, A.; Martikainen, K.; Sieminski, M.; Partinen, M. Parkinson's disease and insomnia. *Neurol. Sci.* **2015**, *36*, 2003–2010. [CrossRef]
11. Shafazand, S.; Wallace, D.M.; Arheart, K.L.; Vargas, S.; Luca, C.C.; Moore, H.; Katzen, H.; Levin, B.; Singer, C. Insomnia, sleep quality, and quality of life in mild to moderate parkinson's disease. *Ann. Am. Thorac. Soc.* **2017**, *14*, 412–419. [CrossRef]
12. Santos-García, D.; de Deus, T.; Cores, C.; Canfield, H.; Paz González, J.M.; Martínez Miró, C.; Valdés Aymerich, L.; Suárez, E.; Jesús, S.; Aguilar, M.; et al. Predictors of global non-motor symptoms burden progression in Parkinson's disease. Results from the COPPADIS Cohort at 2-year follow-up. *J. Pers. Med.* **2021**, *11*, 626. [CrossRef] [PubMed]
13. Ivan, I.-F.; Irincu, V.-L.; Diaconu, Ş.; Falup-Pecurariu, O.; Ciopleiaş, B.; Falup-Pecurariu, C. Gastro-intestinal dysfunctions in Parkinson's disease (Review). *Exp. Ther. Med.* **2021**, *22*, 1083. [CrossRef] [PubMed]
14. Suzuki, K.; Okuma, Y.; Uchiyama, T.; Miyamoto, M.; Sakakibara, R.; Shimo, Y.; Hattori, N.; Kuwabara, S.; Yamamoto, T.; Kaji, Y.; et al. Impact of sleep-related symptoms on clinical motor subtypes and disability in Parkinson's disease: A multicentre cross-sectional study. *J. Neurol. Neurosurg. Psychiatry* **2017**, *88*, 953–959. [CrossRef] [PubMed]
15. Falup-Pecurariu, C.; Diaconu, Ş. Sleep dysfunction in Parkinson's disease. *Int. Rev. Neurobiol.* **2017**, *133*, 719–742. [CrossRef] [PubMed]
16. Paus, S.; Brecht, H.M.; Köster, J.; Seeger, G.; Klockgether, T.; Wüllner, U. Sleep attacks, daytime sleepiness, and dopamine agonists in Parkinson's disease. *Mov. Disord.* **2003**, *18*, 659–667. [CrossRef] [PubMed]
17. Doufas, A.G.; Panagiotou, O.A.; Panousis, P.; Wong, S.S.; Ioannidis, J.P. Insomnia from drug treatments: Evidence from meta-analyses of randomized trials and concordance with prescribing information. *Mayo Clin. Proc.* **2017**, *92*, 72–87. [CrossRef]
18. Chaudhuri, K.R.; Martinez-Martin, P.; Schapira, A.H.V.; Stocchi, F.; Sethi, K.; Odin, P.; Brown, R.G.; Koller, W.; Barone, P.; MacPhee, G.; et al. International multicenter pilot study of the first comprehensive self-completed nonmotor symptoms questionnaire for Parkinson's disease: The NMSQuest study. *Mov. Disord.* **2006**, *21*, 916–923. [CrossRef]
19. Shen, Y.; Huang, J.Y.; Li, J.; Liu, C.F. Excessive daytime sleepiness in Parkinson's disease: Clinical implications and management. *Chin. Med. J.* **2018**, *34*, 180–198. [CrossRef]
20. Johns, M.W. A new method for measuring daytime sleepiness: The Epworth sleepiness scale. *Sleep* **1991**, *14*, 540–545. [CrossRef]
21. Högl, B.; Arnulf, I.; Comella, C.; Ferreira, J.; Iranzo, A.; Tilley, B.; Trenkwalder, C.; Poewe, W.; Rascol, O.; Sampaio, C.; et al. Scales to assess sleep impairment in Parkinson's disease: Critique and recommendations. *Mov. Disord.* **2010**, *25*, 2704–2716. [CrossRef]
22. Huang, J.; Zhuo, W.; Zhang, Y.; Sun, H.; Chen, H.; Zhu, P.; Pan, X.; Yang, J.; Wang, L. Cognitive function characteristics of Parkinson's disease with sleep disorders. *Parkinson's Dis.* **2017**, *79*, 368–376. [CrossRef]
23. Nasreddine, Z.S.; Phillips, N.A.; Bédirian, V.; Charbonneau, S.; Whitehead, V.; Collin, I.; Cummings, J.L.; Chertkow, H. The montreal cognitive assessment, MoCA: A brief screening tool for mild cognitive impairment. *J. Am. Geriatr. Soc.* **2005**, *53*, 695–699. [CrossRef] [PubMed]
24. Hoops, S.; Nazem, S.; Siderowf, A.D.; Duda, J.E.; Xie, S.X.; Stern, M.B.; Weintraub, D. Validity of the MoCA and MMSE in the detection of MCI and dementia in Parkinson disease. *Neurology* **2009**, *73*, 1738–1745. [CrossRef] [PubMed]
25. Fiorenzato, E.; Weis, L.; Falup-Pecurariu, C.; Diaconu, S.; Siri, C.; Reali, E.; Pezzoli, G.; Bisiacchi, P.; Antonini, A.; Biundo, R. Montreal Cognitive Assessment (MoCA) and Mini-Mental State Examination (MMSE) performance in progressive supranuclear palsy and multiple system atrophy. *J. Neural Transm.* **2016**, *123*, 1435–1442. [CrossRef] [PubMed]
26. Johnson-Greene, D. Dementia Rating Scale-2 (DRS-2) By P.J. Jurica, C.L. Leitten, and S. Mattis: Psychological assessment resources, 2001. *Arch. Clin. Neuropsychol.* **2004**, *19*, 145–147. [CrossRef]
27. Pagonabarraga, J.; Kulisevsky, J.; Llebaria, G.; García-Sánchez, C.; Pascual-Sedano, B.; Gironell, A. Parkinson's disease-cognitive rating scale: A new cognitive scale specific for Parkinson's disease. *Mov. Disord.* **2008**, *23*, 998–1005. [CrossRef]
28. Ibáñez, V.; Silva, J.; Cauli, O. A survey on sleep questionnaires and diaries. *Sleep Med.* **2018**, *42*, 90–96. [CrossRef]

29. Stavitsky, K.; Saurman, J.L.; McNamara, P.; Cronin-Golomb, A. Sleep in Parkinson's disease: A comparison of actigraphy and subjective measures. *Parkinsonism Relat. Disord.* 2010, *16*, 280–283. [CrossRef]
30. Videnovic, A.; Klerman, E.B.; Wang, W.; Marconi, A.; Kuhta, T.; Zee, P.C. Timed light therapy for sleep and daytime sleepiness associated with Parkinson disease a randomized clinical trial. *JAMA Neurol.* 2017, *74*, 411–418. [CrossRef]
31. Bollu, P.C.; Kaur, H. Sleep medicine: Insomnia and sleep. *Mo. Med.* 2019, *116*, 68–75.
32. Wade, R.; Pachana, N.A.; Mellick, G.; DIssanayaka, N. Factors related to sleep disturbances for individuals with Parkinson's disease: A regional perspective. *Int. Psychogeriatr.* 2020, *32*, 827–838. [CrossRef]
33. Sobreira-Neto, M.A.; Pena-Pereira, M.A.; Sobreira, E.S.T.; Chagas, M.H.N.; de Almeida, C.M.O.; Fernandes, R.M.F.; Tumas, V.; Eckeli, A.L. Chronic insomnia in patients with Parkinson disease: Which associated factors are relevant? *J. Geriatr. Psychiatry Neurol.* 2020, *33*, 22–27. [CrossRef] [PubMed]
34. Xue, F.; Wang, F.Y.; Mao, C.J.; Guo, S.P.; Chen, J.; Li, J.; Wang, Q.J.; Bei, H.Z.; Yu, Q.; Liu, C.F. Analysis of nocturnal hypokinesia and sleep quality in Parkinson's disease. *J. Clin. Neurosci.* 2018, *54*, 96–101. [CrossRef]
35. Bhidayasiri, R.; Trenkwalder, C. Getting a good night sleep? The importance of recognizing and treating nocturnal hypokinesia in Parkinson's disease. *Parkinsonism Relat. Disord.* 2018, *50*, 10–18. [CrossRef]
36. Mao, C.J.; Yang, Y.P.; Chen, J.P.; Wang, F.; Chen, J.; Zhang, J.R.; Zhang, H.J.; Zhuang, S.; Xiong, Y.T.; Gu, C.C.; et al. Poor nighttime sleep is positively associated with dyskinesia in Parkinson's disease patients. *Parkinsonism Relat. Disord.* 2018, *48*, 68–73. [CrossRef]
37. Dhawan, V.; Dhoat, S.; Williams, A.J.; DiMarco, A.; Pal, S.; Forbes, A.; Tobías, A.; Martinez-Martin, P.; Chaudhuri, K.R. The range and nature of sleep dysfunction in untreated Parkinson's disease (PD). A comparative controlled clinical study using the Parkinson's disease sleep scale and selective polysomnography. *J. Neurol. Sci.* 2006, *248*, 158–162. [CrossRef]
38. Norlinah, M.I.; Afidah, K.N.; Noradina, A.T.; Shamsul, A.S.; Hamidon, B.B.; Sahathevan, R.; Raymond, A.A. Sleep disturbances in Malaysian patients with Parkinson's disease using polysomnography and PDSS. *Parkinsonism Relat. Disord.* 2009, *15*, 670–674. [CrossRef]
39. Cai, G.E.; Luo, S.; Chen, L.N.; Lu, J.P.; Huang, Y.J.; Ye, Q.Y. Sleep fragmentation as an important clinical characteristic of sleep disorders in Parkinson's disease: A preliminary study. *Chin. Med. J.* 2019, *132*, 1788–1795. [CrossRef]
40. Vaughan, C.P.; Bliwise, D.L. Sleep and nocturia in older adults. *Sleep Med. Clin.* 2018, *13*, 107–116. [CrossRef]
41. Chung, S.; Bohnen, N.I.; Albin, R.L.; Frey, K.A.; Müller, M.L.T.M.; Chervin, R.D. Insomnia and sleepiness in Parkinson disease: Associations with symptoms and comorbidities. *J. Clin. Sleep Med.* 2013, *9*, 1131–1137. [CrossRef]
42. Fu, Y.T.; Mao, C.J.; Ma, L.J.; Zhang, H.J.; Wang, Y.; Li, J.; Huang, J.Y.; Liu, J.Y.; Liu, C.F. Pain correlates with sleep disturbances in Parkinson's disease patients. *Pain Pract.* 2018, *18*, 29–37. [CrossRef] [PubMed]
43. Martinez-Martin, P.; Rizos, A.M.; Wetmore, J.B.; Antonini, A.; Odin, P.; Pal, S.; Sophia, R.; Carroll, C.; Martino, D.; Falup-Pecurariu, C.; et al. Relationship of nocturnal sleep dysfunction and pain subtypes in Parkinson's disease. *Mov. Disord. Clin. Pract.* 2019, *6*, 57–64. [CrossRef] [PubMed]
44. Chaudhuri, K.R.; Rizos, A.; Trenkwalder, C.; Rascol, O.; Pal, S.; Martino, D.; Carroll, C.; Paviour, D.; Falup-Pecurariu, C.; Kessel, B.; et al. King's Parkinson's disease pain scale, the first scale for pain in PD: An international validation. *Mov. Disord.* 2015, *30*, 1623–1631. [CrossRef]
45. Kay, D.B.; Tanner, J.J.; Bowers, D. Sleep disturbances and depression severity in patients with Parkinson's disease. *Brain Behav.* 2018, *8*, e00967. [CrossRef]
46. Rana, A.Q.; Qureshi, A.R.M.; Kachhvi, H.B.; Rana, M.A.; Chou, K.L. Increased likelihood of anxiety and poor sleep quality in Parkinson's disease patients with pain. *J. Neurol. Sci.* 2016, *369*, 212–215. [CrossRef]
47. Rana, A.Q.; Qureshi, A.R.M.; Shamli Oghli, Y.; Saqib, Y.; Mohammed, B.; Sarfraz, Z.; Rana, R. Decreased sleep quality in Parkinson's patients is associated with higher anxiety and depression prevalence and severity, and correlates with pain intensity and quality. *Neurol. Res.* 2018, *40*, 696–701. [CrossRef]
48. Ferini-Strambi, L.; Carli, G.; Casoni, F.; Galbiati, A. Restless legs syndrome and Parkinson disease: A causal relationship between the two disorders? *Front. Neurol.* 2018, *9*, 551. [CrossRef] [PubMed]
49. Bonakis, A.; Androutsou, A.; Koloutsou, M.E.; Vagiakis, E. Restless Legs Syndrome masquerades as chronic insomnia. *Sleep Medicine* 2020, *75*, 106–111. [CrossRef]
50. Allen, R.P.; Picchietti, D.L.; Garcia-Borreguero, D.; Ondo, W.G.; Walters, A.S.; Winkelman, J.W.; Zucconi, M.; Ferri, R.; Trenkwalder, C.; Lee, H.B. Restless legs syndrome/Willis-Ekbom disease diagnostic criteria: Updated International Restless Legs Syndrome Study Group (IRLSSG) consensus criteria—History, rationale, description, and significance. *Sleep Med.* 2014, *15*, 860–873. [CrossRef] [PubMed]
51. Walters, A.S.; LeBrocq, C.; Dhar, A.; Hening, W.; Rosen, R.; Allen, R.P.; Trenkwalder, C.; The International Restless Legs Syndrome Study Group. Validation of the International Restless Legs Syndrome Study Group rating scale for restless legs syndrome. *Sleep Med.* 2003, *4*, 121–132. [CrossRef] [PubMed]
52. Björnsdóttir, E.; Janson, C.; Gíslason, T.; Sigurdsson, J.F.; Pack, A.I.; Gehrman, P.; Benediktsdóttir, B. Insomnia in untreated sleep apnea patients compared to controls. *J. Sleep Res.* 2012, *21*, 131–138. [CrossRef] [PubMed]
53. Krell, S.B.; Kapur, V.K. Insomnia complaints in patients evaluated for obstructive sleep apnea. *Sleep Breath.* 2005, *9*, 104–110. [CrossRef] [PubMed]

54. Sobreira-Neto, M.A.; Pena-Pereira, M.A.; Sobreira, E.S.T.; Chagas, M.H.N.; Fernandes, R.M.F.; Tumas, V.; Eckeli, A.L. High frequency of sleep disorders in Parkinson's disease and its relationship with quality of life. *Eur. Neurol.* **2017**, *78*, 330–337. [CrossRef] [PubMed]
55. Sobreira-Neto, M.A.; Pena-Pereira, M.A.; Sobreira, E.S.T.; Chagas, M.H.N.; De Almeida, C.M.O.; Fernandes, R.M.F.; Tumas, V.; Eckeli, A.L. Obstructive sleep apnea and Parkinson's disease: Characteristics and associated factors. *Arq. Neuro-Psiquiatr.* **2019**, *77*, 609–616. [CrossRef]
56. St Louis, E.K.; Boeve, B.F. REM sleep behavior disorder: Diagnosis, clinical implications, and future directions. *Mayo Clin. Proc.* **2017**, *92*, 1723–1736. [CrossRef]
57. Kamble, N.; Yadav, R.; Lenka, A.; Kumar, K.; Nagaraju, B.C.; Pal, P.K. Impaired sleep quality and cognition in patients of Parkinson's disease with REM sleep behavior disorder: A comparative study. *Sleep Med.* **2019**, *62*, 1–5. [CrossRef]
58. Diaconu, Ș.; Falup-Pecurariu, O.; Țînț, D.; Falup-Pecurariu, C. REM sleep behaviour disorder in Parkinson's disease (Review). *Exp. Ther. Med.* **2021**, *22*, 812. [CrossRef]
59. Zhang, X.; Song, Z.; Ye, J.; Fu, Y.; Wang, J.; Su, L.; Zhu, X.; Zhang, M.; Cheng, Y.; Wu, W.; et al. Polysomnographic and neuropsychological characteristics of rapid eye movement sleep behavior disorder patients. *Brain Behav.* **2019**, *9*, e01220. [CrossRef]
60. Goetz, C.G.; Tilley, B.C.; Shaftman, S.R.; Stebbins, G.T.; Fahn, S.; Martinez-Martin, P.; Poewe, W.; Sampaio, C.; Stern, M.B.; Dodel, R.; et al. Movement disorder society-sponsored revision of the unified Parkinson's disease rating scale (MDS-UPDRS): Scale presentation and clinimetric testing results. *Mov. Disord.* **2008**, *23*, 2129–2170. [CrossRef]
61. Chaudhuri, K.R.; Martinez-Martin, P.; Brown, R.G.; Sethi, K.; Stocchi, F.; Odin, P.; Ondo, W.; Abe, K.; MacPhee, G.; MacMahon, D.; et al. The metric properties of a novel non-motor symptoms scale for Parkinson's disease: Results from an international pilot study. *Mov. Disord.* **2007**, *22*, 1901–1911. [CrossRef]
62. Chaudhuri, K.R.; Schrag, A.; Weintraub, D.; Rizos, A.; Rodriguez-Blazquez, C.; Mamikonyan, E.; Martinez-Martin, P. The movement disorder society nonmotor rating scale: Initial validation study. *Mov. Disord.* **2020**, *35*, 116–133. [CrossRef] [PubMed]
63. Chaudhuri, K.R.; Pal, S.; DiMarco, A.; Whately-Smith, C.; Bridgman, K.; Mathew, R.; Pezzela, F.R.; Forbes, A.; Högl, B.; Trenkwalder, C. The Parkinson's disease sleep scale: A new instrument for assessing sleep and nocturnal disability in Parkinson's disease. *J. Neurol. Neurosurg. Psychiatry* **2002**, *73*, 629–635. [CrossRef] [PubMed]
64. Martinez-Martin, P.; Visser, M.; Rodriguez-Blazquez, C.; Marinus, J.; Chaudhuri, K.R.; van Hilten, J.J. SCOPA-sleep and PDSS: Two scales for assessment of sleep disorder in Parkinson's disease. *Mov. Disord.* **2008**, *23*, 1681–1688. [CrossRef] [PubMed]
65. Martínez-Martín, P.; Salvador, C.; Menéndez-Guisasola, L.; González, S.; Tobías, A.; Almazán, J.; Chaudhuri, K.R. Parkinson's disease sleep scale: Validation study of a Spanish version. *Mov. Disord.* **2004**, *19*, 1226–1232. [CrossRef]
66. Abe, K.; Hikita, T.; Sakoda, S. Sleep disturbances in Japanese patients with Parkinson's disease—Comparing with patients in the UK. *J. Neurol. Sci.* **2005**, *234*, 73–78. [CrossRef]
67. Margis, R.; Donis, K.; Schönwald, S.V.; Fagondes, S.C.; Monte, T.; Martín-Martínez, P.; Chaudhuri, K.R.; Kapczinski, F.; Rieder, C.R.M. Psychometric properties of the Parkinson's disease sleep scale—Brazilian version. *Parkinsonism Relat. Disord.* **2009**, *15*, 495–499. [CrossRef]
68. Pierantozzi, M.; Placidi, F.; Liguori, C.; Albanese, M.; Imbriani, P.; Marciani, M.G.; Mercuri, N.B.; Stanzione, P.; Stefani, A. Rotigotine may improve sleep architecture in Parkinson's disease: A double-blind, Randomized, Placebo-controlled polysomnographic study. *Sleep Med.* **2016**, *21*, 140–144. [CrossRef]
69. Trenkwalder, C.; Kohnen, R.; Högl, B.; Metta, V.; Sixel-Döring, F.; Frauscher, B.; Hülsmann, J.; Martinez-Martin, P.; Chaudhuri, K.R. Parkinson's disease sleep scale—Validation of the revised version PDSS-2. *Mov. Disord.* **2011**, *26*, 644–652. [CrossRef]
70. Suzuki, K.; Miyamoto, T.; Miyamoto, M.; Suzuki, S.; Numao, A.; Watanabe, Y.; Tatsumoto, M.; Sakuta, H.; Watanabe, Y.; Fujita, H.; et al. Evaluation of cutoff scores for the Parkinson's disease sleep scale-2. *Acta Neurol. Scand.* **2015**, *131*, 426–430. [CrossRef]
71. Horváth, K.; Aschermann, Z.; Ács, P.; Deli, G.; Janszky, J.; Karádi, K.; Komoly, S.; Faludi, B.; Kovács, N. Test-retest validity of Parkinson's disease sleep scale 2nd version (PDSS-2). *J. Parkinson's Dis.* **2014**, *4*, 687–691. [CrossRef]
72. Martinez-Martin, P.; Wetmore, J.B.; Rodríguez-Blázquez, C.; Arakaki, T.; Bernal, O.; Campos-Arillo, V.; Cerda, C.; Estrada-Bellmann, I.; Garretto, N.; Ginsburg, L.; et al. The Parkinson's Disease Sleep Scale–2 (PDSS-2): Validation of the spanish version and its relationship with a roommate-based version. *Mov. Disord. Clin. Pract.* **2019**, *6*, 294–301. [CrossRef]
73. Arnaldi, D.; Cordano, C.; De Carli, F.; Accardo, J.; Ferrara, M.; Picco, A.; Tamburini, T.; Brugnolo, A.; Abbruzzese, G.; Nobili, F. Parkinson's disease sleep scale 2: Application in an Italian population. *Neurol. Sci.* **2016**, *37*, 283–288. [CrossRef] [PubMed]
74. Zhang, J.; Peng, R.; Du, Y.; Mou, Y.; Li, N.; Cheng, L. Reliability and validity of Parkinson's disease sleep scale-Chinese version in the south west of China. *Natl. Med. J. China* **2016**, *96*, 3294–3299. [CrossRef]
75. Radziunas, A.; Deltuva, V.P.; Tamasauskas, A.; Gleizniene, R.; Pranckeviciene, A.; Petrikonis, K.; Bunevicius, A. Brain MRI morphometric analysis in Parkinson's disease patients with sleep disturbances. *BMC Neurol.* **2018**, *18*, 88. [CrossRef] [PubMed]
76. Chaudhuri, R.K.; Martinez-Martin, P.; Antonini, A.; Brown, R.G.; Friedman, J.H.; Onofrj, M.; Surmann, E.; Ghys, L.; Trenkwalder, C. Rotigotine and specific non-motor symptoms of Parkinson's disease: Post hoc analysis of RECOVER. *Parkinsonism Relat. Disord.* **2013**, *19*, 660–665. [CrossRef] [PubMed]
77. Marinus, J.; Visser, M.; Van Hilten, J.J.; Lammers, G.J.; Stiggelbout, A.M. Assessment of sleep and sleepiness in parkinson disease. *Sleep* **2003**, *26*, 1049–1054. [CrossRef] [PubMed]

78. Patel, N.; Lewitt, P.; Neikrug, A.B.; Kesslak, P.; Coate, B.; Ancoli-Israel, S. Nighttime sleep and daytime sleepiness improved with pimavanserin during treatment of Parkinson's disease psychosis. *Clin. Neuropharmacol.* **2018**, *41*, 210–215. [CrossRef] [PubMed]
79. Buysse, D.J.; Reynolds, C.F.; Monk, T.H.; Berman, S.R.; Kupfer, D.J. The Pittsburgh sleep quality index: A new instrument for psychiatric practice and research. *Psychiatry Res.* **1989**, *28*, 193–213. [CrossRef]
80. Backhaus, J.; Junghanns, K.; Broocks, A.; Riemann, D.; Hohagen, F. Test-retest reliability and validity of the Pittsburgh Sleep Quality Index in primary insomnia. *J. Psychosom. Res.* **2002**, *53*, 737–740. [CrossRef]
81. Kurtis, M.M.; Balestrino, R.; Rodriguez-Blazquez, C.; Forjaz, M.J.; Martinez-Martin, P. A review of scales to evaluate sleep disturbances in movement disorders. *Front. Neurol.* **2018**, *9*, 369. [CrossRef]
82. Mao, Z.; Liu, C.; Ji, S.; Yang, Q.; Ye, H.; Han, H.; Xue, Z. Clinical characteristics of sleep disorders in patients with Parkinson's disease. *J. Huazhong Univ. Sci. Technol. [Med. Sci.]* **2017**, *37*, 100–104. [CrossRef]
83. Medeiros, C.A.M.; Carvalhedo De Bruin, P.F.; Lopes, L.A.; Magalhães, M.C.; De Lourdes Seabra, M.; Sales De Bruin, V.M. Effect of exogenous melatonin on sleep and motor dysfunction in Parkinson's disease: A randomized, double blind, placebo-controlled study. *J. Neurol.* **2007**, *254*, 459–464. [CrossRef]
84. Hadoush, H.; Al-Sharman, A.; Khalil, H.; Banihani, S.A.; Al-Jarrah, M. Sleep quality, depression, and quality of life after bilateral anodal transcranial direct current stimulation in patients with Parkinson's disease. *Med. Sci. Monit. Basic Res.* **2018**, *24*, 198–205. [CrossRef]
85. Martin, J.L.; Hakim, A.D. Wrist actigraphy. *Chest* **2011**, *139*, 1514–1527. [CrossRef]
86. Harvey, A.G.; Tang, N.K.Y. (Mis)perception of sleep in insomnia: A puzzle and a resolution. *Psychol. Bull.* **2012**, *138*, 77–101. [CrossRef]
87. Happe, S.; Klösch, G.; Lorenzo, J.; Kunz, D.; Penzel, T.; Röschke, J.; Himanen, S.L.; Gruber, G.; Zeitlhofer, J. Perception of sleep: Subjective versus objective sleep parameters in patients with Parkinson's disease in comparison with healthy elderly controls—Sleep perception in Parkinson's disease and controls. *J. Neurol.* **2005**, *252*, 936–943. [CrossRef]
88. Marino, M.; Li, Y.; Rueschman, M.N.; Winkelman, J.W.; Ellenbogen, J.M.; Solet, J.M.; Dulin, H.; Berkman, L.F.; Buxton, O.M. Measuring sleep: Accuracy, sensitivity, and specificity of wrist actigraphy compared to polysomnography. *Sleep* **2013**, *36*, 1747–1755. [CrossRef]
89. Mccall, C.; Mccall, W.V. Comparison of actigraphy with polysomnography and sleep logs in depressed insomniacs. *J. Sleep Res.* **2012**, *21*, 122–127. [CrossRef]
90. Withrow, D.; Roth, T.; Koshorek, G.; Roehrs, T. Relation between ambulatory actigraphy and laboratory polysomnography in insomnia practice and research. *J. Sleep Res.* **2019**, *28*, e12854. [CrossRef]
91. Williams, J.M.; Taylor, D.J.; Slavish, D.C.; Gardner, C.E.; Zimmerman, M.R.; Patel, K.; Reichenberger, D.A.; Francetich, J.M.; Dietch, J.R.; Estevez, R. Validity of actigraphy in young adults with insomnia. *Behav. Sleep Med.* **2020**, *18*, 91–106. [CrossRef]
92. Klingelhoefer, L.; Rizos, A.; Sauerbier, A.; McGregor, S.; Martinez-Martin, P.; Reichmann, H.; Horne, M.; Chaudhuri, K.R. Night-time sleep in Parkinson's disease—the potential use of Parkinson's KinetiGraph: A prospective comparative study. *Eur. J. Neurol.* **2016**, *23*, 1275–1288. [CrossRef] [PubMed]
93. Sundgren, M.; Andréasson, M.; Svenningsson, P.; Noori, R.-M.; Johansson, A. Does information from the Parkinson KinetiGraph™ (PKG) influence the neurologist's treatment decisions?—An observational study in routine clinical care of people with Parkinson's disease. *J. Pers. Med.* **2021**, *11*, 519. [CrossRef] [PubMed]
94. Kotschet, K.; Johnson, W.; McGregor, S.; Kettlewell, J.; Kyoong, A.; O'Driscoll, D.M.; Turton, A.R.; Griffiths, R.I.; Horne, M.K. Daytime sleep in Parkinson's disease measured by episodes of immobility. *Parkinsonism Relat. Disord.* **2014**, *20*, 578–583. [CrossRef] [PubMed]
95. Knudson, M.; Thomsen, T.H.; Kjaer, T.W. Comparing objective and subjective measures of Parkinson's disease using the Parkinson's KinetiGraph. *Front. Neurol.* **2020**, *11*, 570833. [CrossRef]
96. Chen, L.; Cai, G.; Weng, H.; Yu, J.; Yang, Y.; Huang, X.; Chen, X.; Ye, Q. More sensitive identification for bradykinesia compared to tremors in Parkinson's disease based on Parkinson's KinetiGraph (PKG). *Front. Aging Neurosci.* **2020**, *12*, 594701. [CrossRef]
97. McGregor, S.; Churchward, P.; Soja, K.; O'Driscoll, D.; Braybrook, M.; Khodakarami, H.; Evans, A.; Farzanehfar, P.; Hamilton, G.; Horne, M. The use of accelerometry as a tool to measure disturbed nocturnal sleep in Parkinson's disease. *NPJ Parkinson's Dis.* **2018**, *4*, 1. [CrossRef]
98. Peerally, T.; Yong, M.H.; Chokroverty, S.; Tan, E.K. Sleep and Parkinson's disease: A review of case-control polysomnography studies. *Mov. Disord.* **2012**, *27*, 1729–1737. [CrossRef]
99. Vaughan, C.P.; Juncos, J.L.; Trotti, L.M.; Johnson, T.M., 2nd; Bliwise, D.L. Nocturia and overnight polysomnography in Parkinson disease. *Neurourol. Urodyn.* **2013**, *32*, 1080–1085. [CrossRef]
100. Eisensehr, I.; v Lindeiner, H.; Jäger, M.; Noachtar, S. REM sleep behavior disorder in sleep-disordered patients with versus without Parkinson's disease: Is there a need for polysomnography? *J. Neurol. Sci.* **2001**, *186*, 7–11. [CrossRef]
101. Littner, M.; Hirshkowitz, M.; Kramer, M.; Kapen, S.; McDowell Anderson, W.; Bailey, D.; Berry, R.B.; Davila, D.; Johnson, S.; Kushida, C.; et al. Practice parameters for using polysomnography to evaluate insomnia: An update. *Sleep* **2003**, *26*, 754–760. [CrossRef]

102. Titova, N.; Chaudhuri, K.R. Personalized medicine in Parkinson's disease: Time to be precise. *Mov. Disord.* **2017**, *32*, 1147–1154. [CrossRef] [PubMed]
103. Titova, N.; Chaudhuri, K.R. Personalized medicine and nonmotor symptoms in Parkinson's disease. *Int. Rev. Neurobiol.* **2017**, *134*, 1257–1281. [CrossRef] [PubMed]

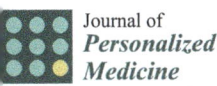

Journal of
Personalized Medicine

Article

Genetic Markers as Risk Factors for the Development of Impulsive-Compulsive Behaviors in Patients with Parkinson's Disease Receiving Dopaminergic Therapy

Anna Fedosova [1], Nataliya Titova [2,3,*], Zarema Kokaeva [1], Natalia Shipilova [2,3], Elena Katunina [2,3] and Eugene Klimov [1,†]

1. Lomonosov Moscow State University, Faculty of Biology, Leninskie Gory, 1, Building 12, 119234 Moscow, Russia; annafedosova@yandex.ru (A.F.); zaremak@inbox.ru (Z.K.); 9395001@mail.ru (E.K.)
2. Pirogov Russian National Research Medical University, Department of Neurology, Neurosurgery and Medical Genetics, Ostrovitianova, 1, 117997 Moscow, Russia; natali.33@mail.ru (N.S.); elkatunina@mail.ru (E.K.)
3. Federal State Budgetary Institution "Federal Center of Brain Research and Neurotechnologies" of the Federal Medical Biological Agency, Department of Neurodegenerative Disorders, Ostrovitianova, 1, Building 10, 117997 Moscow, Russia
* Correspondence: nattitova@yandex.ru; Tel.: +7-903-2428-792
† Deceased on 8 July 2021.

Abstract: Impulsive–compulsive and related behavioral disorders (ICD) are drug-induced non-motor symptoms of Parkinson's disease (PD). Recently research has focused on evaluating whether ICD could be predicted and managed using a pharmacogenetic approach based on dopaminergic therapies, which are the main risk factors. The aim of our study was to evaluate the role of candidate genes such as *DBH, DRD2, MAOA, BDNF, COMT, SLC6A4, SLC6A3, ACE, DRD1* gene polymorphisms in the pathogenesis of ICD in PD. We compared patients with PD and ICD ($n = 49$), patients with PD without ICD ($n = 36$) and a healthy control group ($n = 365$). ICD was diagnosed using the QUIP questionnaires and specific diagnostic criteria for subtypes of ICD. Genotyping was conducted using a number of PCR techniques and SNaPshot. Statistical analysis was performed using WinPepi and APSampler v3.6 software. PCA testing was conducted using RStudio software v1.4.1106-5. The following substitutions showed statistically significant correlations with PD and ICD: *DBH* (rs2097629, rs1611115), *DRD2* (rs6275, rs12364283, rs1076560), *ACE* (rs4646994), *DRD1* (rs686), *BDNF* (rs6265), these associations are novel in Russian PD patients. Our findings suggest that polymorphisms in *DBH, BDNF, DRD2, ACE* genes in Russian subjects are associated with an increased risk of ICD development.

Keywords: Parkinson's disease (PD); impulsive-compulsive disorders (ICD); dopaminergic therapy; genetic markers; pharmacogenetic; polymorphisms

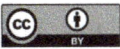

1. Introduction

Parkinson's disease (PD) is a syndromic condition and is phenotypically associated with a range of motor and nonmotor symptoms (NMS) [1]. Various types of disease-related and drug-induced NMS are recognized and impulsive-compulsive disorders (ICD) that include hypersexuality, compulsive overeating, compulsive shopping, pathological gambling, punding, hobbyism and dopamine dysregulation syndrome are challenging dopaminergic therapy related NMS of key clinical significance [2–5]. The subtle and initial symptoms of ICD are often overlooked in clinical practice, since they are quite difficult to recognize at early stages. Early recognition is important as studies suggest that ICD related abnormal behaviors significantly worsen the parameters of daily activities and quality of life of patients with PD worsening psychological stress, depression, anxiety and sleep disorders. Unrecognized and untreated, these disorders can lead to devastating consequences, including financial collapse and bankrupcy, divorce, dismissal from work, disruption of social activities, unsanitary living conditions and somatic complications. The estimated frequency of ICD in PD patients varies greatly in different studies—from 3.5% to 42.8% [3,6,7] due to the use of different study designs, questionnaires, scales, as well as different cultural, social, ethnic and economic characteristics of the patients. There is a clear association between the use of dopaminergic therapy (especially dopamine receptor agonists) and ICD development. Other risk factors for the development of ICD include male gender, young age, early PD development, history of ICD, substance and alcohol abuse, bipolar disorder, depression, smoking, and being unmarried [3,8–12].

Genetic factors are thought to play a certain role in the development of ICD. The involved genes are those encoding receptors or transporters involved in dopamine metabolism, or genes that regulate the activity of enzymes involved in the breakdown pathways of the main neurotransmitters, i.e., dopamine, serotonin, norepinephrine, glutamate [2,13–20]. As an example, addictive behavior in early PD has been linked to *DRD3* variant [18].

Our central hypothesis is based on other research addressing genetic risk factors for ICD using candidate genetic panel-based predictability of ICD in PD and most suggest that related gene products with ICD link are involved in the dopamine metabolizing pathways.

We hypothesized that some proposed ICD markers could be used as a pre-diagnostic marker prior to overt clinical manifestations of the disease. These data could then help to manage and personalize therapy at early stages of PD when there is minimal neuronal degradation.

The study was aimed at evaluating the role of *DBH, DRD2, MAOA, BDNF, COMT, SLC6A4, SLC6A3, ACE, DRD1* gene polymorphisms in the development of ICD in PD patients receiving dopaminergic therapy. To the best of our knowledge, it was the first genetic study evaluating ICD in Russian PD patients.

2. Materials and Methods

2.1. Patients

The 386 PD patients were examined over the period from 2015 to 2018. PD diagnosis was made based on the UK Parkinson's Disease Society Brain Bank clinical diagnostic criteria [21]. The inclusion and exclusion criteria were used for patient enrolment to the study. The inclusion criteria were as follows: age over 40 years, the use of dopaminergic therapy, the patient's informed written consent to participate in the study. For the control group, the inclusion criterion was the history of treatment with dopamine receptor agonists (DA) for at least 3 years. The exclusion criteria were as follows: dementia of any grade (based on the DSM-IV criteria [American Psychiatric Association, 2000], MMSE total score < 24).

The screening survey for the detection of ICD in PD patients was conducted using QUIP-Short and QUIP-Full questionnaires [22,23].

These questionnaires revealed ICD related symptoms in 78 (20.2%) subjects. Subsequently, specific diagnostic criteria were applied to confirm each subtype of ICD. Pathological gambling and compulsive overeating were confirmed based on the DSM-IV diagnostic criteria; compulsive shopping—based on the criteria developed by S. McElroy et al. [24]; hypersexuality—based on the criteria developed by V. Voon et al. [25]; punding and hobbyism—based on the criteria developed by A. Evans et al. [26], dopamine dysregulation syndrome—based on the criteria developed by G. Giovannoni et al. [27]. Thus, the main group included patients who had been found to have ICD based on the QUIP screening survey and the use of comprehensive diagnostic criteria ($n = 49$; PD + ICD; PD1). The control group included 36 PD patients who did not demonstrate abnormal behaviors or ICD (PD2). Demographic and clinical data of the patients are shown in Table 1. The population sample in this study is ethnically homogeneous and represent a white Caucasian population.

Table 1. Demographic and clinical characteristics of the study groups.

Parameters described	PD + ICD, PD1, $n = 49$	PD2, $n = 36$
Mean age, years	65.8 ± 8	70.6 ± 5.9
Number of subjects male	23	18
Number of subjects female	26	18
Education duration, years	15.9 ± 3	15.8 ± 3.6
Duration of the disease, years	6.6 ± 4.94	7.53 ± 4.9
Hoehn and Yahr stage	2.2 ± 0.5	2.5 ± 0.5
UPDRS, total score	33.4 ± 11.9	36.3 ± 12.2
LEDD, mg/day	731.5 ± 454	762.4 ± 342.1
Duration of the use of dopaminergic therapy, years	6.6 ± 4.94	7.53 ± 4.9
Breakdown of the types of dopaminergic therapy	Levodopa + DA ($n = 13$; 26.5%), Levodopa + DA + amantadine ($n = 13$; 26.5%), DA monotherapy ($n = 7$; 14.3%), Levodopa monotherapy ($n = 4$; 8.25%), DA + amantadine ($n = 4$; 8.25%), Levodopa + COMT inhibitor + DA + amantadine ($n = 3$; 6.1%), Levodopa + amantadine ($n = 2$; 4.1%), Levodopa + COMT inhibitor + DA ($n = 1$; 2%), Levodopa + MAO-B inhibitor ($n = 1$; 2%), Levodopa + DA + amantadine + MAO-B inhibitor ($n = 1$; 2%).	Levodopa + DA + amantadine ($n = 14$; 38.9%), Levodopa + DA ($n = 12$; 33.3%), DA + amantadine ($n = 5$; 13.9%), DA monotherapy ($n = 4$; 11.1%), Levodopa + COMT inhibitor + DA + amantadine ($n = 1$; 2.8%).

UPDRS = Unified Parkinson's disease rating scale; LEDD = levodopa equivalent daily dose; DA = dopamine agonists; COMT inhibitor = catechol-O-methyltransferase inhibitor; MAO-B inhibitor = monoamine Oxidase B inhibitor.

2.2. Ethical Principles

The study was conducted in accordance with the requirements of the World Medical Association (WMA)'s Declaration of Helsinki. All patients gave their written informed consent to participate in the study.

2.3. Methods

Laboratory tests included collection of venous blood samples in PD patients of the main group ($n = 49$; PD + ICD) and the control group ($n = 36$). Blood samples were stored in vacuum tubes with EDTA K2/K3 specially designed for laboratory whole blood studies. EDTA fillers (ethylenediaminacetic acid) bind calcium ions, creating stable complexes and was used as an anticoagulant in this study. Blood sampling was performed at N.I. Pirogov Municipal Clinical Hospital No.1 (N.I. Pirogov Russian National Research Medical University) and a consultative medical office for patients with extrapyramidal symptoms of catchment of the District Neurology Department of Central Administrative District of Moscow City.

Population control group blood samples ($n = 365$; control) were provided by blood transfusion station on condition of anonymity. The population control aim is needed to provide a natural baseline for mutation frequencies. The estimated number of PD patients in Russia is approximately 210,000 people (prevalence of 30–140/100,000) and thus it is necessary to provide control data as far as possible so as to account for natural variations. We used a fully health screened blood donor group where all the donors had passed a rigorous medical examination with exclusion of those with family history of neurodegenerative disorders, PD, dementia as well as any behavioral or mental health issues.

Genotype frequencies of selected gene substitutions were estimated:
- ACE (rs4646994)

- BDNF (rs2049046, rs6265)
- COMT (rs4680)
- DBH (rs141116007, rs2097629, rs1611115)
- DRD1 (rs686)
- DRD2 (rs1799732, rs6275, rs2283265, rs12364283, rs1076560)
- MAOA (VNTR)
- SLC6A3 (rs27072)
- SLC6A4 (rs38130034)

2.3.1. DNA Isolation

DNA was isolated from whole blood samples using columns according to the manufacturer's instructions (IG Spin DNA Prep 100 kit, manufactured by Isogen Laboratory LLC, Russia).

2.3.2. PCR Testing

The allelic analysis was conducted using polymerase chain reaction (PCR)-based techniques: PCR, PCR-RFLP (the combination of the polymerase chain reaction with the restriction fragment length polymorphism analysis), real-time PCR, and SNaPshot (single nucleotide polymorphism genotyping using allele-specific PCR and fluorescence melting curves) [28]. The sequences of primers (manufactured by DNA-Synthesis LLC, Moscow, Russia) are shown in Supplementary Material Tables S1 and S2.

PCR testing was carried out using HS Taq DNA polymerase and ScreenMix-HS test kits (manufactured by Evrogen, Moscow, Russia), and the T100 device (Bio-Rad Laboratories, Inc, Hercules, CA, USA). The following PCR cycling parameters were used: 94 °C–3 min; 40–45 cycles: 94 °C—20 s, To °C—15 s, 72 °C—30 s; 72 °C—5 min, where To is the primer annealing temperature (see Supplementary Material Tables S1 and S2).

Real-time PCR was conducted using qPCRmix-HS and qPCRmix-HS SYBR test kits (manufactured by Evrogen, Moscow, Russia) and the StepOnePlus Real Time PCR System device (Applied Biosystems, Waltham, MA, USA). The fluorescence detection was performed at FAM/VIC channels.

2.3.3. Restriction Analysis

The restriction analysis of PCR products was conducted in the conditions described by the restriction endonuclease manufacturer (SibEnzyme Ltd., Novosibirsk, Russia). The table describing restriction endonucleases used and DNA fragments obtained is presented in Supplementary Material Table S3.

2.4. Statistical Analysis

A two-tailed Fisher exact test (Fi) was used to reliably compare small samples during the assessment of gene substitution association. The calculations were performed using WinPepi software, v.11.65 (http://www.brixtonhealth.com/pepi4windows.html) (accessed on 23 August 2016) [29]. The results with Fisher's p-value < 0.05 were considered statistically significant. The mode of inheritance (dominant or recessive) was determined in accordance with the Akaike information criterion.

The groups of PD patients with ICD symptoms while on dopaminergic therapy, PD patients not experiencing impulse control disorders, and the population control group were used for comparative analysis.

The following groups were compared: PD1 versus PD2, PD1 versus control, PD2 versus control, PD1 + PD2 versus control.

The detection of complex genotypes associated with a trait was conducted using APSampler v3.6 [30] polygenic data analysis software based on common statistical tests (Fisher's exact test, Bonferroni adjustment for p-value and FDR) as well as the permutation test algorithm, which allowed to analyze associations in small samples.

2.5. Principal Component Analysis

PCA was applied to ensure best visualization of differences in a data set with many variables. The data set is adjusted to the new coordinate system in such a way that the most significant variance is detected at the first coordinate, and each subsequent coordinate is orthogonal to the last one and has a smaller variance. Thus, a set of X correlated variables for Y samples is transformed into a set of p uncorrelated principal components for the same samples. The analysis was conducted using RStudio software.

3. Results

3.1. Association between the Genetic Markers in PD Patients without ICD (PD2 Group)

The association between PD without ICD and patient genotypes was evaluated by statistical analysis using the WinPepi software. The mode of inheritance was determined using the Akaike information criterion. The mode with the lowest p-value according to the Fisher's test was considered the correct one. All data obtained for SNP genes evaluated are shown in Table 2.

Table 2. Summary table of statistical analysis for the group of patients with Parkinson's disease (PD) without impulsive-compulsive disorder (ICD) (PD2) vs. population control group.

Gene	Substitution		PD2	Control	Chi, p	Fi (p)	OR	CI95%
DBH	rs141116007	II + ID	26	282	1.017	0.294	0.67	0.30–1.64
		DD	10	73	0.313		1.49	0.61–3.36
BDNF	rs2049046	AA	7	50	0.847	0.327	1.51	0.53–3.76
		AT + TT	29	312	0.358		0.66	0.27–1.90
DRD2	rs1799732	CC	15	18	1.911	0.189	1.83	0.71–4.68
		CD + DD	21	46	0.167		0.55	0.21–1.42
MAOA	VNTR	SS + SL	20	129	3.309	0.076	1.89	0.89–4.05
		LL	16	195	0.069		0.53	0.25–1.12
DRD2	rs6275	TT	18	34	43.706	2.9×10^{-8}	9.00	3.97–20.14
		CT + CC	18	306	3.8×10^{-11}		0.11	0.05–0.25
DBH	rs2097629	AA	6	114	5.995	0.016	0.34	0.11–0.86
		AG + GG	30	192	0.014		2.97	1.17–8.97
BDNF	rs6265	AA + AG	16	94	8.308	6.7×10^{-3}	2.83	1.27–6.29
		GG	16	266	3.9×10^{-3}		0.35	0.16–0.79
DBH	rs1611115	TT + CT	26	328	11.256	2.8×10^{-3}	0.27	0.11–0.68
		CC	10	34	7.9×10^{-4}		3.71	1.46–8.77
COMT	rs4680	AA + AG	22	147	3.773	0.063	0.48	0.22–1.11
		GG	14	45	0.052		2.08	0.90–4.65
DRD2	rs2283265	TT + CT	34	161	0.572	0.610	0.53	0.08–5.78
		CC	2	5	0.449		1.89	0.17–12.13
DRD2	rs12364283	TT	30	100	6.877	0.012	3.30	1.25–10.19
		CT + CC	6	66	8.7×10^{-3}		0.30	0.10–0.80
DRD2	rs1076560	TT + CT	14	40	3.305	0.095	2.00	0.86–4.53
		CC	22	126	0.069		0.50	0.22–1.16
SLC6A4	rs38130034	TT	13	43	2.762	0.140	1.89	0.81–4.28
		CT + CC	23	144	0.097		0.53	0.23–1.24

Table 2. Cont.

Gene	Substitution		PD2	Control	Chi, p	Fi (p)	OR	CI95%
ACE	rs4646994	II + ID	26	228	0.367	0.708	1.27	0.57–3.05
		DD	10	111	0.545		0.79	0.33–1.77
SLC6A3	rs27072	CC	24	86	2.634	0.139	1.86	0.83–4.36
		CT + TT	12	80	0.105		0.54	0.23–1.21
DRD1	rs686	CC	0	23	5.629	0.017	0.00	0.0000–0.7362
		CT + TT	36	143	0.018		∞	1.3583–∞

VNTR = variable number of tandem repeats; Fi = Fisher's test criteria; OR = odds ratio; 95% CI = 95% confidence interval.

Our study demonstrated statistically significant results for several substitutions (Table 2):

- rs2097629 substitution in the *DBH* gene (9q34.2, 1434 + 1579A > G, 3' region) is associated with the disease. Analysis of allele frequencies of this substitution also showed an association of the G allele with PD ($p = 0.016$, OR = 2.97, CI95% [1.17–8.97]). The mode of inheritance was found to be dominant.
- rs1611115 substitution in the *DBH* gene (9q34.2, 1021T > C, 5' region) is associated with the disease. Analysis of the frequencies of alleles of this substitution also showed an association of the allele with PD ($p = 2.8 \times 10^{-3}$, OR = 3.71, CI95% [1.46–8.77]). The mode of inheritance was found to be recessive.
- rs6265 substitution in the *BDNF* gene (11p14.1, 196G > A, Val66Met, Exon 2) it is associated with the disease. Analysis of allele frequencies of this substitution also showed an association of Allele A with PD ($p = 6.7 \times 10^{-3}$, OR = 2.83, CI95% [1.27–6.29]). The mode of inheritance was found to be dominant.
- rs6275 substitution in the *DRD2* gene (11q23.2, 939T > C, His313His, Exon 7) is associated with the disease. Analysis of allele frequencies of this substitution also showed an association of the T allele with PD ($p = 2.9 \times 10^{-8}$, OR = 9.00, CI95% [3.97–20.14]). The mode of inheritance was found to be recessive.
- rs12364283 substitution in the *DRD2* gene (11q23.2, 4047A > G, 5' region) is associated with the disease. Analysis of allele frequencies of this substitution also showed an association of the T allele with PD ($p = 0.012$, OR = 3.30, CI95% [1.25–10.19]). The mode of inheritance was found to be recessive.
- rs686 substitution in the *DRD1* gene (5q35.1, 7464G > A, 3' region) is associated with the disease. Analysis of allele frequencies of this substitution also showed an association of Allele A with PD ($p = 0.017$, OR = ∞, CI95% [1.3583–∞]). The mode of inheritance was found to be dominant.

A polygenic analysis was conducted to evaluate the predisposition to PD in the group of patients versus the population control group. The analysis was carried out based on the genotypes of 36 PD patients and 365 residents of Moscow and the Moscow region (population control group) assessed for six polymorphic sites of four candidate genes. The results of the polygenic analysis are shown in Tables 3 and 4. Combinations of genotypes or individual genotypes and alleles were considered statistically significant if the *p*-value (Westfall–Young) was <0.001.

A total of four complex genotypes were found to meet our parameters (OR > 1). In three of four cases, the rs6275 TT substitution genotype was found in the *DRD2* gene, which resulted in about seven-fold increase in the risk of PD development (Table 3).

Two protective variants were determined during the complex genotype analysis. In both cases, the *DRD2* rs6275:C allele is present, which is associated with about seven-fold decreased risk of PD development (Table 4).

Table 3. Results of analysis of complex genotype associations in PD2 group patients. An increased risk of PD development.

Informative Allelic Pattern	Genotype Carriers		Fi (p)	OR	CI95%
	PD2	Control			
DBH_rs2097629:G; DRD1_rs686:G; DRD2_rs12364283:A,A	75.0%	29.7%	6.38×10^{-7}	7.10	3.11–16.21
DBH_rs2097629:G; DRD2_rs6275:T,T	44.4%	8.6%	1.42×10^{-6}	8.51	3.62–20.04
BDNF_rs6265:A; DRD2_rs6275:T,T	36.4%	4.3%	1.92×10^{-6}	12.57	4.45–35.49
DRD2_rs6275:T,T	50%	12.3%	2.24×10^{-6}	7.15	3.20–15.97

Fi = Fisher's test criteria; OR = odds ratio; 95% CI = 95% confidence interval; p (Westfall–Young) < 0.001.

Table 4. Results of analysis of complex genotype associations in PD2 group patients A decreased risk of PD development.

Informative Allelic Pattern	Genotype Carriers		Fi (p)	OR	CI95%
	PD2	Control			
BDNF_rs6265:G; DRD2_rs6275:C	45.5%	86.9%	9.51×10^{-7}	0.13	0.055–0.29
DRD2_rs6275:C	50%	87.7%	2.24×10^{-6}	0.14	0.063–0.31

Fi = Fisher's test criteria; OR = odds ratio; 95% CI = 95% confidence interval; p (Westfall–Young) < 0.001.

3.2. Association between the Genetic Markers and ICD in PD Patients (PD1 Group)

The association between PD patient genotypes and ICD development was evaluated by statistical analysis that included comparison of genotypes in the following groups: PD + ICD versus control group and PD + ICD versus PD without ICD group (used as a control group in this case). The mode of inheritance was determined using the Akaike information criterion. The mode with the lowest p-value according to the Fisher's test was considered the correct one. All data obtained for SNP genes evaluated are shown in Table 5.

Table 5. Summary table of statistical analysis for PD patients with ICD (PD1) vs. population control group.

Gene	Substitution		PD1	Control	Chi, p	Fi (p)	OR	CI95%
DBH	rs141116007	II + ID	38	282	0.312	0.580	0.82	0.39–1.81
		DD	12	73	0.576		1.22	0.55–2.53
BDNF	rs2049046	AA	11	50	2.335	0.138	1.76	0.76–3.79
		AT + TT	39	312	0.126		0.57	0.26–1.32
DRD2	rs1799732	CC	20	18	2.506	0.156	1.89	0.79–4.52
		CD + DD	27	46	0.113		0.53	0.22–1.26
MAOA	VNTR	SS + SL	27	129	3.585	0.065	1.77	0.93–3.39
		LL	23	195	0.058		0.56	0.29–1.07
DRD2	rs6275	TT	13	34	10.528	3.8×10^{-3}	3.16	1.40–6.81
		CT + CC	37	306	1.1×10^{-3}		0.32	0.15–0.72
DBH	rs2097629	AA + AG	39	263	2.110	0.199	0.58	0.27–1.36
		GG	11	43	0.146		1.73	0.74–3.76
BDNF	rs6265	AA + AG	27	94	23.224	5.7×10^{-6}	4.49	2.24–9.18
		GG	17	266	1.4×10^{-6}		0.22	0.11–0.45
DBH	rs1611115	TT	14	209	15.644	1.1×10^{-4}	0.28	0.14–0.56
		CT + CC	36	153	7.6×10^{-5}		3.51	1.77–7.29

Table 5. Cont.

Gene	Substitution		PD1	Control	Chi, p	Fi (p)	OR	CI95%
COMT	rs4680	AA	10	52	0.446	0.575	0.77	0.32–1.73
		AG + GG	35	140	0.504		1.30	0.58–3.16
DRD2	rs2283265	TT	26	118	2.893	0.105	0.56	0.27–1.17
		CT + CC	19	48	0.089		1.80	2.74–25.02
DRD2	rs12364283	TT	37	100	7.512	7.7×10^{-3}	3.05	1.29–8.04
		CT + CC	8	66	6.1×10^{-3}		0.33	0.12–0.78
DRD2	rs1076560	TT + CT	19	40	5.774	0.024	2.30	1.08–4.83
		CC	26	126	0.016		0.43	0.21–0.93
SLC6A4	rs38130034	TT	15	43	2.068	0.179	1.67	0.76–3.56
		CT + CC	30	144	0.150		0.60	0.28–1.31
ACE	rs4646994	II + ID	38	228	5.513	0.024	2.64	1.12–7.22
		DD	7	111	0.019		0.38	0.14–0.90
SLC6A3	rs27072	CC + CT	43	149	1.452	0.377	2.45	0.55–22.65
		TT	2	17	0.228		0.41	0.04–1.83
DRD1	rs686	CC + CT	39	137	0.438	0.653	1.38	0.51–4.34
		TT	6	29	0.508		0.73	0.23–1.96

VNTR = variable number of tandem repeats; Fi = Fisher's test criteria; OR = odds ratio; 95% CI = 95% confidence interval.

Our study demonstrated statistically significant results for several substitutions (Table 5):

- rs1611115 substitution in the *DBH* gene (9q34.2, 1021T > C, 5' region) is associated with the disease. Analysis of the frequencies of alleles of this substitution also showed an association of the allele with PD ($p = 2.8 \times 10^{-3}$, OR = 3.71, CI95% [1.46–8.77]). The mode of inheritance was found to be dominant.
- rs6265 substitution in the *BDNF* gene (11p14.1, 196G > A, Val66Met, Exon 2) it is associated with the disease. Analysis of allele frequencies of this substitution also showed an association of Allele A with PD ($p = 6.7 \times 10^{-3}$, OR = 2.83, CI95% [1.27–6.29]). The mode of inheritance was found to be dominant.
- rs6275 substitution in the *DRD2* gene (11q23.2, 939T > C, His313His, Exon 7) is associated with the disease. Analysis of allele frequencies of this substitution also showed an association of the T allele with PD ($p = 2.9 \times 10^{-8}$, OR = 9.00, CI95% [3.97–20.14]). The mode of inheritance was found to be dominant.
- rs12364283 substitution in the *DRD2* gene (11q23.2, 4047A > G, 5' region) is associated with the disease. Analysis of allele frequencies of this substitution also showed an association of the T allele with PD ($p = 0.012$, OR = 3.30, CI95% [1.25–10.19]). The mode of inheritance was found to be recessive.
- rs1076560 substitution in the *DRD2* gene (11q23.2, 67314C > A, Intron 6) is associated with the disease. Analysis of allele frequencies of this substitution also showed an association of the T allele with PD ($p = 0.012$, OR = 3.30, CI95% [1.25–10.19]). The mode of inheritance was found to be dominant.
- rs4646994 substitution in *ACE* gene (11q23.2, I/D 289bp, Intron 16) is associated with the disease. Analysis of allele frequencies of this substitution also showed an association of the T allele with PD ($p = 0.024$, OR = 2.64, CI95% [1.12–7.22]). The mode of inheritance was found to be dominant.

A polygenic analysis was conducted to evaluate the predisposition to ICD in the group of patients versus the population control group. The analysis was carried out based on the genotypes of 45 PD patients and 365 residents of Moscow and the Moscow region (population control group) assessed for six polymorphic sites of four candidate genes. The results of the polygenic analysis are shown in Tables 6 and 7. Combinations of genotypes or individual genotypes and alleles were considered statistically significant if the *p*-value (Westfall–Young) was <0.001.

Table 6. The result of analysis of complex genotypes in patients with ICD. An increased risk of ICD development.

Informative Allelic Pattern	Genotype Carriers		Fi (*p*)	OR	CI95%
	PD1	Control			
ACE_rs4646994:I; BDNF_rs6265:A; DRD2_rs1076560:A	25.6%	0.006%	2.68×10^{-7}	55.17	6.80–447.57
BDNF_rs6265:A; DRD2_rs1076560:A	28.2%	2.5%	3.28×10^{-6}	15.42	4.58–51.86
BDNF_rs6265:A; DBH_rs1611115:T	43.2%	12.4%	1.89×10^{-5}	5.36	2.51–11.44
BDNF_rs6265:G; DBH_rs1611115:T	72.7%	37.3%	2.63×10^{-5}	4.49	2.15–9.37

Fi = Fisher's test criteria; OR = odds ratio; 95% CI = 95% confidence interval; *p* (Westfall–Young) < 0.001.

Table 7. The result of analysis of complex genotypes in patients with ICD A decreased risk of ICD development.

Informative Allelic Pattern	Genotype Carriers		Fi (*p*)	OR	CI95%
	PD1	Control			
BDNF_rs6265:G; DBH_rs1611115:C,C	22.3%	60.8%	5.73×10^{-6}	0.19	0.09–0.41
BDNF_rs6265:G,G; DRD2_rs6275:C	27.3%	64.6%	9.77×10^{-6}	0.21	0.10–0.43

Fi = Fisher's test criteria; OR = odds ratio; 95% CI = 95% confidence interval; *p* (Westfall–Young) < 0.001.

A total of four complex genotypes were found to be associated with ICD (OR > 1). In three of four cases, there is a *BDNF_rs6265:A* allele, which makes a significant contribution to the development of ICD in PD patients receiving long-term dopaminergic therapy (Table 6).

Two protective variants were determined during the complex genotype analysis. In both cases, a *BDNF_rs6265:G* allele is present (Table 7).

Only the following genotype combinations were found to be statistically significant in the analysis of PD1 versus PD2 groups: CT + CC, rs6275 in the *DRD2* gene (11q23, 939T > C, His313His, Exon 7). The analysis of prevalence of this substitution demonstrated a correlation between the C allele with PD + ICD (*p* = 0.026, OR = 2.85, CI95% [1.04–7.81]). The mode of inheritance was found to be dominant.

No additional statistical analysis was conducted in respect of a single *DRD2* gene when comparing PD + ICD (PD1) versus PD without ICD (PD2, control).

3.3. Principal Component Analysis

Principal component analysis (PCA) was conducted using R-Studio software based on genotype data in 49 patients of the PD + ICD group, 36 PD patients without ICD and 201 patients from the population control group. The following substitutions demonstrating statistically significant correlation with the disease development were selected for the analysis: *DBH* (rs2097629, rs1611115), *DRD2* (rs6275, rs12364283, rs1076560), *ACE* (rs4646994), *DRD1* (rs686), *BDNF* (rs6265).

PCA allowed to identify three statistically significant clusters that corresponded to the baseline data.

The greatest differences in the groups of PD patients and the control group were observed in respect of *DBH*, *DRD2*, *BDNF* gene substitutions. The heterogeneity of the PD group was due to the diverse effects of *DRD2* gene substitutions on the disease development (Figure 1).

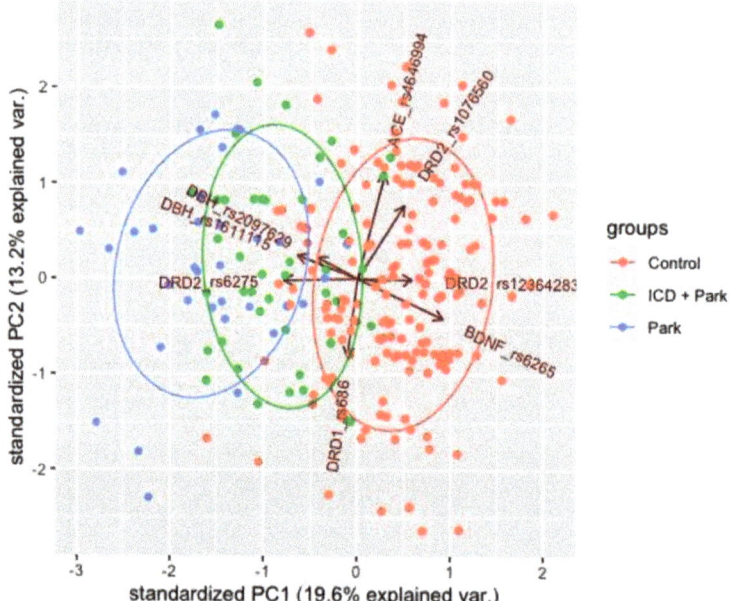

Figure 1. PCA results. PC1, PC2 are the principal components that explain 19.6% and 13.2% of the variance, i.e., the percentages of the total spread in points that falls on each of the new coordinates. Each sample has its own coordinates on the multidimensional plane. These coordinates consist of all possible vectors of the effects of DBH substitutions *DBH* (rs2097629, rs1611115), *DRD2* (rs6275, rs12364283, rs1076560), *ACE* (rs4646994), *DRD1* (rs686), *BDNF* (rs6265). In the obtained coordinate system, the samples are distributed into three clusters corresponding to the original data groups. *DBH*, *DRD2*, *BDNF* gene substitutions demonstrate the greatest impacts on the distribution of control, PD1 and PD + ICD (PD2) groups. The heterogeneity of the PD groups (PD1 + PD2) was due to the diverse effects of *DRD2* gene substitutions on the disease development.

These findings are supported by the analysis of associations between the genetic markers and ICD in PD patients.

4. Discussion

Our study reports the key findings that variants rs1611115 *DBH*, rs6265 *BDNF*, rs6275 *DRD2* rs12364283 *DRD2*, rs1076560 *DRD2*, rs4646994 *ACE* are associated with an increased ICD risk among PD patients. To the best of our knowledge, we believe that this is the first report of clinical genetic testing conducted in patients with PD and ICD in Russia. We will now discuss individual aspects of these findings.

4.1. Association between the Genetic Markers and PD

A range of genetic markers have been associated with behavioral and other drug induced nonmotor issues in PD. For instance, the *DRD2* rs1799732 and *DRD3* rs6280 gene polymorphisms have been linked to levodopa induced gastrointestinal symptoms [19]. Post-traumatic stress disorder as well as sleep dysfunction arising from chronic stress have also been linked to SNP *DRD2* density and *DRD2* gene polymorphisms [31,32]. In PD, ICD is widely regarded as a drug induced behavioural issue and we now discuss relevant and related genetic basis.

The *DBH* gene encodes a protein of the same name that is responsible for the conversion of dopamine to norepinephrine. The *DBH* gene sequence includes a coding DBH antisense RNA 1—DBH-AS1 region; this non-coding protein transcript may regulate the

DBH gene translation. The dominant G allele of the rs2097629 substitution was shown to be associated with the PD development ($p = 0.016$) with OR = 2.97, 95% CI [1.17–8.97]). This substitution located in 3′ region of the gene has been postulated to produce a negative effect on dopamine metabolism by reducing the dopamine beta-hydroxylase synthesis [33]. The 5′ region of the gene includes a rs1611115 substitution [31], the recessive Allele C of which is also implicated in the pathogenesis of PD ($p = 2.8 \times 10^{-3}$) with OR = 3.71, 95% CI [1.46–8.77]. This substitution significantly regulates the enzyme plasma activity [34]. In this regard, the impaired function of the dopaminergic system increases the risk of PD development.

We also interrogated the BDNF gene which encodes a protein that is active in the spinal cord and the brain and regulates the growth, differentiation and functioning of neurons. The dominant Allele A of the rs6265 substitution increases the risk of PD development ($p = 6.7 \times 10^{-3}$), with OR = 2.83, 95% CI [1.27–6.29]. This substitution is located in Exon 2 of the BDNF gene and leads to the Val66Met amino acid substitution. The Met allele is associated with abnormal intracellular packaging of the BDNF precursor and a decrease in the cell production of mature BDNF [35]. The rs6265 substitution is also associated with obsessive-compulsive disorder (OCD), attention-deficit/hyperactivity disorder, anxiety disorders and could be operative via functional alterations within the hippocampus and prefrontal cortex [36]. Moreover, this substitution is also associated with the development of Alzheimer's disease as it causes progressive memory loss and cognitive impairment [37].

The DRD2 gene encodes the dopamine receptor, which is a G-coupled protein located on the surface of neurons and inhibiting dopamine-induced adenylate cyclase activity [32]. TT genotype of the rs6275 substitution increases the risk of PD development ($p = 2.9 \times 10^{-8}$) with OR = 9.00, 95% CI [3.97–20.14]. The C allele is dominant, and the T allele is recessive. This substitution is located in Exon 7 of the dopamine D2 receptor encoding gene and the T allele affects the stability of the DRD2 transcript and its translation efficiency [38]. The major effect is expected on the presynaptic membrane, where the D2 dopamine receptor activates the dopamine reuptake. With a decrease in the amount of DRD2 on the presynaptic membrane, dopamine accumulation in the synaptic cleft should be expected. This may result in excessive activation of the downstream dopamine receptors and an increased response on the dopamine release. The TT genotype is likely to result in a decreased reuptake from the synapse due to imbalance of the number of D2 dopamine receptors and dopamine, which can lead to striatal dopamine depletion. The 5′ region of the gene includes a rs12364283 substitution, the recessive Allele A of which is associated with the PD development ($p = 0.012$) with OR = 3.30, 95% CI [1.25–10.19]. This substitution has been found to be associated with behavioral disorders and possibly also with pathogenesis of PD [39] D1 receptor gene (DRD1) is located at 5q35.1 and has two exons. DRD1 is one of the most common dopaminergic receptors in the central nervous system. This gene is involved in social cognition, attention, reinforcement learning, executive functioning, working memory, and neuropsychiatric disorders such as alcohol addiction and pathological gambling [40]. The rs686 polymorphism is located in the 3′ untranslated region of this gene, the dominant Allele A of which increases the risk of PD development ($p = 0.017$), with an estimate of OR = ∞, 95% CI [1.36–∞]. This polymorphism leads to allele-specific effects on the differential expression of the DRD1 gene, while the C allele shows lower activity compared to the T allele, which is due to the fact that this SNP is located in the miR-504 binding region [40].

4.2. Analysis of Complex Genotype Associations in PD Patients

The analysis of complex genotype associations in PD patients was carried out in APSampler software designed to analyze composite genetic biomarkers associated with polygenic disease phenotypes. All associated substitutions: rs2097629, rs1611115, rs6265, rs6275, rs12364283, rs686 were included in the analysis.

We were able to identify a total of 4 PD-associated complex genotypes that were assessed using a permutation test. In three of four cases, the rs6275:T substitution genotype was found in the *DRD2* gene, which resulted in about 9-fold increase in the risk of PD development. Furthermore, a rs2097629:G allele of the *DBH* gene was revealed in two of four cases, which resulted in about three-fold increase in the risk of PD development. It is worth noting that the rs6275:C allele of the *DRD2* gene demonstrates obvious protective properties in relation to PD. Thus, the study showed that the *DBH* and *DRD2* genes had the most pronounced effects on the PD development. No obvious correlations were revealed between the rs2097629 substitution of the *DBH* gene and the PD symptoms, however, it may be assumed that there is an increased risk of the disease as a result of a decrease in the enzyme synthesis in combination with other factors. No data are available on the correlation between the PD development and the rs6275 substitution in the *DRD2* gene.

4.3. Association between the Genetic Markers and ICD in PD Patients

The *BDNF* gene encodes a protein that is active in the spinal cord and the brain. Its main function is to regulate the growth, differentiation and functioning of neurons. The dominant Allele A of the rs6265 substitution increases the risk of ICD development ($p = 5.7 \times 10^{-6}$), with an estimate of OR = 4.49, 95% CI [2.24–9.18]. This substitution is located in Exon 2 of the *BDNF* gene, and leads to the Val66Met amino acid substitution. The Met allele is associated with abnormal intracellular packaging of the BDNF precursor and a decrease in the cell production of mature BDNF [35]. The association between the rs6265 substitution with OCD, attention-deficit/hyperactivity disorder, anxiety disorders, Parkinson's disease is well-known, and we reasonably conclude that as the substitution is associated with behavioral disorders, it can be assumed that this polymorphism is associated with ICD.

The TT genotype of the rs6275 substitution in this gene increases the risk of ICD development ($p = 3.8 \times 10^{-3}$), with OR = 3.16, 95% CI [1.40–6.81]. The C allele is dominant, and the T allele is recessive. As it was mentioned before, this substitution is located in Exon 7 of the dopamine D2 receptor encoding gene and the T allele affects the stability of the DRD2 transcript and its translation efficiency [38]. The T allele effect may be expressed in a decrease in the amount of DRD2 on the presynaptic membrane, dopamine accumulation in the synaptic cleft should be expected. The TT genotype is likely to result in excessive activation of the downstream dopamine receptors and an increased response on the dopamine release. The 5' region of the gene includes a rs12364283 substitution, the recessive Allele A of which is associated with the ICD development ($p = 7.7 \times 10^{-3}$) with OR = 3.05, 95% CI [1.29–8.04]. There have been reports on correlation between this substitution and the development of behavioral disorders and dependencies [41], which suggests an association with ICD. The Intron 6 of the *DRD2* gene includes a rs1076560 substitution, the dominant Allele A of which demonstrated a correlation with ICD ($p = 0.024$) with OR = 2.30, 95% CI [1.08–4.83]. There have been reports on the correlation between this substitution and the development of alcohol abuse and drug addiction [42].

The *DBH* gene encodes a protein of the same name that is responsible for the conversion of dopamine to norepinephrine. Dopamine being a key neurotransmitter, having impaired balance in PD patients, was of great interest in our study. The 5' region of the gene includes a rs1611115 substitution, the recessive Allele C of which is associated with the ICD development ($p = 1.1 \times 10^{-4}$) with OR = 3.51, 95% CI [1.77–7.29]. This substitution significantly regulates the enzyme plasma activity [34]. In this regard, the impaired function of the dopaminergic system increases the risk of ICD development.

The *ACE* gene, located at 17q23.3, encodes the angiotensin conversion enzyme (peptidyl dipeptidase A). This enzyme is responsible for cleavage of some proteins of the renin-angiotensin system, which regulates blood pressure and the fluid and electrolyte balance in the body [43]. The functional polymorphism rs4646994 is present in Intron 16 in the form of insertion (I) and/or deletion (D) of a sequence of Alu repeats with a length of 289 bp (rs4646994). The dominant Allele I is associated with the ICD development ($p = 0.024$) with OR = 2.64, 95% CI [1.12–7.22]. The I/D polymorphism may affect the *ACE* gene expression and/or the ACE function. Angiotensin II is known to activate several signaling pathways, including mitogen-activated protein kinase (MAPK), phosphoinositide-3-kinase (PI3K)/AKT, and cAMP-dependent protein kinase pathways that play a role in regulating cell growth and differentiation, cytoplasmic protein reorganization, and cell cycle regulation [44].

4.4. Analysis of Complex Genotype Associations in PD Patients with ICD

The analysis of complex genotype associations in PD patients was carried out in APSampler software designed to analyze composite genetic biomarkers associated with polygenic disease phenotypes. All associated substitutions: rs1611115, rs6265, rs6275, rs12364283, rs1076560, rs4646994 were included in the analysis.

We were able to identify a total of 4 ICD-associated complex genotypes that were assessed using a permutation test. In three of four cases, there is a *BDNF*_rs6265: A allele, which makes a significant contribution to the development of ICD in PD patients receiving long-term dopaminergic therapy. This allele can independently result in a four-fold increase in the risk of ICD development. However, the *BDNF*_rs6265: G allele demonstrates protective properties in respect of ICD development. An *DRD2*_rs1076560: A allele that was observed in two of four cases and was associated with an increased risk of the disease is of interest for complex genotype analysis. The *DBH*_rs1611115:T allele was found in two of four cases, which independently resulted in about four-fold increase in the risk of the disease.

The *BDNF* rs6265 was shown to correlated with the development of OCD, ADHD and behavioral disorders, which confirms a possible association with ICD (19582215). The *DRD2* rs1076560 substitution might be associated with the development of alcohol abuse and drug addiction, which makes it possible to assume a correlation with the development of ICD as an abnormal behavior. The *DBH* rs1611115 polymorphism is significantly associated with cognitive functions, which explains the probable correlation with ICD [45].

4.5. Association between the Genetic Markers and ICD in PD Patients

CT and CC substitutions (rs6275) of the *DRD2* gene increase the risk of ICD development in PD patients ($p = 0.026$) with OR = 2.85; 95% CI [1.04–7.81]. The C allele is dominant, and the T allele is recessive.

The comparison of PD + ICD (49) group and PD group (36) as the internal control showed that the rs6275 substitution in the *DRD2* gene suggested a correlation between the CT and CC genotypes and the PD + ICD phenotype (OR = 2.85), i.e., Allele C has a dominant mode of inheritance for the PD + ICD sample. There is an association between the TT genotype and PD + ICD phenotype (OR = 3.16) (recessive mode of inheritance) as evidenced by the comparison of PD + ICD group versus the population control. There is also a significant association between the TT genotype with the recessive mode of inheritance (OR = 9.00) as evidenced by the comparison of PD without ICD group versus the population control.

The OR values show that the presence of the TT genotype plays a crucial role in the development of PD without related disorders whereas the development of ICD depends more on the presence of the C allele. The presence of a recessive T allele (TT genotype) was observed when comparing PD patients with the control group. The C or T substitutions lead to changes in RNA splicing, which result in altered proportions of the long and short DRD2 receptor isoforms, respectively. The C allele is often a wild-type allele, which has a positive effect on the stability of the DRD2 transcript and the translation efficiency [38]. Normal activity of the *DRD2* gene in PD patients leads to a more effective response to dopamine therapy. Therefore, it can be assumed that PD itself is not the cause of ICD development, and that ICD symptoms may manifest as a result of the use of dopaminergic therapy.

5. Conclusions

In summary, we have shown that variants rs1611115 *DBH*, rs6265 *BDNF*, rs6275 *DRD2* rs12364283 *DRD2*, rs1076560 *DRD2*, rs4646994 *ACE* are associated with an increased ICD risk among PD patients. To the best of our knowledge, this is the first report of clinical genetic testing and identification of risk factors for ICD conducted in patients with PD and ICD in Russia. These results would need to be replicated by further studies with a larger population and other ethnic groups as we recognize that the sample size of this study was small although the statistical power was sufficient for analyses. We also acknowledge that our control population group, taken from a biobank of a healthy screened blood transfusion service was not specifically screened for ICD. This fact is a possible limitation towards the conclusions reached. However, as mentioned previously we used a fully health screened blood donor group where all the donors had passed a rigorous medical examination, and those with family history of neurodegenerative disorders, dementia as well any behavioral or mental health issues were excluded. This would mean that those with family history of PD were excluded and furthermore, exclusion of those with significant mental health issues or behavioral disorders would mean that intrusive ICD would have been likely to have been screened out as well.

Special attention should be drawn to rs6275 *DRD2* gene polymorphism. Our data suggest that this specific polymorphism is associated with a strong clinical genetic risk factor for the development of ICD in PD patients and may therefore enable pharmacogenetic strategies to aid personalized treatment while also enabling possible prophylaxis [46]. This issue is also highly relevant in the view of the increasing frequency of "dopamine agonist phobia" which has been recently reported [47]. These studies also contribute to our better understanding of the role of dopaminergic transmission and signaling in the mesocorticolimbic dopaminergic system and the involvement of other neurotransmitter systems in the mechanisms of ICD development. A possible long-term gain may be that the proposed genetic risk factors for ICD development might be used as a biomarker of neurotransmitter dysfunction based nonmotor subtypes of PD [48], allowing a personalized approach to PD therapy [49,50].

Supplementary Materials: The following are available online at https://www.mdpi.com/article/10.3390/jpm11121321/s1, Table S1: characteristics of primers and PCR conditions, Table S2: characteristics of primers and probes, PCR—real-time conditions, Table S3: restrictases and restriction fragments.

Author Contributions: Conceptualization, N.T., E.K. (Elena Katunina) and E.K. (Eugene Klimov); data curation, A.F., Z.K., N.S. and E.K. (Eugene Klimov); formal analysis, A.F. and E.K. (Eugene Klimov); investigation, A.F., Z.K. and N.S.; methodology, N.T., E.K. (Elena Katunina) and E.K. (Eugene Klimov); project administration, E.K. (Elena Katunina) and E.K. (Eugene Klimov); resources, N.T. and E.K. (Eugene Klimov); supervision, N.T., E.K. (Elena Katunina) and E.K. (Eugene Klimov); writing—original draft, A.F.; writing—review and editing, A.F., N.T. and E.K. (Eugene Klimov). All authors have read and agreed to the published version of the manuscript.

Funding: The study was funded in part by a career development grant for NT from Parkinson's disease nonmotor group (PDNMG) and was carried out within the framework of the scientific project of the state assignment of Moscow State University No. 121032500088-4.

Institutional Review Board Statement: The study was conducted according to the guidelines of the Declaration of Helsinki, and approved by the Ethics Committee of Pirogov Russian National Research Medical University (Protocol Code: 150, date of approval: 14 December 2015).

Informed Consent Statement: Informed consent was obtained from all subjects involved in the study.

Data Availability Statement: The data presented in this study are available on request from the corresponding author. The data are not publicly available due to country specific and ethical committee regulations.

Acknowledgments: The authors thank the patients who agree to take part in the study. We wish to pay our gratitude and our tribute to our co-author and colleague, Eugene Klimov, who passed away on 8 July 2021. He was a dedicated scientist with a passion for research and a soulful curator, without whom this work could not be possible. We also thank K Ray Chaudhuri (Kings College, London) for a review of the manuscript.

Conflicts of Interest: The authors declare no conflict of interest.

References

1. Titova, N.; Padmakumar, C.; Lewis, S.J.G.; Chaudhuri, K.R. Parkinson's: A syndrome rather than a disease? *J. Neural Transm.* **2017**, *124*, 907–914. [CrossRef] [PubMed]
2. Magistrelli, L.; Ferrari, M.; Furgiuele, A.; Milner, A.V.; Contaldi, E.; Comi, C.; Marino, F. Polymorphisms of Dopamine Receptor Genes and Parkinson's Disease: Clinical Relevance and Future Perspectives. *Int. J. Mol. Sci.* **2021**, *22*, 3781. [CrossRef]
3. Vilas, D.; Pont-Sunyer, C.; Tolosa, E. Impulse control disorders in Parkinson's disease. *Parkinsonism Relat. Disord.* **2012**, *18* (Suppl. 1), S80–S84. [CrossRef]
4. Antonini, A.; Barone, P.; Bonuccelli, U.; Annoni, K.; Asgharnejad, M.; Stanzione, P. ICARUS study: Prevalence and clinical features of impulse control disorders in Parkinson's disease. *J. Neurol. Neurosurg. Psychiatry* **2017**, *88*, 317–324. [CrossRef]
5. Kim, J.; Kim, M.; Kwon, D.Y.; Seo, W.K.; Kim, J.H.; Baik, J.S.; Koh, S.B. Clinical characteristics of impulse control and repetitive behavior disorders in Parkinson's disease. *J. Neurol.* **2013**, *260*, 429–437. [CrossRef] [PubMed]
6. Sarathchandran, P.; Soman, S.; Sarma, G.; Krishnan, S.; Kishore, A. Impulse control disorders and related behaviors in Indian patients with Parkinson's disease. *Mov. Disord.* **2013**, *28*, 1901–1902. [CrossRef] [PubMed]
7. Weintraub, D.; Potenza, M.N. Impulse control disorders in Parkinson's disease. *Curr. Neurol. Neurosci. Rep.* **2006**, *6*, 302–306. [CrossRef] [PubMed]
8. Voon, V.; Hassan, K.; Zurowski, M.; de Souza, M.; Thomsen, T.; Fox, S.; Lang, A.E.; Miyasaki, J. Prevalence of repetitive and reward-seeking behaviors in Parkinson's disease. *Neurology* **2006**, *67*, 1254–1257. [CrossRef] [PubMed]
9. Weintraub, D.; Koester, J.; Potenza, M.N.; Siderowf, A.D.; Stacy, M.; Voon, V.; Whetteckey, J.; Wunderlich, G.R.; Lang, A.E. Impulse control disorders in Parkinson's disease: A cross-sectional study of 3090 patients. *Arch. Neurol.* **2010**, *67*, 589–595. [CrossRef]
10. Zhang, Y.; He, A.Q.; Li, L.; Chen, W.; Liu, Z.G. Clinical characteristics of impulse control and related disorders in Chinese Parkinson's disease patients. *BMC Neurol.* **2017**, *17*, 98. [CrossRef] [PubMed]
11. Bhattacharjee, S. Impulse control disorders in Parkinson's disease: Review of pathophysiology, epidemiology, clinical features, management, and future challenges. *Neurol. India* **2018**, *66*, 967–975. [CrossRef] [PubMed]
12. Latella, D.; Maggio, M.G.; Maresca, G.; Saporoso, A.F.; Le Cause, M.; Manuli, A.; Milardi, D.; Bramanti, P.; De Luca, R.; Calabrò, R.S. Impulse control disorders in Parkinson's disease: A systematic review on risk factors and pathophysiology. *Neurol. Sci.* **2019**, *398*, 101–106. [CrossRef] [PubMed]
13. Brewer, J.A.; Potenza, M.N. The neurobiology and genetics of impulse control disorders: Relationships to drug addictions. *Biochem. Pharm.* **2008**, *75*, 63–75. [CrossRef] [PubMed]
14. Comings, D.E.; Gade-Andavolu, R.; Gonzalez, N.; Wu, S.; Muhleman, D.; Chen, C.; Koh, P.; Farwell, K.; Blake, H.; Dietz, G.; et al. The additive effect of neurotransmitter genes in pathological gambling. *Clin. Genet.* **2001**, *60*, 107–116. [CrossRef] [PubMed]
15. Lee, J.Y.; Lee, E.K.; Park, S.S.; Lim, J.Y.; Kim, H.J.; Kim, J.S.; Jeon, B.S. Association of DRD3 and GRIN2B with impulse control and related behaviors in Parkinson's disease. *Mov. Disord.* **2009**, *24*, 1803–1810. [CrossRef] [PubMed]
16. Cilia, R.; Benfante, R.; Asselta, R.; Marabini, L.; Cereda, E.; Siri, C.; Pezzoli, G.; Goldwurm, S.; Fornasari, D. Tryptophan hydroxylase type 2 variants modulate severity and outcome of addictive behaviors in Parkinson's disease. *Parkinsonism Relat. Disord.* **2016**, *29*, 96–103. [CrossRef] [PubMed]
17. Zainal Abidin, S.; Tan, E.L.; Chan, S.C.; Jaafar, A.; Lee, A.X.; Abd Hamid, M.H.; Abdul Murad, N.A.; Pakarul Razy, N.F.; Azmin, S.; Ahmad Annuar, A.; et al. DRD and GRIN2B polymorphisms and their association with the development of impulse control behaviour among Malaysian Parkinson's disease patients. *BMC Neurol.* **2015**, *15*, 59. [CrossRef] [PubMed]
18. Castro-Martínez, X.H.; García-Ruiz, P.J.; Martínez-García, C.; Martínez-Castrillo, J.C.; Vela, L.; Mata, M.; Hoenicka, J. Behavioral addictions in early-onset Parkinson disease are associated with DRD3 variants. *Parkinsonism Relat. Disord.* **2018**, *49*, 100–103. [CrossRef]
19. Rieck, M.; Schumacher-Schuh, A.; Altmann, V.; Callegari-Jacques, S.M.; Rieder, C.R.M.; Hutz, M.H. Association between DRD2 and DRD3 gene polymorphisms and gastrointestinal symptoms induced by levodopa therapy in Parkinson's disease. *Pharm. J.* **2018**, *18*, 196–200. [CrossRef] [PubMed]
20. Krishnamoorthy, S.; Rajan, R.; Banerjee, M.; Kumar, H.; Sarma, G.; Krishnan, S.; Sarma, S.; Kishore, A. Dopamine D3 receptor Ser9Gly variant is associated with impulse control disorders in Parkinson's disease patients. *Parkinsonism Relat. Disord.* **2016**, *30*, 13–17. [CrossRef] [PubMed]
21. Todt, U.; Netzer, C.; Toliat, M.; Heinze, A.; Goebel, I.; Nürnberg, P.; Göbel, H.; Freudenberg, J.; Kubisch, C. New genetic evidence for involvement of the dopamine system in migraine with aura. *Hum. Genet.* **2009**, *125*, 265–279. [CrossRef] [PubMed]
22. Zabetian, C.P.; Anderson, G.M.; Buxbaum, S.G.; Elston, R.C.; Ichinose, H.; Nagatsu, T.; Kim, K.S.; Kim, C.H.; Malison, R.T.; Gelernter, J.; et al. A quantitative-trait analysis of human plasma–dopamine β-hydroxylase activity: Evidence for a major functional polymorphism at the DBH locus. *Am. J. Hum. Genet.* **2001**, *68*, 515–522. [CrossRef] [PubMed]
23. Chen, Z.Y.; Patel, P.D.; Sant, G.; Meng, C.X.; Teng, K.K.; Hempstead, B.L.; Lee, F.S. Variant brain-derived neurotrophic factor (BDNF)(Met66) alters the intracellular trafficking and activity-dependent secretion of wild-type BDNF in neurosecretory cells and cortical neurons. *J. Neurosci.* **2004**, *24*, 4401–4411. [CrossRef]
24. Cheng, L.; Ge, Q.; Xiao, P.; Sun, B.; Ke, X.; Bai, Y.; Lu, Z. Association study between BDNF gene polymorphisms and autism by three-dimensional gel-based microarray. *Int. J. Mol. Sci.* **2009**, *10*, 2487–2500. [CrossRef] [PubMed]

25. Boots, E.A.; Schultz, S.A.; Clark, L.R.; Racine, A.M.; Darst, B.F.; Koscik, R.L.; Carlsson, C.M.; Gallagher, C.L.; Hogan, K.J.; Bendlin, B.B.; et al. BDNF Val66Met predicts cognitive decline in the Wisconsin Registry for Alzheimer's Prevention. *Neurology* **2017**, *88*, 2098–2106. [CrossRef]
26. Duan, J.; Wainwright, M.S.; Comeron, J.M.; Saitou, N.; Sanders, A.R.; Gelernter, J.; Gejman, P.V. Synonymous mutations in the human dopamine receptor D2 (DRD2) affect mRNA stability and synthesis of the receptor. *Hum. Mol. Genet.* **2003**, *12*, 205–216. [CrossRef]
27. Davis, C.; Levitan, R.D.; Yilmaz, Z.; Kaplan, A.S.; Carter, J.C.; Kennedy, J.L. Binge eating disorder and the dopamine D2 receptor: Genotypes and sub-phenotypes. *Prog. Neuropsychopharmacol. Biol. Psychiatry* **2012**, *38*, 328–335. [CrossRef] [PubMed]
28. Jiménez, K.M.; Pereira-Morales, A.J.; Forero, D.A. A functional polymorphism in the DRD1 gene, that modulates its regulation by miR-504, is associated with depressive symptoms. *Psychiatry Investig.* **2018**, *15*, 402–406. [CrossRef] [PubMed]
29. Nelson, E.C.; Heath, A.C.; Lynskey, M.T.; Agrawal, A.; Henders, A.K.; Bowdler, L.M.; Todorov, A.A.; Madden, P.A.; Moore, E.; Degenhardt, L.; et al. PTSD risk associated with a functional DRD2 polymorphism in heroin-dependent cases and controls is limited to amphetamine-dependent individuals. *Addict. Biol.* **2014**, *19*, 700–707. [CrossRef] [PubMed]
30. Lucht, M.; Samochowiec, A.; Samochowiec, J.; Jasiewicz, A.; Grabe, H.J.; Geissler, I.; Rimmbach, C.; Rosskopf, D.; Grzywacz, A.; Wysiecka, J.P.; et al. Influence of DRD2 and ANKK1 genotypes on apomorphine-induced growth hormone (GH) response in alcohol-dependent patients. *Prog. Neuropsychopharmacol. Biol. Psychiatry* **2010**, *34*, 45–49. [CrossRef]
31. Zhang, K.; Wang, L.; Cao, C.; Li, G.; Fang, R.; Liu, P.; Luo, S.; Zhang, X.; Liberzon, I. A DRD2/ANNK1-COMT Interaction, Consisting of Functional Variants, Confers Risk of Post-traumatic Stress Disorder in Traumatized Chinese. *Front. Psychiatry* **2018**, *9*, 170. [CrossRef]
32. Jiang, Y.; Liu, B.; Wu, C.; Gao, X.; Lu, Y.; Lian, Y.; Liu, J. Dopamine Receptor D2 Gene (DRD2) Polymorphisms, Job Stress, and Their Interaction on Sleep Dysfunction. *Int. J. Environ. Res. Public Health* **2020**, *17*, 8174. [CrossRef]
33. Sayed-Tabatabaei, F.A.; Oostra, B.A.; Isaacs, A.; van Duijn, C.M.; Witteman, J.C. ACE polymorphisms. *Circ. Res.* **2006**, *98*, 1123–1133. [CrossRef] [PubMed]
34. Zmorzynski, S.; Szudy-Szczyrek, A.; Popek-Marciniec, S.; Korszen-Pilecka, I.; Wojcierowska-Litwin, M.; Luterek, M.; Chocholska, S.; Styk, W.; Swiderska-Kołacz, G.; Januszewska, J.; et al. ACE insertion/deletion polymorphism (rs4646994) is associated with the increased risk of multiple myeloma. *Front. Oncol.* **2019**, *9*, 44. [CrossRef]
35. Kieling, C.; Genro, J.P.; Hutz, M.H.; Rohde, L.A. The−1021 C/T DBH polymorphism is associated with neuropsychological performance among children and adolescents with ADHD. *Am. J. Med. Genet. B Neuropsychiatr. Genet.* **2008**, *147B*, 485–490. [CrossRef]
36. Gibb, W.R. Accuracy in the clinical diagnosis of parkinsonian syndromes. *Postgrad. Med. J.* **1988**, *64*, 345–351. [CrossRef]
37. Weintraub, D.; Hoops, S.; Shea, J.A.; Lyons, K.E.; Pahwa, R.; Driver-Dunckley, E.D.; Adler, C.H.; Potenza, M.N.; Miyasaki, J.; Siderowf, A.D.; et al. Validation of the questionnaire for impulsive-compulsive disorders in Parkinson's disease. *Mov. Disord.* **2009**, *24*, 1461–1467. [CrossRef] [PubMed]
38. Weintraub, D.; Mamikonyan, E.; Papay, K.; Shea, J.A.; Xie, S.X.; Siderowf, A. Questionnaire for impulsive-compulsive disorders in Parkinson's Disease–Rating Scale. *Mov. Disord.* **2012**, *27*, 242–247. [CrossRef]
39. McElroy, S.L.; Keck, P.E., Jr.; Pope, H.G., Jr.; Smith, J.M.; Strakowski, S.M. Compulsive buying: A report of 20 cases. *J. Clin. Psychiatry* **1994**, *55*, 242–248. [PubMed]
40. Voon, V. Repetition, repetition, and repetition: Compulsive and punding behaviors in Parkinson's disease. *Mov. Disord.* **2004**, *19*, 367–370. [CrossRef]
41. Evans, A.H.; Katzenschlager, R.; Paviour, D.; O'Sullivan, J.D.; Appel, S.; Lawrence, A.D.; Lees, A.J. Punding in Parkinson's disease: Its relation to the dopamine dysregulation syndrome. *Mov. Disord.* **2004**, *19*, 397–405. [CrossRef] [PubMed]
42. Giovannoni, G.; O'Sullivan, J.D.; Turner, K.; Manson, A.J.; Lees, A.J. Hedonistic homeostatic dysregulation in patients with Parkinson's disease on dopamine replacement therapies. *J. Neurol. Neurosurg. Psychiatry* **2000**, *68*, 423–428. [CrossRef] [PubMed]
43. Papp, A.C.; Pinsonneault, J.K.; Cooke, G.; Sadée, W. Single nucleotide polymorphism genotyping using allele-specific PCR and fluorescence melting curves. *Biotechniques* **2003**, *34*, 1068–1072. [CrossRef]
44. Abramson, J.H. WINPEPI updated: Computer programs for epidemiologists, and their teaching potential. *Epidemiol. Perspect. Innov.* **2011**, *8*, 1–9. [CrossRef] [PubMed]
45. Favorov, A.V.; Andreewski, T.V.; Sudomoina, M.A.; Favorova, O.O.; Parmigiani, G.; Ochs, M.F. A Markov chain Monte Carlo technique for identification of combinations of allelic variants underlying complex diseases in humans. *Genetics* **2005**, *171*, 2113–2121. [CrossRef]
46. Titova, N.; Chaudhuri, K.R. Personalized Medicine and Nonmotor Symptoms in Parkinson's Disease. *Int. Rev. Neurobiol.* **2017**, *134*, 1257–1281. [CrossRef]
47. Rota, S.; Boura, I.; Batzu, L.; Titova, N.; Jenner, P.; Falup-Pecurariu, C.; Chaudhuri, K.R. 'Dopamine agonist Phobia' in Parkinson's disease: When does it matter? Implications for non-motor symptoms and personalized medicine. *Expert Rev. Neurother.* **2020**, *20*, 953–965. [CrossRef]
48. Titova, N.; Qamar, M.A.; Chaudhuri, K.R. Biomarkers of Parkinson's Disease: An Introduction. *Int. Rev. Neurobiol.* **2017**, *132*, 183–196. [CrossRef]

49. Titova, N.; Jenner, P.; Chaudhuri, K.R. The Future of Parkinson's Treatment—Personalised and Precision Medicine. *Eur. Neurol. Rev.* **2017**, *12*, 15. [CrossRef]
50. Marras, C.; Chaudhuri, K.R.; Titova, N.; Mestre, T.A. Therapy of Parkinson's Disease Subtypes. *Neurotherapeutics* **2020**, *17*, 1366–1377. [CrossRef]

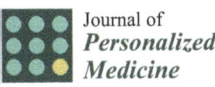

Review

Are Parkinson's Disease Patients the Ideal Preclinical Population for Alzheimer's Disease Therapeutics?

Thomas F. Tropea and Alice Chen-Plotkin *

Department of Neurology, Perelman School of Medicine, University of Pennsylvania, Philadelphia, PA 19104, USA; thomas.tropea@pennmedicine.upenn.edu
* Correspondence: chenplot@pennmedicine.upenn.edu; Tel.: +1-215-573-7193

Abstract: Concomitant neuropathological hallmarks of Alzheimer's Disease (AD) are common in the brains of people with Parkinson's disease (PD). Furthermore, AD biomarkers are associated with cognitive decline and dementia in PD patients during life. Here, we highlight the considerable overlap between AD and PD, emphasizing neuropathological, biomarker, and mechanistic studies. We suggest that precision medicine approaches may successfully identify PD patients most likely to develop concomitant AD. The ability to identify PD patients at high risk for future concomitant AD in turn provides an ideal cohort for trials of AD-directed therapies in PD patients, aimed at delaying or preventing cognitive symptoms.

Keywords: Parkinson's disease; Alzheimer's disease; clinical trial; precision medicine

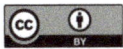

The symptoms of Alzheimer's disease (AD) and Parkinson's disease (PD), the two most common neurodegenerative diseases, present a decade or more after the disease process takes hold. Neuroprotective clinical trials in AD increasingly target early or at-risk groups to prevent or delay the onset of disease, yet therapies that clearly impact the cognitive course remain elusive. Identifying the ideal group of people to target in AD neuroprotective studies remains of key importance.

PD affects over 6 million people worldwide, or 1–3% of people over age 65 [1–3], already making it the second most common neurodegenerative disease, with numbers that are growing [4,5]. Bradykinesia plus tremor or rigidity make up the cardinal symptoms of PD [6], although mood, cognition, sleep, and autonomic function are also often affected [7]. Dementia, one of the most devastating complications in PD, is associated with worse outcomes and increased mortality [8,9]. People with PD develop dementia at a higher rate than age-matched peers without PD [10]. Specifically, PD dementia (PDD) affects as many as 83% of PD patients long-term [11] and is typically preceded by a prodromal cognitive state of mild cognitive impairment (PD-MCI) [12]. Neuropathologically, PD is characterized by neuronal inclusions composed of misfolded alpha-synuclein (aSyn) that exist in Lewy bodies [13]. However, PD neuropathology does not exist in isolation; as many as 70% of postmortem brain samples from people diagnosed with PD in life have a secondary neuropathological diagnosis of AD [14,15], defining PD as an AD risk state.

PD differs from AD in its clinical and neuropathological characteristics. AD is an insidiously progressive cognitive disorder and the most common cause of dementia, affecting an estimated 50 million people worldwide [16]. In the preclinical stage, neuroimaging and molecular changes associated with AD are observed, albeit without clinical signs or symptoms of cognitive impairment or dementia. The prodromal phase is associated with changes in cognitive function without functional or social impairment [17]. The preclinical changes and prodromal phase can begin as many as 20 years prior to the onset of dementia. Dementia secondary to AD typically begins in the 7th decade of life and is characterized by impairments in memory, language, problem-solving, and other domains of cognition [18]. Postmortem examination of AD cases shows significant cortical and medial temporal lobe atrophy, and the neuropathological diagnosis is established by the presence of plaques containing aggregated amyloid-β_{1-42} (Aβ) peptides and neurofibrillary tangles of hyper-phosphorylated tau [19].

To date, clinical trials studying compounds aimed at slowing or reversing the course of established MCI or dementia secondary to AD have largely been underwhelming. One of the reasons for these disappointing results might be that the clinical syndrome appears near the end of the pathological cascade [20]. Most studies have targeted groups with MCI defined by genetic, neuroimaging, and biomarker characteristics to have early AD pathology for enrollment in AD neuroprotection trials (Table 1). Yet, even this approach may miss a critically early time point in AD pathogenesis, beyond which interventions will have minimal clinical impact. How, then, might we identify individuals at an earlier stage—a cognitively normal cohort with *incipient* AD pathology—without casting such a wide net as to be impractical, if not altogether infeasible?

Table 1. Alzheimer's Disease Clinical Trials in Preclinical or Prodromal Participants.

Study Drug	Mechanism of Action	Sponsor	Enrollment Criteria	Ref
Studies enrolling at-risk or preclinical stage human participants				
Atabecestat	BACE Inhibitor	Janssen	APOE E4 genotype.	[21]
Celecoxib	Selective COX-2 inhibitor	Pfizer	Cognitively normal with a family history of AD.	[22]
Crenezumab	Aβ monoclonal antibody	Hoffmann-La Roche	PSEN1 E280A mutation carriers.	[23,24]
Gantenerumab	Aβ monoclonal antibody	Hoffmann-La Roche	APP, presenilin-1, or presenilin-2 carriers.	[25]
Simvastatin	HMG-CoA reductase inhibitor	Merck	Cognitively normal with a family history of AD.	[26]
Solenezumab	Aβ monoclonal antibody	Eli Lilly	APP, presenilin-1, or presenilin-2 carriers.	[25]
Studies enrolling prodromal human participants				
Aducanumab	Aβ monoclonal antibody	Biogen	MCI with positive amyloid PET.	[27]
Atabecestat	BACE Inhibitor	Janssen	MCI with pathological CSF Aβ or positive amyloid PET.	[28]
BI 409306	Phosphodiesterase-9A inhibitor	Boehringer Ingelheim	MCI.	[29]
Crenezumab	Aβ monoclonal antibody	Hoffmann-La Roche	Pathological CSF Aβ or positive amyloid PET.	[23,24]
Donanemab	Aβ monoclonal antibody	Eli Lilly	MCI with positive amyloid PET.	[30]
Elenbecestat	BACE inhibitor	Biogen, Eisai	MCI.	[31]
Exenatide	Glucagon-like peptide-1 agonist	Astra Zeneca	MCI.	NA
Gantenerumab	Aβ monoclonal antibody	Hoffmann-La Roche	MCI with pathological CSF Aβ.	[25,32]
JNJ-63733657	Tau monoclonal antibody	Janssen	Subjective cognitive decline and positive tau PET.	[33]
Pepinemab	Semaphorin 4D monoclonal antibody	Vaccinex	MCI with pathological CSF Aβ or positive amyloid PET.	[34]
Semorinemab	Tau monocloncal antibody	Genentech	MCI with pathological CSF Aβ or positive amyloid PET.	[35]
Simvastatin	HMG-CoA reductase inhibitor	Merck	MCI.	[36]
Solenezumab	Aβ monoclonal antibody	Eli Lilly	MCI with positive amyloid PET.	[37,38]
Verubecestat	BACE inhibitor	Merck	MCI with positive amyloid PET.	[39]

BACE = β-site amyloid precursor protein cleaving enzyme. Aβ = amyloid-β. MCI = mild cognitive impairment. PET = positron emission tomography.

We argue here that individuals with early PD may be exactly the cognitively normal, high-AD-risk population in which interventions are likely to impact cognitive course in a clinically meaningful way. In making our case, we review the considerable overlap between AD and PD, emphasizing neuropathological, biomarker, and mechanistic studies. We then highlight precision medicine approaches to identify people with PD at highest risk of AD, in order to support the feasibility of viewing PD as an ideal preclinical cohort to target AD neuropathology in disease-modifying clinical trials.

1. AD Pathology Is Common in PD Brains and Is Associated with Worse Cognitive Performance during Life

The neuropathological hallmark of PD is the aSyn-containing neuronal Lewy body inclusion. However, co-occurring AD pathology is common among all Lewy body disorder cases, which includes PD, PD with dementia (PDD), and dementia with Lewy bodies (DLB), Figure 1), although exact figures differ between studies. Among published cases with a primary neuropathological Lewy body disorder diagnosis, nearly all have some amount of concomitant tau pathology, with one third of them showing a moderate to severe degree of tau pathology. Roughly 50–70% demonstrated sufficient concomitant Aβ plaques and tau neurofibrillary tangles to warrant a secondary neuropathological diagnosis of AD [14,15]. Moreover, the severity of AD pathology among different brain regions is proportional to the aSyn burden in those regions [40]. Furthermore, tau and aSyn co-aggregate in the same neuronal populations in the amygdala and entorhinal cortex and lesser in the prefrontal cortex [41]. Thus, human neuropathological studies suggest synergy between aSyn, tau, and Aβ with some regional and cellular specificity.

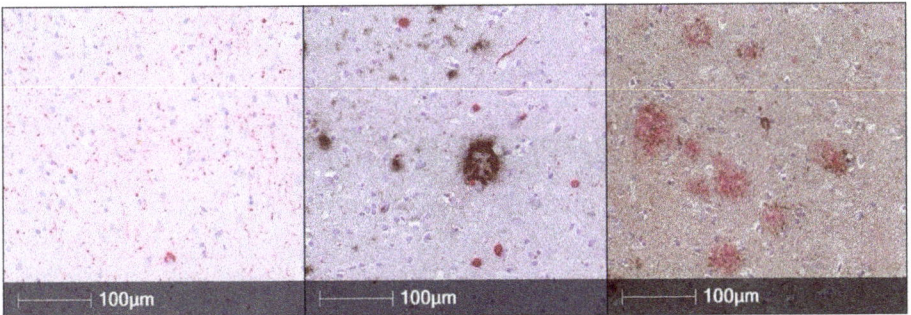

Figure 1. Immunohistochemical sections (160×) demonstrating Lewy Body aSyn (red) pathology in the anterior cingulate cortex (**Left**), concomitant Aβ (brown) and aSyn (red) in the anterior cingulate cortex (**middle**), and Aβ (red) and tau neurofibrillary tangles (brown) in the middle frontal cortex (**Right**). Reprinted with Permission from Dai et al, 2020 [42].

In vivo positron emission tomography (PET) neuroimaging with amyloid specific tracers have helped to describe amyloid pathology at different stages in living PD patients. In early, untreated, cognitively normal PD cases from the Parkinson's Progression Markers Initiative (PPMI), cerebral amyloid [^{18}F] Florbetaben uptake is present in ~20% of cases [43], similar to neurologically normal published cohorts at the same age [44]. Throughout the course of PD, amyloid positivity increases as cognition declines. Indeed, Pittsburgh Compound B (PiB) positivity indicating amyloid deposition is at its lowest in PD with mild cognitive impairment (~5%) and higher in PD cases with dementia (~34%). In cases with DLB, with diffuse neocortical aSyn pathology early in the disease, PiB positivity is at its highest (68%) [45]. Although variability exists between amyloid PET tracers, amyloid appears to accumulate as PD progresses, following patterns of aSyn pathology. Pathological tau PET imaging studies have been more challenging due to off-target binding of available tracers. However, retention of the 3R/4R tau tracer ^{18}F-flortaucepir in Lewy body disease cases is intermediate between healthy controls and AD, is higher in temporal-parietal regions in cases with higher cerebrospinal fluid (CSF) amyloid levels, and is associated with higher CSF tau levels and a higher severity of neuropathological tau [40].

The location and severity of aSyn pathology associates with clinical features that patients exhibit during life. That is, PD patients with aSyn pathology found not only in the brainstem but also throughout the limbic system and cortex are more likely to have cognitive impairment than PD patients with less extensive aSyn pathology [46]. People with PD and concomitant AD have more severe motor dysfunction, a higher burden of depression, faster rate of cognitive progression, shorter interval from motor to cognitive symptom onset, impaired language performance, higher rate of nursing home admittance, and higher mortality risk, compared to PD patients without AD pathology [46–48]. Specifically, temporal lobe tau burden has been independently associated with antemortem deficits in confrontation naming [40,49]. The combination of aSyn and AD copathology confers a worse prognosis associated with worse cognitive function and higher mortality risk.

2. AD Associated Biomarkers of Neurodegeneration, Tau, and Alpha-Synuclein Associate with Cognitive Performance in PD Cohorts

To obtain a glimpse of the underlying neuropathological process, in vivo biomarker studies are important tools, as they can be obtained from biofluids during life, and patients can be observed after the biofluids have been collected. This approach has been informative in AD, through the development and standardization of CSF and plasma-based biomarkers (Aβ, total tau, phosphorylated tau, and neurofilament light [NFL]) [50]. These biochemical biomarkers are highly specific for underlying axonal degeneration (t-tau and NFL) [51–53], Aβ-containing plaques (Aβ) [54], and NFT pathology (p-tau) [55]. Indeed, diagnostic criteria employing these biomarkers have been proposed in the AD field [56], and clinical trials in AD use CSF-based biomarkers as entry criteria [57].

Numerous studies have examined AD biomarkers as predictors of dementia in PD. For example, lower baseline CSF Aβ level was shown to predict a faster rate of cognitive decline in a study of 45 cognitively normal PD patients. When compared to subjects above a cutoff value of 192 pg/mL, those with lower Aβ levels had a greater annual decline by 5.85 points on the Mattis Dementia Rating Scale-2 (DRS) [58]. Lower CSF Aβ was also associated with a higher risk of cognitive impairment within 3 years of disease duration in the PPMI cohort [59]. Unlike Aβ, CSF t-tau is not associated with cognitive outcome in PD, while phospho-tau results have been mixed, with some studies showing association with cognitive impairment and others not demonstrating such a relationship [58,60]. Although NFL is not specific to AD, higher plasma NFL levels are associated with cognitive impairment in PD [61]. Beyond biochemical biomarkers, the *APOE* E4 allele remains the strongest genetic risk factor for late onset AD. In PD, carrying one or two *APOE* E4 alleles is also associated with an increased risk for dementia in PD and a faster rate of cognitive decline [62,63]. Furthermore, structural MRI correlates of AD captured in the Spatial Pattern of Abnormality for Recognition of Early Alzheimer's (SPARE-AD) index associate with cognitive impairment and predict a faster rate of cognitive decline in PD [62]. Thus, cognitive impairment in PD associates with biomarkers of underlying Aβ pathology and axonal degeneration as well as genetic risk of AD, suggesting that AD-related pathophysiology is at least partially causal for the cognitive decline that occurs in the majority of individuals with PD.

3. In Vitro, Cell-Based, and Animal Models Provide Evidence for AD Pathogenic Mechanisms in PD

In vitro studies have long suggested synergy between the key pathological proteins implicated in AD and PD, especially tau and aSyn (reviewed in [64,65]). In particular, Jensen et al. reported over 20 years ago that tau and aSyn can physically interact through pulldowns in human brain lysates [66]. Subsequently, Giasson et al. demonstrated that aSyn induced the fibrillization of tau in vitro and that co-incubation of tau and aSyn accelerated the fibrillization of both proteins [67].

More recently, the discovery that pathological forms of both tau and aSyn may template the misfolding of non-pathological tau and aSyn and that these pathological tau and aSyn species may then propagate from cell to cell has led to new data supporting synergy between AD and PD pathogenic processes in cellular and animal models [68]. For example, Bassil et al. recently showed that co-inoculation of pathological conformations of aSyn and tau into mouse brain increased the formation of tau aggregates, and the absence of endogenous aSyn reduced the formation and spread of tau aggregates [69].

Thus, in vitro, cell-based, and animal models support the premise that the presence of aSyn may accelerate the development and spread of at least tau, and possibly AD, pathology.

4. Precision Medicine Approaches Can Enrich for Those PD Individuals Most Likely to Develop Concomitant AD Pathology

As summarized in the preceding sections, PD individuals who develop cognitive impairment are more likely to carry the *APOE* E4 genotype, more likely to have low CSF Aβ and high CSF and plasma NFL, and more likely to have positive amyloid PET scans. If we turn these associations on their heads and ask, instead, whether the presence of these AD biomarkers can enrich or identify those PD individuals who are most likely to have concomitant AD pathology, the answer that is emerging is very promising.

Specifically, in a neuropathological study of 208 LBD cases from Penn, structured as discovery and replication cohorts, with validation in an additional 70 LBD cases from 20 centers in the National Alzheimer's Coordinating Center (NACC) database, we have shown that genotypes at just three single nucleotide polymorphisms (SNPs), along with age at LBD onset, can be used to calculate a risk score for concomitant AD pathology. PD individuals with AD risk scores in the highest quintile, in turn, were fourfold more likely to have concomitant AD pathology than those in the lowest two quintiles. Importantly, the absolute rate of concomitant AD pathology ranged from 60% to 80% in the highest quintile of AD risk among Penn LBD cases [42]. Put simply, this study suggests that a blood test obtained at any time in PD disease course may be able to identify a sizeable group of individuals with 60–80% chance of having concomitant AD at death. If we infer, based on rates of amyloid positivity by PET imaging in newly diagnosed PD cohorts or PD individuals with minimal cognitive symptoms, that only a small minority of PD individuals have incipient amyloid pathology at these early stages, there is great potential to identify very high-risk PD individuals who are not yet amyloid positive.

While fourfold enrichment for PD individuals destined to have concomitant AD pathology at death is promising, this may still fall short of the levels of certainty needed to enroll a cognitively normal PD group in higher-risk trials aimed at targeting AD-related pathogenic mechanisms. However, a strategy in which (1) minimally invasive blood draws are used to perform genetics-based risk calculation, enriching for a cohort in which (2) AD biochemical biomarker levels (from the CSF or, increasingly, from the plasma) may further hone accuracy, yielding a subgroup in which (3) PET imaging is used to detect the earliest phases of amyloid deposition, is already feasible. Such a strategy is also likely to yield a sizeable group of PD individuals at high enough risk for AD pathology to warrant that targeted intervention.

5. Concluding Remarks

We close with a few observations that may further strengthen the case for viewing "precision-medicine-identified" PD individuals as an ideal preclinical cohort for AD-directed therapies. First, in contrast to current strategies following high-genetic-risk groups in the general population (e.g., carriers of *APOE* E4 alleles), timelines are compressed, and a starting point for thinking about intervention—the time of PD diagnosis—is clearly indicated. Second, we believe that for individuals who already have a neurodegenerative disease diagnosis (PD), willingness to accept the risks inherent in any experimental therapeutic may differ from those with no neurological signs or symptoms. Finally, compared to individuals with established AD (including, for example, those who would fall under the wide-ranging use cases for the recently FDA-approved amyloid-targeting drug aducanumab), cognitively normal PD patients stand to benefit enormously from arresting the course of cognitive decline.

Author Contributions: Conceptualization, T.F.T. and A.C.-P.; Writing—Original Draft Preparation, T.F.T. and A.C.-P.; Writing—Review and Editing, T.F.T. and A.C.-P. All authors have read and agreed to the published version of the manuscript.

Funding: Thomas F. Tropea is funded by the NIH (K23-NS11416). Alice Chen-Plotkin is funded by the NIH (RO1 NS115139, U19 AG062418, P30 AG010124, RO1 NS082265), a Biomarkers Across Neurodegenerative Diseases (BAND) grant from the Michael J. Fox Foundation/Alzheimer's Association/Weston Institute, the AHA-Allen Institute, and the Chan Zuckerberg Initiative Neurodegeneration Challenge. Alice Chen-Plotkin is additionally supported by the Parker Family Chair.

Acknowledgments: We would like to thank our patients and their families.

Conflicts of Interest: The authors declare no conflict of interest.

References

1. Tanner, C.M.; Goldman, S.M. Epidemiology of Movement-Disorders. *Curr. Opin. Neurol.* **1994**, *7*, 340–345. [CrossRef] [PubMed]
2. Nussbaum, R.L.; Ellis, C.E. Alzheimer's Disease and Parkinson's Disease. *N. Engl. J. Med.* **2003**, *348*, 1356–1364. [CrossRef] [PubMed]
3. de Lau, L.M.; Breteler, M.M. Epidemiology of Parkinson's disease. *Lancet Neurol.* **2006**, *5*, 525–535. [CrossRef]
4. Dorsey, E.R.; Constantinescu, R.; Thompson, J.P.; Biglan, K.M.; Holloway, R.G.; Kieburtz, K.; Marshall, F.J.; Ravina, B.M.; Schifitto, G.; Siderowf, A.; et al. Projected number of people with Parkinson disease in the most populous nations, 2005 through 2030. *Neurology* **2007**, *68*, 384–386. [CrossRef] [PubMed]
5. Marras, C.; Beck, J.C.; Bower, J.H.; Roberts, E.; Ritz, B.; Ross, G.W.; Abbott, R.D.; Savica, R.; Van Den Eeden, S.K.; Willis, A.W.; et al. Prevalence of Parkinson's disease across North America. *NPJ Park. Dis.* **2018**, *4*. [CrossRef]
6. Postuma, R.B.; Berg, D.; Stern, M.; Poewe, W.; Olanow, C.W.; Oertel, W.; Obeso, J.; Marek, K.; Litvan, I.; Lang, A.E.; et al. MDS clinical diagnostic criteria for Parkinson's disease. *Mov. Disord.* **2015**, *30*, 1591–1601. [CrossRef]
7. Martinez-Martin, P.; Rodriguez-Blazquez, C.; Kurtis, M.M.; Chaudhuri, K.R. The impact of non-motor symptoms on health-related quality of life of patients with Parkinson's disease. *Mov. Disord.* **2011**, *26*, 399–406. [CrossRef]
8. Kudlicka, A.; Clare, L.; Hindle, J.V. Quality of life, health status and caregiver burden in Parkinson's disease: Relationship to executive functioning. *Int. J. Geriatr. Psychiatry* **2014**, *29*, 68–76. [CrossRef]
9. Vossius, C.; Larsen, J.P.; Janvin, C.; Aarsland, D. The economic impact of cognitive impairment in Parkinson's disease. *Mov. Disord.* **2011**, *26*, 1541–1544. [CrossRef]
10. Aarsland, D.; Andersen, K.; Larsen, J.P.; Lolk, A.; Nielsen, H.; Kragh-Sørensen, P. Risk of dementia in Parkinson's disease: A community-based, prospective study. *Neurology* **2001**, *56*, 730–736. [CrossRef]
11. Hely, M.A.; Reid, W.G.J.; Adena, M.A.; Halliday, G.M.; Morris, J.G.L. The Sydney Multicenter Study of Parkinson's disease: The inevitability of dementia at 20 years. *Mov. Disord.* **2008**, *23*, 837–844. [CrossRef] [PubMed]
12. Litvan, I.; Aarsland, D.; Adler, C.H.; Goldman, J.G.; Kulisevsky, J.; Mollenhauer, B.; Rodriguez-Oroz, M.C.; Tröster, A.I.; Weintraub, D. MDS task force on mild cognitive impairment in Parkinson's disease: Critical review of PD-MCI. *Mov. Disord.* **2011**, *26*, 1814–1824. [CrossRef]
13. Spillantini, M.G.; Goedert, M. Synucleinopathies: Past, present and future. *Neuropathol. Appl. Neurobiol.* **2016**, *42*, 3–5. [CrossRef] [PubMed]
14. Robinson, J.L.; Lee, E.B.; Xie, S.X.; Rennert, L.; Suh, E.; Bredenberg, C.; Caswell, C.; Van Deerlin, V.M.; Yan, N.; Yousef, A.; et al. Neurodegenerative disease concomitant proteinopathies are prevalent, age-related and APOE4-associated. *Brain* **2018**, *141*, 2181–2193. [CrossRef] [PubMed]
15. Smith, C.; Malek, N.; Grosset, K.; Cullen, B.; Gentleman, S.; Grosset, D.G. Neuropathology of dementia in patients with Parkinson's disease: A systematic review of autopsy studies. *J. Neurol. Neurosurg. Psychiatry* **2019**, *90*, 1234–1243. [CrossRef] [PubMed]
16. Alzheimer's Disease International. *World Alzheimer Report 2018—The State of the Art of Dementia Research: New Frontiers*; Alzheimer's Disease International: London, UK, 2018; pp. 1–82.
17. Sperling, R.A.; Aisen, P.S.; Beckett, L.A.; Bennett, D.A.; Craft, S.; Fagan, A.M.; Iwatsubo, T.; Jack, C.R.; Kaye, J.; Montine, T.J.; et al. Toward defining the preclinical stages of Alzheimer's disease: Recommendations from the National Institute on Aging-Alzheimer's Association workgroups on diagnostic guidelines for Alzheimer's disease. *Alzheimer's Dement.* **2011**, *7*, 280–292. [CrossRef]
18. 2021 Alzheimer's disease facts and figures. *Alzheimer's Dement.* **2021**, *17*, 327–406. [CrossRef]
19. Montine, T.J.; Phelps, C.H.; Beach, T.G.; Bigio, E.H.; Cairns, N.J.; Dickson, D.W.; Duyckaerts, C.; Frosch, M.P.; Mirra, S.S.; Nelson, P.T.; et al. National Institute on Aging-Alzheimer's Association guidelines for the neuropathologic assessment of Alzheimer's disease: A practical approach NIH Public Access. *Acta Neuropathol.* **2012**, *123*, 1–11. [CrossRef]
20. Kang, J.H.; Korecka, M.; Figurski, M.J.; Toledo, J.B.; Blennow, K.; Zetterberg, H.; Waligorska, T.; Brylska, M.; Fields, L.; Shah, N.; et al. The Alzheimer's Disease Neuroimaging Initiative 2 Biomarker Core: A review of progress and plans. *Alzheimer's Dement.* **2015**, *11*, 772–791. [CrossRef]
21. Novak, G.; Streffer, J.R.; Timmers, M.; Henley, D.; Brashear, H.R.; Bogert, J.; Russu, A.; Janssens, L.; Tesseur, I.; Tritsmans, L.; et al. Long-term safety and tolerability of atabecestat (JNJ-54861911), an oral BACE1 inhibitor, in early Alzheimer's disease spectrum patients: A randomized, double-blind, placebo-controlled study and a two-period extension study. *Alzheimers. Res. Ther.* **2020**, *12*, 58. [CrossRef]
22. Leoutsakos, J.-M.S.; Muthen, B.O.; Breitner, J.C.S.; Lyketsos, C.G. ADAPT Research Team Effects of non-steroidal anti-inflammatory drug treatments on cognitive decline vary by phase of pre-clinical Alzheimer disease: Findings from the randomized controlled Alzheimer's Disease Anti-inflammatory Prevention Trial. *Int. J. Geriatr. Psychiatry* **2012**, *27*, 364–374. [CrossRef]
23. A Study of Crenezumab Versus Placebo to Evaluate the Efficacy and Safety in Participants with Prodromal to Mild Alzheimer's Disease (AD) (CREAD 2). Available online: https://clinicaltrials.gov/ct2/show/NCT02670083 (accessed on 15 June 2021).

24. Tariot, P.N.; Lopera, F.; Langbaum, J.B.; Thomas, R.G.; Hendrix, S.; Schneider, L.S.; Rios-Romenets, S.; Giraldo, M.; Acosta, N.; Tobon, C.; et al. The Alzheimer's Prevention Initiative Autosomal-Dominant Alzheimer's Disease Trial: A study of crenezumab versus placebo in preclinical PSEN1 E280A mutation carriers to evaluate efficacy and safety in the treatment of autosomal-dominant Alzheimer's disease, including a placebo-treated noncarrier cohort. *Alzheimer's Dement.* **2018**, *4*, 150–160. [CrossRef]
25. Dominantly Inherited Alzheimer Network Trial: An Opportunity to Prevent Dementia. A Study of Potential Disease Modifying Treatments in Individuals at Risk for or With a Type of Early Onset Alzheimer's Disease Caused by a Genetic Mutation. Available online: https://clinicaltrials.gov/ct2/show/NCT01760005 (accessed on 15 June 2021).
26. Carlsson, C.M.; Gleason, C.E.; Hess, T.M.; Moreland, K.A.; Blazel, H.M.; Koscik, R.L.; Schreiber, N.T.N.; Johnson, S.C.; Atwood, C.S.; Puglielli, L.; et al. Effects of simvastatin on cerebrospinal fluid biomarkers and cognition in middle-aged adults at risk for Alzheimer's disease. *J. Alzheimer's Dis.* **2008**, *13*, 187–197. [CrossRef] [PubMed]
27. Sevigny, J.; Chiao, P.; Bussière, T.; Weinreb, P.H.; Williams, L.; Maier, M.; Dunstan, R.; Salloway, S.; Chen, T.; Ling, Y.; et al. The antibody aducanumab reduces Aβ plaques in Alzheimer's disease. *Nature* **2016**, *537*, 50–56. [CrossRef] [PubMed]
28. Timmers, M.; Streffer, J.R.; Russu, A.; Tominaga, Y.; Shimizu, H.; Shiraishi, A.; Tatikola, K.; Smekens, P.; Börjesson-Hanson, A.; Andreasen, N.; et al. Pharmacodynamics of atabecestat (JNJ-54861911), an oral BACE1 inhibitor in patients with early Alzheimer's disease: Randomized, double-blind, placebo-controlled study. *Alzheimers. Res. Ther.* **2018**, *10*, 85. [CrossRef] [PubMed]
29. Frölich, L.; Wunderlich, G.; Thamer, C.; Roehrle, M.; Garcia, M.; Dubois, B. Evaluation of the efficacy, safety and tolerability of orally administered BI 409306, a novel phosphodiesterase type 9 inhibitor, in two randomised controlled phase II studies in patients with prodromal and mild Alzheimer's disease. *Alzheimer's Res. Ther.* **2019**, *11*, 18. [CrossRef] [PubMed]
30. Lowe, S.L.; Willis, B.A.; Hawdon, A.; Natanegara, F.; Chua, L.; Foster, J.; Shcherbinin, S.; Ardayfio, P.; Sims, J.R. Donanemab (LY3002813) dose-escalation study in Alzheimer's disease. *Alzheimer's Dement.* **2021**, *7*, e12112. [CrossRef]
31. Lynch, S.Y.; Kaplow, J.; Zhao, J.; Dhadda, S.; Luthman, J.; Albala, B. P4-389: Elenbecestat, E2609, a bace inhibitor: Results from a phase-2 study in subjects with mild cognitive impairment and mild-to-moderate dementia due to alzheimer's disease. *Alzheimer's Dement.* **2018**, *14*, P1623–P1623. [CrossRef]
32. Ostrowitzki, S.; Lasser, R.A.; Dorflinger, E.; Scheltens, P.; Barkhof, F.; Nikolcheva, T.; Ashford, E.; Retout, S.; Hofmann, C.; Delmar, P.; et al. A phase III randomized trial of gantenerumab in prodromal Alzheimer's disease. *Alzheimer's Res. Ther.* **2017**, *9*, 95. [CrossRef]
33. A Study of JNJ-63733657 in Participants With Early Alzheimer's Disease—Full Text View—ClinicalTrials.gov. Available online: https://clinicaltrials.gov/ct2/show/NCT04619420?term=JNJ-63733657&draw=2&rank=1 (accessed on 15 June 2021).
34. SEMA4D Blockade Safety and Brain Metabolic Activity in Alzheimer's Disease (AD) (SIGNAL-AD). Available online: https://clinicaltrials.gov/ct2/show/NCT04381468 (accessed on 15 June 2021).
35. PRESS RELEASE AC Immune Reports Top Line Results from TAURIEL Phase 2 Trial Evaluating Semorinemab in Early Alzheimer's Disease. Available online: https://ir.acimmune.com/static-files/7296e650-85ea-4151-aca5-6f63ec71653c (accessed on 15 June 2021).
36. Serrano-Pozo, A.; Vega, G.L.; Lütjohann, D.; Locascio, J.J.; Tennis, M.K.; Deng, A.; Atri, A.; Hyman, B.T.; Irizarry, M.C.; Growdon, J.H. Effects of simvastatin on cholesterol metabolism and Alzheimer disease biomarkers. *Alzheimer Dis. Assoc. Disord.* **2010**, *24*, 220–226. [CrossRef]
37. Clinical Trial of Solanezumab for Older Individuals Who May be at Risk for Memory Loss—Full Text View—ClinicalTrials.gov. Available online: https://clinicaltrials.gov/ct2/show/NCT02008357?term=solanezumab&draw=2&rank=5 (accessed on 15 June 2021).
38. A Study of Solanezumab (LY2062430) in Participants With Prodromal Alzheimer's Disease—Full Text View—ClinicalTrials.gov. Available online: https://clinicaltrials.gov/ct2/show/NCT02760602?term=solanezumab&draw=2&rank=1 (accessed on 15 June 2021).
39. Egan, M.F.; Kost, J.; Voss, T.; Mukai, Y.; Aisen, P.S.; Cummings, J.L.; Tariot, P.N.; Vellas, B.; van Dyck, C.H.; Boada, M.; et al. Randomized Trial of Verubecestat for Prodromal Alzheimer's Disease. *N. Engl. J. Med.* **2019**, *380*, 1408–1420. [CrossRef] [PubMed]
40. Coughlin, D.; Xie, S.X.; Liang, M.; Williams, A.; Peterson, C.; Weintraub, D.; McMillan, C.T.; Wolk, D.A.; Akhtar, R.S.; Hurtig, H.I.; et al. Cognitive and Pathological Influences of Tau Pathology in Lewy Body Disorders. *Ann. Neurol.* **2019**, *85*, 259–271. [CrossRef]
41. Colom-Cadena, M.; Gelpi, E.; Charif, S.; Belbin, O.; Blesa, R.; Martí, M.J.; Clarimon, J.; Lleó, A. Confluence of α-Synuclein, Tau, and β-Amyloid Pathologies in Dementia With Lewy Bodies. *J. Neuropathol. Exp. Neurol.* **2013**, *72*, 1203–1212. [CrossRef]
42. Dai, D.L.; Tropea, T.F.; Robinson, J.L.; Suh, E.; Hurtig, H.; Weintraub, D.; Van Deerlin, V.; Lee, E.B.; Trojanowski, J.Q.; Chen-Plotkin, A.S. ADNC-RS, a clinical-genetic risk score, predicts Alzheimer's pathology in autopsy-confirmed Parkinson's disease and Dementia with Lewy bodies. *Acta Neuropathol.* **2020**, *140*, 449–461. [CrossRef]
43. Fiorenzato, E.; Biundo, R.; Cecchin, D.; Frigo, A.C.; Kim, J.; Weis, L.; Strafella, A.P.; Antonini, A. Brain Amyloid Contribution to Cognitive Dysfunction in Early-Stage Parkinson's Disease: The PPMI Dataset. *J. Alzheimer's Dis.* **2018**, *66*, 229–237. [CrossRef]
44. Roberts, R.O.; Aakre, J.A.; Kremers, W.K.; Vassilaki, M.; Knopman, D.S.; Mielke, M.M.; Alhurani, R.; Geda, Y.E.; Machulda, M.M.; Coloma, P.; et al. Prevalence and outcomes of amyloid positivity among persons without dementia in a longitudinal, population-based setting. *JAMA Neurol.* **2018**, *75*, 970–979. [CrossRef] [PubMed]
45. Petrou, M.; Dwamena, B.A.; Foerster, B.R.; Maceachern, M.P.; Bohnen, N.I.; Müller, M.L.; Albin, R.L.; Frey, K.A. Amyloid deposition in Parkinson's disease and cognitive impairment: A systematic review. *Mov. Disord.* **2015**, *30*, 928–935. [CrossRef] [PubMed]

46. Irwin, D.J.; Grossman, M.; Weintraub, D.; Hurtig, H.I.; Duda, J.E.; Xie, S.X.; Lee, E.B.; Van Deerlin, V.M.; Lopez, O.L.; Kofler, J.K.; et al. Neuropathological and genetic correlates of survival and dementia onset in synucleinopathies: A retrospective analysis. *Lancet Neurol.* **2017**, *16*, 55. [CrossRef]
47. Lemstra, A.W.; De Beer, M.H.; Teunissen, C.E.; Schreuder, C.; Scheltens, P.; Van Der Flier, W.M.; Sikkes, S.A.M. Concomitant AD pathology affects clinical manifestation and survival in dementia with Lewy bodies. *J. Neurol. Neurosurg. Psychiatry* **2017**, *88*, 113–118. [CrossRef]
48. Howard, E.; Irwin, D.J.; Rascovsky, K.; Nevler, N.; Shellikeri, S.; Tropea, T.F.; Spindler, M.; Deik, A.; Chen-Plotkin, A.; Siderowf, A.; et al. Cognitive Profile and Markers of Alzheimer Disease-Type Pathology in Patients With Lewy Body Dementias. *Neurology* **2021**, *96*, 1855–1864. [CrossRef]
49. Peavy, G.M.; Edland, S.D.; Toole, B.M.; Hansen, L.A.; Galasko, D.R.; Mayo, A.M. Phenotypic differences based on staging of Alzheimer's neuropathology in autopsy-confirmed dementia with Lewy bodies. *Park. Relat. Disord.* **2016**, *31*, 72–78. [CrossRef] [PubMed]
50. Weiner, M.W.; Veitch, D.P.; Aisen, P.S.; Beckett, L.A.; Cairns, N.J.; Cedarbaum, J.; Green, R.C.; Harvey, D.; Jack, C.R.; Jagust, W.; et al. 2014 Update of the Alzheimer's Disease Neuroimaging Initiative: A review of papers published since its inception. *Alzheimer's Dement.* **2015**, *11*, e1–e120. [CrossRef] [PubMed]
51. Wallin, Å.K.; Blennow, K.; Zetterberg, H.; Londos, E.; Minthon, L.; Hansson, O. CSF biomarkers predict a more malignant outcome in Alzheimer disease. *Neurology* **2010**, *74*, 1531–1537. [CrossRef] [PubMed]
52. Zetterberg, H.; Skillbäck, T.; Mattsson, N.; Trojanowski, J.Q.; Portelius, E.; Shaw, L.M.; Weiner, M.W.; Blennow, K. Association of cerebrospinal fluid neurofilament light concentration with Alzheimer disease progression. *JAMA Neurol.* **2016**, *73*, 60–67. [CrossRef]
53. Olsson, B.; Portelius, E.; Cullen, N.C.; Sandelius, Å.; Zetterberg, H.; Andreasson, U.; Höglund, K.; Irwin, D.J.; Grossman, M.; Weintraub, D.; et al. Association of Cerebrospinal Fluid Neurofilament Light Protein Levels with Cognition in Patients with Dementia, Motor Neuron Disease, and Movement Disorders. *JAMA Neurol.* **2019**, *76*, 318–325. [CrossRef] [PubMed]
54. Strozyk, D.; Blennow, K.; White, L.R.; Launer, L.J. CSF Aß 42 levels correlate with amyloid-neuropathology in a population-based autopsy study. *Neurology* **2003**, *60*, 652–656. [CrossRef]
55. Olsson, B.; Lautner, R.; Andreasson, U.; Öhrfelt, A.; Portelius, E.; Bjerke, M.; Hölttä, M.; Rosén, C.; Olsson, C.; Strobel, G.; et al. CSF and blood biomarkers for the diagnosis of Alzheimer's disease: A systematic review and meta-analysis. *Lancet Neurol.* **2016**, *15*, 673–684. [CrossRef]
56. Jack, C.R.; Bennett, D.A.; Blennow, K.; Carrillo, M.C.; Dunn, B.; Haeberlein, S.B.; Holtzman, D.M.; Jagust, W.; Jessen, F.; Karlawish, J.; et al. NIA-AA Research Framework: Toward a biological definition of Alzheimer's disease. *Alzheimer's Dement.* **2018**, *14*, 535–562. [CrossRef]
57. Sperling, R.A.; Rentz, D.M.; Johnson, K.A.; Karlawish, J.; Donohue, M.; Salmon, D.P.; Aisen, P. The A4 study: Stopping AD before symptoms begin? *Sci. Transl. Med.* **2014**, *6*, 228fs13. [CrossRef]
58. Siderowf, A.; Xie, S.X.; Hurtig, H.; Weintraub, D.; Duda, J.; Chen-Plotkin, A.; Shaw, L.M.; Van Deerlin, V.; Trojanowski, J.Q.; Clark, C. CSF amyloid β 1-42 predicts cognitive decline in Parkinson disease. *Neurology* **2010**, *75*, 1055–1061. [CrossRef]
59. Terrelonge, M.; Marder, K.S.; Weintraub, D.; Alcalay, R.N. CSF β-Amyloid 1-42 Predicts Progression to Cognitive Impairment in Newly Diagnosed Parkinson Disease. *J. Mol. Neurosci.* **2016**, *58*, 88–92. [CrossRef] [PubMed]
60. Hall, S.; Surova, Y.; Öhrfelt, A.; Blennow, K.; Zetterberg, H.; Hansson, O. Longitudinal Measurements of Cerebrospinal Fluid Biomarkers in Parkinson's Disease. *Mov. Disord.* **2016**, *31*, 898–905. [CrossRef]
61. Lin, C.-H.; Li, C.-H.; Yang, K.-C.; Lin, F.-J.; Wu, C.-C.; Chieh, J.-J.; Chiu, M.-J. Blood NfL: A biomarker for disease severity and progression in Parkinson disease. *Neurology* **2019**, *93*, e1104–e1111. [CrossRef]
62. Tropea, T.F.; Xie, S.X.; Rick, J.; Chahine, L.M.; Dahodwala, N.; Doshi, J.; Davatzikos, C.; Shaw, L.M.; Van Deerlin, V.; Trojanowski, J.Q.; et al. APOE, thought disorder, and SPARE-AD predict cognitive decline in established Parkinson's disease. *Mov. Disord.* **2018**, *33*, 289–297. [CrossRef] [PubMed]
63. Guo, Y.; Liu, F.-T.; Hou, X.-H.; Li, J.-Q.; Cao, X.-P.; Tan, L.; Wang, J.; Yu, J.-T. Predictors of cognitive impairment in Parkinson's disease: A systematic review and meta-analysis of prospective cohort studies. *J. Neurol.* **2021**, *268*, 2713–2722. [CrossRef] [PubMed]
64. Moussaud, S.; Jones, D.R.; Moussaud-Lamodière, E.L.; Delenclos, M.; Ross, O.A.; McLean, P.J. Alpha-synuclein and tau: Teammates in neurodegeneration? *Mol. Neurodegener.* **2014**, *9*, 43. [CrossRef] [PubMed]
65. Yan, X.; Uronen, R.-L.; Huttunen, H.J. The interaction of α-synuclein and Tau: A molecular conspiracy in neurodegeneration? *Semin. Cell Dev. Biol.* **2020**, *99*, 55–64. [CrossRef]
66. Jensen, P.H.; Hager, H.; Nielsen, M.S.; Hojrup, P.; Gliemann, J.; Jakes, R. alpha-synuclein binds to Tau and stimulates the protein kinase A-catalyzed tau phosphorylation of serine residues 262 and 356. *J. Biol. Chem.* **1999**, *274*, 25481–25489. [CrossRef]
67. Giasson, B.I.; Forman, M.S.; Higuchi, M.; Golbe, L.I.; Graves, C.L.; Kotzbauer, P.T.; Trojanowski, J.Q.; Lee, V.M.Y.M.-Y. Initiation and synergistic fibrillization of tau and alpha-synuclein. *Science* **2003**, *300*, 636–640. [CrossRef]
68. Guo, J.L.; Lee, V.M.Y. Cell-to-cell transmission of pathogenic proteins in neurodegenerative diseases. *Nat. Med.* **2014**, *20*, 130–138. [CrossRef]
69. Bassil, F.; Meymand, E.S.; Brown, H.J.; Xu, H.; Cox, T.O.; Pattabhiraman, S.; Maghames, C.M.; Wu, Q.; Zhang, B.; Trojanowski, J.Q.; et al. α-Synuclein modulates tau spreading in mouse brains. *J. Exp. Med.* **2021**, *218*, e20192193. [CrossRef] [PubMed]

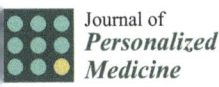

Viewpoint

Personalised Advanced Therapies in Parkinson's Disease: The Role of Non-Motor Symptoms Profile

Valentina Leta [1,2,†], Haidar S. Dafsari [3,†], Anna Sauerbier [1,2,3], Vinod Metta [1,2], Nataliya Titova [4,5], Lars Timmermann [6], Keyoumars Ashkan [7], Michael Samuel [2], Eero Pekkonen [8], Per Odin [9], Angelo Antonini [10], Pablo Martinez-Martin [11], Miriam Parry [1,2], Daniel J. van Wamelen [1,2,12] and K. Ray Chaudhuri [1,2,*]

1. Department of Basic and Clinical Neurosciences, Institute of Psychiatry, Psychology & Neuroscience, King's College London, London SE5 9RT, UK; valentina.1.leta@kcl.ac.uk (V.L.); anna.sauerbier@uk-koeln.de (A.S.); vinod.metta@nhs.net (V.M.); miriamparry@nhs.net (M.P.); daniel.van_wamelen@kcl.ac.uk (D.J.v.W.)
2. Parkinson's Foundation Centre of Excellence, King's College Hospital, London SE5 9RS, UK; m.samuel@nhs.net
3. Department of Neurology, Faculty of Medicine, University of Cologne, 50937 Cologne, Germany; haidar.dafsari@uk-koeln.de
4. Department of Neurology, Neurosurgery and Medical Genetics, Federal State Autonomous Educational Institution of Higher Education «N.I. Pirogov Russian National Research Medical University», Ministry of Health of the Russian Federation, 117997 Moscow, Russia; nattitova@yandex.ru
5. Department of Neurodegenerative Diseases, Federal State Budgetary Institution «Federal Center of Brain and Neurotechnologies», Ministry of Health of the Russian Federation, 117997 Moscow, Russia
6. Department of Neurology, University Hospital of Giessen and Marburg, Campus Marburg, 35043 Marburg, Hessen, Germany; lars.timmermann@uk-gm.de
7. Neurosurgical Department, King's College Hospital Foundation Trust, London SE5 9RS, UK; k.ashkan@nhs.net
8. Department of Neurology, University of Helsinki, 00029 HUS Helsinki, Finland; eero.pekkonen@hus.fi
9. Division of Neurology, Department of Clinical Sciences Lund, Lund University, P663+Q9 Lund, Sweden; per.odin@med.lu.se
10. Parkinson and Movement Disorders Unit, Department of Neuroscience, University of Padua, 35138 Padua, Italy; angelo.antonini@unipd.it
11. Centre for Networked Biomedical Research in Neurodegenerative Diseases (CIBERNED), Carlos III Institute of Health, 28031 Madrid, Spain; pmm650@hotmail.com
12. Department of Neurology, Donders Institute for Brain, Cognition and Behaviour, Radboud University Medical Centre, 6500HB Nijmegen, The Netherlands
* Correspondence: ray.chaudhuri@kcl.ac.uk; Tel.: +44-20-3299-8807
† These authors contributed equally to this work.

Abstract: Device-aided therapies, including levodopa-carbidopa intestinal gel infusion, apomorphine subcutaneous infusion, and deep brain stimulation, are available in many countries for the management of the advanced stage of Parkinson's disease (PD). Currently, selection of device-aided therapies is mainly focused on patients' motor profile while non-motor symptoms play a role limited to being regarded as possible exclusion criteria in the decision-making process for the delivery and sustenance of a successful treatment. Differential beneficial effects on specific non-motor symptoms of the currently available device-aided therapies for PD are emerging and these could hold relevant clinical implications. In this viewpoint, we suggest that specific non-motor symptoms could be used as an additional anchor to motor symptoms and not merely as exclusion criteria to deliver bespoke and patient-specific personalised therapy for advanced PD.

Keywords: Parkinson's disease; device-aided therapies; non-motor symptoms; personalised medicine; apomorphine; levodopa-carbidopa intestinal gel; deep brain stimulation

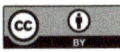

1. Advanced Parkinson's Disease: The Clinical Scenario

Parkinson's disease (PD) is a heterogenous syndromic disorder with a complex natural history, spanning prodromal to palliative stages [1,2]. While early motor phases of PD can be effectively managed by oral and transdermal dopamine replacement therapies, treatment of the more advanced phases remains a challenge, partly complicated by the requirement to choose which device-aided therapies (DAT) to offer to which patients, including levodopa-carbidopa intestinal gel infusion (LCIG) with or without entacapone, subcutaneous apomorphine infusion (APO), and deep brain stimulation (DBS). An optimal therapeutic choice is important as advanced PD is associated with motor and non-motor complications which may be refractory to standard oral/transdermal therapy negatively affecting quality of life [3–6]. International consensus and standard guidelines have attempted to address ideal DAT selection, but the latter still remains an unmet need [7–9]. A recent initiative based on an international Delphi-panel approach identified key motor, non-motor, and functional indicators of advanced PD [10], externally validated in the OBSERVE-PD study [11]. This has led to the development of the '5-2-1' paradigm ($\geq$5-times oral levodopa doses/day, $\geq$2 h of 'off' symptoms/day, $\geq$1 h of troublesome dyskinesia/day) to identify motor aspects of advanced PD and ensure timely referral for DAT initiation [10]. The interim analysis of DUOGLOBE, an observational study evaluating the long-term effectiveness of LCIG in patients with advanced PD, showed that only 20% of patients met all of the 5-2-1 criteria, but 98% met at least one criterion, highlighting the need for further refinement and personalisation of DAT selection [12].

A clinically relevant issue is the debate on whether earlier (than currently adopted in clinical practice) initiation of DAT may be beneficial for patients with PD. The EARLYSTIM study as well as the post-hoc analysis of the GLORIA registry have explored an earlier introduction of DBS and LCIG, respectively, but appropriate timing of DAT initiation largely remains an area of debate [13–15]. Moreover, older patients ($\geq$75 years), for whom DBS is often not considered because of risk-benefit uncertainty, may nonetheless benefit from a modified approach involving DBS of several nuclei [16]. Another emergent debate is focused on how non-motor symptoms (NMS) may guide DAT selection for patients with PD as a positive inclusion criterion, rather than being used purely as an exclusion criterion, e.g., severe depression as a contraindication for DBS and severe hallucinations for APO.

Finally, also in relation to initiatives of providing earlier initiation of DAT in patients with PD, the relatively high costs of DAT need to be taken into account. Here, the societal impact of advanced PD is considerable as the 20% most affected patients are responsible for around 70% of secondary care costs [17]. The costs of DAT can be considerable, but NMS have not been taken into account in cost-effectiveness analyses [18]. This is a relevant observation as NMS contribute at least equally, if not more, to quality of life as motor symptoms [19,20]. Additionally, motor fluctuations, the most common indication for DAT, are often accompanied by non-motor fluctuations, adding to perceived quality of life [21,22]. Thus, it seems reasonable to include NMS in the decision to initiate DAT in patients with PD, especially for those with only moderate motor symptoms but severe non-motor burden [23].

Therefore, in this viewpoint, we will focus on the emerging role of the non-motor profile integral to the choice and outcomes of personalised medicine [1] when delivering DAT in PD. We aim to delineate the emerging field of non-motor indications for DAT and discuss possible implications for clinical practice.

2. Current Use of Non-Motor Symptoms in Device-Aided Therapies Selection

NMS have been proposed as criteria to consider for use of DAT; however, they are not considered in most country-based guidelines by licensing authorities or are merely used as exclusion criteria. The latter has been reviewed as part of the NAVIGATE PD initiative [7], for instance, and NMS constitute both relative and absolute contraindications for certain DAT while data suggests NMS could be improved by DAT. An absolute contraindication (in most countries) for all DAT is severe dementia, whereas non-motor aspects representing relative contraindications are more diverse. For APO and LCIG these include impulse control disorder and dopamine dysregulation syndrome, along with mild to moderate cognitive dysfunction; for DBS the main non-motor contraindications are severe depression and clinically relevant cognitive impairments [7,24]. Moreover, presence of symptomatic orthostatic hypotension, excessive daytime sleepiness, and severe hallucinations could be considered exclusion criteria for APO [25].

3. Device-Aided Therapies and Differential Effect on Non-Motor Symptoms

While therapeutic decisions and research on DAT have largely focused on the influence and effect on motor symptoms, NMS are an integral feature of PD and, therefore, should play an active part in the decision-making process to select the ideal DAT for patients with PD [7,10]. Although APO, LCIG and bilateral subthalamic nucleus (STN) DBS have been available for many years for the treatment of PD in many countries, head-to-head comparative studies are limited. Following on from the original EuroInf study [26], the EuroInf 2 study is the first and only study concurrently comparing all three DAT [27]. Although open-label in its design, it offers Class IIb evidence on the differential effects of these DAT on NMS measured by the NMS scale (NMSS) total burden and its domain's scores. In agreement with other studies, all three therapeutic options confirmed an improvement in motor complications, Hoehn and Yahr stage and quality of life [26–32]. Although all three DAT decreased total NMS burden, interestingly, each treatment appeared to have a bias towards specific NMS thus providing some early indications of varied responsiveness to each therapy. For instance, in this cohort of 173 patients, APO decreased the attention/memory domain scores, while bilateral STN-DBS and LCIG did to a lesser extent which was not statically significant. Nonetheless, it needs to be acknowledged that patients with cognitive problems would be excluded a priori from receiving DBS. Similarly, in this study patients receiving APO had higher NMSS attention/memory baseline scores compared to the other groups, leaving more room for improvement. Data on patients with severe attention/memory problems are not available. On the other hand, DBS and LCIG appeared to reduce the urinary and gastrointestinal domains scores, respectively. All three treatment options decreased the mood/apathy and miscellaneous domains scores, the latter including weight changes, altered thermoregulation and olfaction as well as unexplained pain. Improvements here were heterogeneous, and while APO reduced weight change-related scores, LCIG and DBS improved most of the symptoms contained within the miscellaneous domain. Aspects of sleep dysfunction and fatigue as measured by the NMSS also improved with both LCIG and bilateral STN-DBS, but not after APO initiation. Finally, there is evidence to suggest that APO and bilateral STN-DBS decrease the perceptual problems and hallucinations domain scores, although typically these are considered contra-indications [10]. The mechanisms behind these associations need to be further elucidated; however, it is possible to argue that, for instance, historical presence of visual hallucinations which are mainly drug-induced, and which might subside after drug withdrawal at the expense of a troublesome motor worsening, might benefit from DAT initiation. Finally, combined DAT-related data is also emerging, and may help us to overcome specific issues [33–38].

3.1. Non-Motor Effects of Deep Brain Stimulation

Important conceptual advances may hold promise in relation to the delivery of personalised medicine and DAT in PD [2]. In addition to the abovementioned EuroInf studies, this is exemplified by several studies that have been conducted on the non-motor effects of DBS, showing improvements in several non-motor areas that have been reviewed elsewhere [39–44]. In brief, a recent meta-analysis, including 48 studies with mainly 12-month follow-up data, suggested post-STN-DBS improvements of depression and anxiety-related symptoms but increased apathy [41]. Another meta-analysis of seven studies with follow-up data ranging from three to 24 months showed post-STN-DBS improvements in sleep quality and restless leg syndrome; however, a high degree of heterogeneity among studies was reported [39,44,45], and few studies have investigated the effect of STN-DBS on REM sleep behaviour disorder [42,46]. Another recently published review summarised post-DBS positive outcomes related to urinary dysfunction (mean bladder volumes at desire and urge point to void), while controversial and limited data are available in relation to sexual, cardiovascular, thermoregulatory and gastrointestinal dysfunction [40]. Finally, even though presence of dementia is a contraindication for DBS, a systematic review of 13 studies showed that although there was a decline in verbal fluency and attention domains of cognition, other cognitive functions remained unchanged over a follow-up period ranging from six months to eight years [43]. It needs to be acknowledged that most included studies had small cohort sizes and heterogenous outcome measures.

Further advancements in relation to personalised medicine with DBS might be achieved by directing neurostimulation to specific parts of the basal ganglia and leveraging their specific connectivity profiles [47–49].

More theoretical approaches, such as adaptive DBS, have been developed as a method where DBS is turned on and off according to a closed-loop feedback signal recorded from the tissue surrounding the stimulating electrode. This may develop into personalised approach if it can show to activate DBS at times of necessity and reduce it at times of quiescence, for example in sleep, with the aim of a more physiological treatment and potentially reducing the frequency for battery replacements in non-rechargeable systems. Presently, limitations to the clinical application of adaptive DBS are: (1) Tremor frequency, beta-band and other oscillations required for the closed-loop feedback arc of adaptive DBS are not recordable in all patients with PD [50]; (2) beta-band activity represents not only pathological alterations, but is also modulated by physiological functions [51,52] (3) pathological tremor frequency and beta-band oscillations may, in some patients, reflect tremor, bradykinesia and rigidity, but not NMS [53]; (4) motor symptoms can fluctuate at different times during the course of the day than non-motor fluctuations [21,22]. As such, situations may arise in which the neurostimulation is not active because tremor frequency and beta-band oscillations cannot be detected, but the patient nonetheless presents with NMS such as pain or depressed mood. Therefore, studies are needed to investigate the effect of adaptive DBS on quality of life and NMS, not only motor symptoms [54].

3.2. Non-Motor Effects of Levodopa-Carbidopa Intestinal Gel Infusion

There is robust evidence on the effect of LCIG on NMS. In 2015, a systematic review identified eight open-label studies confirming that LCIG improved total NMS burden after a follow up period ranging from six to 25 months, with specific positive effects on sleep and autonomic dysfunction, and particularly gastrointestinal issues measured by the NMSS [55]. Additionally, more recent reviews have highlighted the non-motor effect of LCIG where a general improvement in the non-motor burden was noted [56,57]. Studies included in these reviews were, among others, the GLORIA registry, whose 24-month follow up data showed a remarkable beneficial effect of LCIG on sleep disturbances, apathy, and gastrointestinal dysfunction as measured by the NMSS [29], and the interim analysis of the DUOGLOBE study, where an overall improvement in the NMS total burden was also shown after only six months [12]. Additional open labels studies with 6-month follow-up data showed a post-LCIG improvement in NMS total burden, including reduction of the cardiovascular, attention/memory, urinary and miscellaneous domains scores of the NMSS [26,58]. Interestingly, the baseline total burden of NMS in PD can predict a robust total non-motor response to LCIG therapy at two years follow up. This observation can underpin DAT selection with an NMS focus, specifically when considering personalised LCIG therapy for instance [59].

3.3. Non-Motor Effects of Apomorphine Subcutaneous Infusion

Although APO has been in use longest compared with DBS and LCIG (APO became available on the European market in the early 1990s), data regarding APO and selection of this device-aided therapy based on patients' non-motor profile is less obvious and the results from the double-blind TOLEDO study are awaited with interest [60]. However, several open-label and case report-based studies show that this treatment can have a beneficial effect on the NMS total burden as well as on specific non-motor areas, and these have been reviewed elsewhere [56,61,62]. In brief, there is evidence suggesting post-APO improvements in depression, anxiety, apathy, perceptual problems, cognitive impairment, sleep dysfunction (insomnia and restless leg syndrome), fatigue, urinary dysfunction (urinary frequency, urgency and nocturia), and gastrointestinal dysfunction (dribbling of saliva) as measured by the NMSS at both 6- and 12-month follow up [26,63]. The reported beneficial effect or tolerability of APO on mild visual hallucinations is of interest given that it is a dopamine D1 and D2 receptor agonist, and suggested underlying mechanisms include the associated reduction in oral medication and/or a psychotropic action of APO, possibly due to the piperidine moiety in its structure [64,65]. In addition, the potential beneficial role of APO on cerebral amyloid deposition is worth considering in relation to its positive modulatory effect on cognition [26,63,66,67].

4. Need for Personalised Treatment in Advanced Parkinson's: Clinical Cases

Taking into account the distinct NMS effects of these three DAT, it can be postulated that the specific non-motor profile of patients with advanced PD may serve as an additional anchor to motor symptoms to deliver personalised medicine. Two illustrative clinical cases are presented in Figure 1 showing the different non-motor profile of two patients with advanced PD evaluated for DAT initiation.

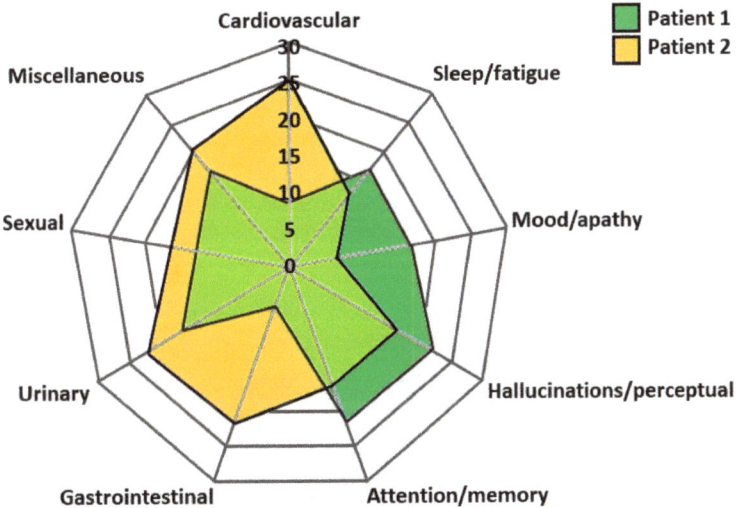

Figure 1. Radar chart of non-motor profile of two patients with advanced Parkinson's disease assessed for initiation of device-aided treatments. The radar chart is based on the Non-Motor Symptoms Scale (NMSS) domains scores obtained as part of routine clinical assessment. While patient 1's non-motor profile is dominated by mild attention/memory issues as well as mild perceptual problems, patient 2's main complaint is dysautonomia, including cardiovascular, urinary and gastrointestinal dysfunction. Numbers represent the NMSS domains scores. The light green area represents the overlap in symptoms between the two patients.

The clinical assessment revealed that both patients suffered from motor complications including troublesome dyskinesia and motor fluctuations refractory to conventional therapies; in addition, the non-motor profile of patient 1 was dominated by mild cognitive decline and non-intrusive perceptual issues, whereas for patient 2, cardiovascular, urinary, and gastrointestinal dysfunction were particularly pronounced. On the basis of these two different non-motor profiles and according to the EuroInf 2 data, it can be argued that APO may represent the best therapeutic option for patient 1, while, for patient 2, APO may not be suitable as it may exacerbate pre-existing cardiovascular problems, including orthostatic hypotension. On the other hand, while LCIG may be useful to improve gastrointestinal symptoms, STN-DBS may be the best option to improve urinary dysfunction for patient 2. As such, it would be important to inquire which one of the two is the most troublesome/severe NMS to better tailor the decision-making process.

Other factors are also implicated in the delivery of personalised DAT in PD [2]. Evaluation of patient age, for instance, represents a key aspect in the assessment for DBS suitability; indeed, age >70 or 75 years is an exclusion criterion for DBS in some centres given the associated higher risk of complications [68]; nevertheless, biological age is more often taken into consideration than chronological age in addition to the fact that the impact of "healthy ageing" is growing [69]. Another relevant aspect of this decision-making process is the evaluation of comorbidities. For instance, poorly controlled diabetic patients with PD have a higher risk of developing skin infections and this should be considered in the evaluation for any DAT [70]. Other comorbidities, such as pre-existing significant and symptomatic peripheral neuropathy needs consideration for LCIG, impulse control disorder and intrusive psychosis (as opposed to mild non-intrusive psychosis) for APO, and severe depression or suicidal trends for DBS [7]. Last but not least, patient personality and preferences need to be taken into account: some active young patients may prefer a more invasive brain surgery than a percutaneous endoscopic gastrostomy in order to avoid carrying a visible infusion pump every day, and for a "quick fix" of dyskinesias and tremor [71]. Body weight has also emerged as an important aspect of the decision-making process [72]. Low body weight patients with advanced PD may develop pain, discomfort and worsening of postural problems with subsequent risk of falls when carrying a heavy infusion pump [73]. The advent of a smaller infusion pump with the new levodopa-carbidopa-entacapone intestinal gel product now licensed for use in Sweden and Germany may represent a significant advance in this respect [74,75]. Whether this new product will have an impact on NMS similar to LCIG remains unexplored. Evaluating the ability of the patient and/or caregiver to handle the medication and the device, as well as daily skin hygiene, is also critical [73].

5. Conclusions

Device-aided therapies are now established worldwide for the management of advanced Parkinson's disease. While the emphasis of device-aided therapies selection remains based on the motor profile of patients with PD, non-motor symptoms have also been shown to play a part in the prognostic aspects of the successful delivery of these therapeutic options and are now included in the diagnostic algorithm of advanced PD. Considering the differential effect on non-motor symptoms of the currently available device-aided therapies, non-motor symptoms are relevant to delivering personalised medicine in Parkinson's disease. We envisage that the identification of different motor and non-motor phenotypes of Parkinson's may guide the delivery of personalised medicine in the advanced stage of the condition, perhaps guided by technology able to predict motor and non-motor responses to device-aided therapies on the basis of the patient-specific pre-intervention symptom's profile. We suggest that non-motor symptoms are an important enabler of the constituents of the "circle of personalised medicine" and offers a chance to deliver bespoke personalised therapy for advanced PD (Figure 2).

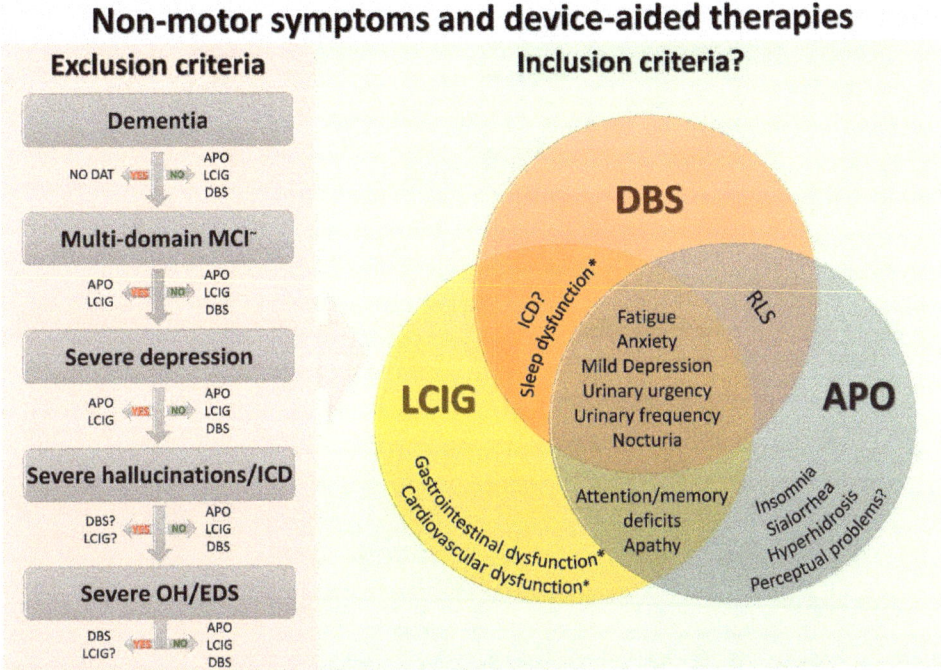

Figure 2. Non-motor enablers for a successful selection of device-aided therapy for patients with advanced Parkinson's disease. The figure shows non-motor exclusion and possible inclusion criteria for a successful patient initiation on device-aided therapies. We emphasise that these conditions should not be considered an absolute contraindication or indication for the device-aided therapies and expert opinion based on multi-disciplinary assessments should have the final say. ~ Multi-domain MCI with a predominant cortical pattern (e.g., memory, language, visuospatial); * Further studies are needed to better clarify which aspect of sleep, gastrointestinal and cardiovascular dysfunction can improve after device-aided therapy initiation. Abbreviations: APO, apomorphine subcutaneous infusion; DAT, device-aided therapies; DBS, Deep brain stimulation; EDS, excessive daytime sleepiness; ICD, Impulse control disorder; LCIG, levodopa-carbidopa intestinal gel infusion; MCI; mild cognitive impairment; NMS, non-motors symptoms; OH, orthostatic hypotension; RLS, Restless legs syndrome.

Author Contributions: Conceptualization, V.L., H.S.D., K.R.C.; writing—original draft preparation, V.L.; writing—review and editing, H.S.D., K.R.C., D.J.v.W., A.S., V.M., N.T., L.T., K.A., M.S., E.P., P.O., A.A., P.M.-M., M.P.; supervision, H.S.D., K.R.C. All authors have read and agreed to the published version of the manuscript.

Funding: The authors did not receive support from any organization for the submitted work.

Institutional Review Board Statement: Not applicable.

Informed Consent Statement: Not applicable.

Data Availability Statement: Not applicable.

Acknowledgments: The views expressed are those of the authors and not necessarily those of the NHS, NIHR or Department of Health. The authors acknowledge the support of the International Parkinson and Movement Disorder Society Non-Motor Parkinson's disease Study Group, the NIHR London South Clinical Research Network and the NIHR Biomedical Research Centre. The authors acknowledge Juliet Staunton for the proofreading of the manuscript. This article represents independent collaborative research performed by staff who are part funded by the NIHR Biomedical Research Centre at South London and Maudsley NHS Foundation Trust and King's College London.

Conflicts of Interest: V.L. reports grants from Parkinson's UK and honoraria for sponsored symposia from UCB, Bial, Invisio, Profile and Britannia Pharmaceuticals, outside the submitted work. H.S.D. was funded by the EU Joint Programme—Neurodegenerative Disease Research (JPND), the Prof. Klaus Thiemann Foundation in the German Society of Neurology, the Felgenhauer Foundation, the KoelnFortune program of the Medical Faculty of the University of Cologne, and has received honoraria by Boston Scientific, Medtronic and Stadapharm, outside the submitted work. A.S. is funded by the Gusyk program and the Advanced Cologne Clinician Scientist program of the Medical Faculty of the University of Cologne and has received funding from the Prof. Klaus Thiemann Foundation, outside the submitted work. L.T. received payments as a consultant for Boston Scientific, honoraria as a speaker on symposia sponsored by UCB, Desitin, Boston Scientific, AbbVIE, Novartis, GlaxoSmithKline und DIAPLAN; the institution of L.T., not L.T. personally received funding by Boston Scientific, the German Research Foundation, the German Ministry of Education and Research and the Deutsche Parkinson Vereinigung, outside the submitted work. K.A. reports educational grant and honoraria from Medtronic and Abbott, outside the submitted work. M.S. has received educational support from Medtronic (paid to the institution), Parkinson's UK (via the UK DBS network), acts as a consultant for Abbott, and received honoraria from The Movement Disorders Society, outside the submitted work. E.P. reports the following disclosures outside the submitted work: consulting neurologist for Finnish Patient Insurance Centre; Standing Member of the MDS Non-Motor Parkinson's Disease, Study Group; Consulting fees: NordicInfu Care AB, Abbvie, Zambon; Member of Advisory board: Abbvie; Lecture fees: Abbott, Abbvie, Nordic Infucare. P.O. has received honoraria for lectures and advice from AbbVie, Bial, Britannia, Kyowa, Nordic Infucare and Zambon, outside the submitted work. P.M.M. has received honoraria from National School of Public Health (ISCIII), Editorial Viguera and Takeda Pharmaceuticals for lecturing in courses; and from the International Parkinson and Movement Disorder Society (IPMDS) for management of the Program on Rating Scales, outside the submitted work. M.P. has received honoraria form AbbVie and Britannia Pharmaceuticals, outside the submitted work. D.J.v.W. received a grant, and consultancy, and speaker fees from Britannia Pharmaceuticals, speaker fees from Bial Pharmaceuticals, and consultancy fees from Invisio Pharma, outside the submitted work. K.R.C. reports advisory board for AbbVie, UCB, GKC, Bial, Cynapsus, Novartis, Lobsor, Stada, Medtronic, Zambon, Profile, Sunovion, Roche, Theravance, Scion, Britannia; honoraria for lectures from AbbVie, Britannia, UCB, Mundipharma, Zambon, Novartis, Boeringer Ingelheim; grants (Investigator Initiated) from Britania Pharmaceuticals, AbbVie, UCB, GKC, Bial; academic grants from EU, IMI EU, Horizon 2020, Parkinson's UK, NIHR, PDNMG, EU (Horizon 2020), Kirby Laing Foundation, NPF, MRC, Wellcome Trust, outside the submitted work.

References

1. Titova, N.; Chaudhuri, K.R. Non-motor Parkinson disease: New concepts and personalised management. *Med. J. Aust.* **2018**, *208*, 404–409. [CrossRef]
2. Titova, N.; Chaudhuri, K.R. Personalized medicine in Parkinson's disease: Time to be precise. *Mov. Disord.* **2017**, *32*, 1147–1154. [CrossRef]
3. Ray Chaudhuri, K.; Poewe, W.; Brooks, D. Motor and Nonmotor Complications of Levodopa: Phenomenology, Risk Factors, and Imaging Features. *Mov. Disord. Off. J. Mov. Disord. Soc.* **2018**, *33*, 909–919. [CrossRef] [PubMed]
4. Leta, V.; Jenner, P.; Chaudhuri, K.R.; Antonini, A. Can therapeutic strategies prevent and manage dyskinesia in Parkinson's disease? An update. *Expert Opin. Drug Saf.* **2019**, *18*, 1203–1218. [CrossRef] [PubMed]
5. Chapuis, S.; Ouchchane, L.; Metz, O.; Gerbaud, L.; Durif, F. Impact of the motor complications of Parkinson's disease on the quality of life. *Mov. Disord. Off. J. Mov. Disord. Soc.* **2005**, *20*, 224–230. [CrossRef] [PubMed]
6. Politis, M.; Wu, K.; Molloy, S.; Bain, P.G.; Chaudhuri, K.R.; Piccini, P. Parkinson's disease symptoms: The patient's perspective. *Mov. Disord. Off. J. Mov. Disord. Soc.* **2010**, *25*, 1646–1651. [CrossRef] [PubMed]
7. Odin, P.; Ray Chaudhuri, K.; Slevin, J.T.; Volkmann, J.; Dietrichs, E.; Martinez-Martin, P.; Krauss, J.K.; Henriksen, T.; Katzenschlager, R.; Antonini, A.; et al. Collective physician perspectives on non-oral medication approaches for the management of clinically relevant unresolved issues in Parkinson's disease: Consensus from an international survey and discussion program. *Parkinsonism Relat. Disord.* **2015**, *21*, 1133–1144. [CrossRef]
8. Lang, A.E.; Houeto, J.L.; Krack, P.; Kubu, C.; Lyons, K.E.; Moro, E.; Ondo, W.; Pahwa, R.; Poewe, W.; Troster, A.I.; et al. Deep brain stimulation: Preoperative issues. *Mov. Disord.* **2006**, *21* (Suppl. S14), S171–S196. [CrossRef]
9. National Instiute for Health and Care Excellence. Parkinson's Disease in Adults [NICE Guideline No. 71]. 2017. Available online: https://www.nice.org.uk/guidance/ng71 (accessed on 6 August 2021).
10. Antonini, A.; Stoessl, A.J.; Kleinman, L.S.; Skalicky, A.M.; Marshall, T.S.; Sail, K.R.; Onuk, K.; Odin, P.L.A. Developing consensus among movement disorder specialists on clinical indicators for identification and management of advanced Parkinson's disease: A multi-country Delphi-panel approach. *Curr. Med. Res. Opin.* **2018**, *34*, 2063–2073. [CrossRef]

11. Fasano, A.; Fung, V.S.C.; Lopiano, L.; Elibol, B.; Smolentseva, I.G.; Seppi, K.; Takáts, A.; Onuk, K.; Parra, J.C.; Bergmann, L.; et al. Characterizing advanced Parkinson's disease: OBSERVE-PD observational study results of 2615 patients. *BMC Neurol.* **2019**, *19*, 50. [CrossRef]
12. Aldred, J.; Anca-Herschkovitsch, M.; Antonini, A.; Bajenaru, O.; Bergmann, L.; Bourgeois, P.; Cubo, E.; Davis, T.L.; Iansek, R.; Kovács, N.; et al. Application of the '5-2-1' screening criteria in advanced Parkinson's disease: Interim analysis of Duoglobe. *Neurodegener. Dis. Manag.* **2020**, *10*, 309–323. [CrossRef]
13. Schuepbach, W.M.; Rau, J.; Knudsen, K.; Volkmann, J.; Krack, P.; Timmermann, L.; Halbig, T.D.; Hesekamp, H.; Navarro, S.M.; Meier, N.; et al. Neurostimulation for Parkinson's disease with early motor complications. *N. Engl. J. Med.* **2013**, *368*, 610–622. [CrossRef] [PubMed]
14. Schuepbach, W.M.M.; Tonder, L.; Schnitzler, A.; Krack, P.; Rau, J.; Hartmann, A.; Halbig, T.D.; Pineau, F.; Falk, A.; Paschen, L.; et al. Quality of life predicts outcome of deep brain stimulation in early Parkinson disease. *Neurology* **2019**, *92*, e1109–e1120. [CrossRef]
15. Antonini, A.; Robieson, W.Z.; Bergmann, L.; Yegin, A.; Poewe, W. Age/disease duration influence on activities of daily living and quality of life after levodopa-carbidopa intestinal gel in Parkinson's disease. *Neurodegener. Dis. Manag.* **2018**, *8*, 161–170. [CrossRef]
16. Dafsari, H.S.; Reker, P.; Silverdale, M.; Reddy, P.; Pilleri, M.; Martinez-Martin, P.; Rizos, A.; Perrier, E.; Weiß, L.; Ashkan, K.; et al. Subthalamic Stimulation Improves Quality of Life of Patients Aged 61 Years or Older with Short Duration of Parkinson's Disease. *Neuromodulation J. Int. Neuromodulation Soc.* **2018**, *21*, 532–540. [CrossRef]
17. Heald, A.H.; Livingston, M.; Stedman, M.; Wyrko, Z. Higher levels of apomorphine and rotigotine prescribing reduce overall secondary healthcare costs in Parkinson's disease. *Int. J. Clin. Pract.* **2016**, *70*, 907–915. [CrossRef]
18. Smilowska, K.; van Wamelen, D.J.; Pietrzykowski, T.; Calvano, A.; Rodriguez-Blazquez, C.; Martinez-Martin, P.; Odin, P.; Chaudhuri, K.R. Cost-Effectiveness of Device-Aided Therapies in Parkinson's Disease: A Structured Review. *J. Parkinson's Dis.* **2021**, *11*, 475–489. [CrossRef] [PubMed]
19. Schapira, A.H.V.; Chaudhuri, K.R.; Jenner, P. Non-motor features of Parkinson disease. *Nat. Rev. Neurosci.* **2017**, *18*, 435–450. [CrossRef]
20. van Wamelen, D.J.; Sauerbier, A.; Leta, V.; Rodriguez-Blazquez, C.; Falup-Pecurariu, C.; Rodriguez-Violante, M.; Rizos, A.; Tsuboi, Y.; Metta, V.; Bhidayasiri, R.; et al. Cross-sectional analysis of the Parkinson's disease Non-motor International Longitudinal Study baseline non-motor characteristics, geographical distribution and impact on quality of life. *Sci. Rep.* **2021**, *11*, 9611. [CrossRef]
21. Storch, A.; Schneider, C.B.; Wolz, M.; Sturwald, Y.; Nebe, A.; Odin, P.; Mahler, A.; Fuchs, G.; Jost, W.H.; Chaudhuri, K.R.; et al. Nonmotor fluctuations in Parkinson disease: Severity and correlation with motor complications. *Neurology* **2013**, *80*, 800–809. [CrossRef] [PubMed]
22. van Wamelen, D.J.; Leta, V.; Ray Chaudhuri, K.; Storch, A. Non-motor Fluctuations in Parkinson's Disease. In *Parkinson's Disease and Movement Disorders*; The Parkinson's Disease and Movement Disorder Society; in press.
23. Ray Chaudhuri, K.; Rojo, J.M.; Schapira, A.H.; Brooks, D.J.; Stocchi, F.; Odin, P.; Antonini, A.; Brown, R.G.; Martinez-Martin, P. A proposal for a comprehensive grading of Parkinson's disease severity combining motor and non-motor assessments: Meeting an unmet need. *PLoS ONE* **2013**, *8*, e57221. [CrossRef]
24. Dafsari, H.S.; Ray-Chaudhuri, K.; Mahlstedt, P.; Sachse, L.; Steffen, J.K.; Petry-Schmelzer, J.N.; Dembek, T.A.; Reker, P.; Barbe, M.T.; Visser-Vandewalle, V.; et al. Beneficial effects of bilateral subthalamic stimulation on alexithymia in Parkinson's disease. *Eur. J. Neurol.* **2019**, *26*, 222-e17. [CrossRef] [PubMed]
25. Carbone, F.; Djamshidian, A.; Seppi, K.; Poewe, W. Apomorphine for Parkinson's Disease: Efficacy and Safety of Current and New Formulations. *CNS Drugs* **2019**, *33*, 905–918. [CrossRef]
26. Martinez-Martin, P.; Reddy, P.; Katzenschlager, R.; Antonini, A.; Todorova, A.; Odin, P.; Henriksen, T.; Martin, A.; Calandrella, D.; Rizos, A.; et al. EuroInf: A multicenter comparative observational study of apomorphine and levodopa infusion in Parkinson's disease. *Mov. Disord.* **2015**, *30*, 510–516. [CrossRef] [PubMed]
27. Dafsari, H.S.; Martinez-Martin, P.; Rizos, A.; Trost, M.; Dos Santos Ghilardi, M.G.; Reddy, P.; Sauerbier, A.; Petry-Schmelzer, J.N.; Kramberger, M.; Borgemeester, R.W.K.; et al. EuroInf 2: Subthalamic stimulation, apomorphine, and levodopa infusion in Parkinson's disease. *Mov. Disord.* **2019**, *34*, 353–365. [CrossRef]
28. Deuschl, G.; Schade-Brittinger, C.; Krack, P.; Volkmann, J.; Schafer, H.; Botzel, K.; Daniels, C.; Deutschlander, A.; Dillmann, U.; Eisner, W.; et al. A randomized trial of deep-brain stimulation for Parkinson's disease. *N. Engl. J. Med.* **2006**, *355*, 896–908. [CrossRef] [PubMed]
29. Antonini, A.; Poewe, W.; Chaudhuri, K.R.; Jech, R.; Pickut, B.; Pirtosek, Z.; Szasz, J.; Valldeoriola, F.; Winkler, C.; Bergmann, L.; et al. Levodopa-carbidopa intestinal gel in advanced Parkinson's: Final results of the GLORIA registry. *Parkinsonism Relat. Disord.* **2017**, *45*, 13–20. [CrossRef] [PubMed]
30. Shalash, A.; Alexoudi, A.; Knudsen, K.; Volkmann, J.; Mehdorn, M.; Deuschl, G. The impact of age and disease duration on the long term outcome of neurostimulation of the subthalamic nucleus. *Parkinsonism Relat. Disord.* **2014**, *20*, 47–52. [CrossRef]
31. De Fabregues, O.; Dot, J.; Abu-Suboh, M.; Hernández-Vara, J.; Ferré, A.; Romero, O.; Ibarria, M.; Seoane, J.L.; Raguer, N.; Puiggros, C.; et al. Long-term safety and effectiveness of levodopa-carbidopa intestinal gel infusion. *Brain Behav.* **2017**, *7*, e00758. [CrossRef]
32. Pietz, K.; Hagell, P.; Odin, P. Subcutaneous apomorphine in late stage Parkinson's disease: A long term follow up. *J. Neurol. Neurosurg. Psychiatry* **1998**, *65*, 709–716. [CrossRef]

33. Regidor, I.; Benita, V.; Del Álamo de Pedro, M.; Ley, L.; Martinez Castrillo, J.C. Duodenal Levodopa Infusion for Long-Term Deep Brain Stimulation-Refractory Symptoms in Advanced Parkinson Disease. *Clin. Neuropharmacol.* **2017**, *40*, 103–107. [CrossRef]
34. Kumar, N.; Murgai, A.; Naranian, T.; Jog, M.; Fasano, A. Levodopa-carbidopa intestinal gel therapy after deep brain stimulation. *Mov. Disord. Off. J. Mov. Disord. Soc.* **2018**, *33*, 334–335. [CrossRef]
35. Elkouzi, A.; Ramirez-Zamora, A.; Zeilman, P.; Barabas, M.; Eisinger, R.S.; Malaty, I.A.; Okun, M.S.; Almeida, L. Rescue levodopa-carbidopa intestinal gel (LCIG) therapy in Parkinson's disease patients with suboptimal response to deep brain stimulation. *Ann. Clin. Transl. Neurol.* **2019**, *6*, 1989–1995. [CrossRef] [PubMed]
36. Bautista, J.M.P.; Oyama, G.; Nuermaimaiti, M.; Sekimoto, S.; Sasaki, F.; Hatano, T.; Nishioka, K.; Ito, M.; Umemura, A.; Ishibashi, Y.; et al. Rescue Levodopa/Carbidopa Intestinal Gel for Secondary Deep Brain Stimulation Failure. *J. Mov. Disord.* **2020**, *13*, 57–61. [CrossRef]
37. Sesar, Á.; Fernández-Pajarín, G.; Ares, B.; Relova, J.L.; Arán, E.; Rivas, M.T.; Gelabert-González, M.; Castro, A. Continuous subcutaneous apomorphine in advanced Parkinson's disease patients treated with deep brain stimulation. *J. Neurol.* **2019**, *266*, 659–666. [CrossRef] [PubMed]
38. Mulroy, E.; Leta, V.; Zrinzo, L.; Foltynie, T.; Chaudhuri, K.R.; Limousin, P. Successful Treatment of Levodopa/Carbidopa Intestinal Gel Associated "Biphasic-like" Dyskinesia with Pallidal Deep Brain Stimulation. *Mov. Disord. Clin. Pract.* **2021**, *8*, 273–274. [CrossRef] [PubMed]
39. Zhang, X.; Xie, A. Improvement of Subthalamic Nucleus Deep Brain Stimulation in Sleeping Symptoms in Parkinson's Disease: A Meta-Analysis. *Parkinsons Dis.* **2019**, *2019*, 6280896. [CrossRef]
40. Bellini, G.; Best, L.A.; Brechany, U.; Mills, R.; Pavese, N. Clinical Impact of Deep Brain Stimulation on the Autonomic System in Patients with Parkinson's Disease. *Mov. Disord. Clin. Pract.* **2020**, *7*, 373–382. [CrossRef]
41. Cartmill, T.; Skvarc, D.; Bittar, R.; McGillivray, J.; Berk, M.; Byrne, L.K. Deep Brain Stimulation of the Subthalamic Nucleus in Parkinson's Disease: A Meta-Analysis of Mood Effects. *Neuropsychol. Rev.* **2021**. [CrossRef] [PubMed]
42. Cavalloni, F.; Debove, I.; Lachenmayer, M.L.; Krack, P.; Pollo, C.; Schuepbach, W.M.M.; Bassetti, C.L.A.; Bargiotas, P. A case series and systematic review of rapid eye movement sleep behavior disorder outcome after deep brain stimulation in Parkinson's disease. *Sleep Med.* **2021**, *77*, 170–176. [CrossRef]
43. Maheshwary, A.; Mohite, D.; Omole, J.A.; Bhatti, K.S.; Khan, S. Is Deep Brain Stimulation Associated With Detrimental Effects on Cognitive Functions in Patients of Parkinson's Disease? A Systematic Review. *Cureus* **2020**, *12*, e9688. [CrossRef] [PubMed]
44. Jost, S.T.; Ray Chaudhuri, K.; Ashkan, K.; Loehrer, P.A.; Silverdale, M.; Rizos, A.; Evans, J.; Petry-Schmelzer, J.N.; Barbe, M.T.; Sauerbier, A.; et al. Subthalamic Stimulation Improves Quality of Sleep in Parkinson Disease: A 36-Month Controlled Study. *J. Parkinson's Dis.* **2021**, *11*, 323–335. [CrossRef]
45. Dafsari, H.S.; Ray-Chaudhuri, K.; Ashkan, K.; Sachse, L.; Mahlstedt, P.; Silverdale, M.; Rizos, A.; Strack, M.; Jost, S.T.; Reker, P.; et al. Beneficial effect of 24-month bilateral subthalamic stimulation on quality of sleep in Parkinson's disease. *J. Neurol.* **2020**, *267*, 1830–1841. [CrossRef] [PubMed]
46. Baumann-Vogel, H.; Imbach, L.L.; Surucu, O.; Stieglitz, L.; Waldvogel, D.; Baumann, C.R.; Werth, E. The Impact of Subthalamic Deep Brain Stimulation on Sleep-Wake Behavior: A Prospective Electrophysiological Study in 50 Parkinson Patients. *Sleep* **2017**, *40*. [CrossRef]
47. Irmen, F.; Horn, A.; Mosley, P.; Perry, A.; Petry-Schmelzer, J.N.; Dafsari, H.S.; Barbe, M.; Visser-Vandewalle, V.; Schneider, G.H.; Li, N.; et al. Left Prefrontal Connectivity Links Subthalamic Stimulation with Depressive Symptoms. *Ann. Neurol.* **2020**, *87*, 962–975. [CrossRef]
48. Petry-Schmelzer, J.N.; Krause, M.; Dembek, T.A.; Horn, A.; Evans, J.; Ashkan, K.; Rizos, A.; Silverdale, M.; Schumacher, W.; Sack, C.; et al. Non-motor outcomes depend on location of neurostimulation in Parkinson's disease. *Brain* **2019**, *142*, 3592–3604. [CrossRef]
49. Dafsari, H.S.; Dos Santos Ghilardi, M.G.; Visser-Vandewalle, V.; Rizos, A.; Ashkan, K.; Silverdale, M.; Evans, J.; Martinez, R.C.R.; Cury, R.G.; Jost, S.T.; et al. Beneficial nonmotor effects of subthalamic and pallidal neurostimulation in Parkinson's disease. *Brain Stimul.* **2020**, *13*, 1697–1705. [CrossRef] [PubMed]
50. Little, S.; Brown, P. What brain signals are suitable for feedback control of deep brain stimulation in Parkinson's disease? *Ann. N. Y. Acad. Sci.* **2012**, *1265*, 9–24. [CrossRef] [PubMed]
51. Florin, E.; Dafsari, H.S.; Reck, C.; Barbe, M.T.; Pauls, K.A.; Maarouf, M.; Sturm, V.; Fink, G.R.; Timmermann, L. Modulation of local field potential power of the subthalamic nucleus during isometric force generation in patients with Parkinson's disease. *Neuroscience* **2013**, *240*, 106–116. [CrossRef]
52. Imbach, L.L.; Baumann-Vogel, H.; Baumann, C.R.; Surucu, O.; Hermsdorfer, J.; Sarnthein, J. Adaptive grip force is modulated by subthalamic beta activity in Parkinson's disease patients. *Neuroimage Clin.* **2015**, *9*, 450–457. [CrossRef]
53. Hoang, K.B.; Cassar, I.R.; Grill, W.M.; Turner, D.A. Biomarkers and Stimulation Algorithms for Adaptive Brain Stimulation. *Front. Neurosci.* **2017**, *11*, 564. [CrossRef]
54. Jost, S.T.; Visser-Vandewalle, V.; Rizos, A.; Loehrer, P.A.; Silverdale, M.; Evans, J.; Samuel, M.; Petry-Schmelzer, J.N.; Sauerbier, A.; Gronostay, A.; et al. Non-motor predictors of 36-month quality of life after subthalamic stimulation in Parkinson disease. *NPJ Parkinsons Dis.* **2021**, *7*, 48. [CrossRef]
55. Wirdefeldt, K.; Odin, P.; Nyholm, D. Levodopa-Carbidopa Intestinal Gel in Patients with Parkinson's Disease: A Systematic Review. *CNS Drugs* **2016**, *30*, 381–404. [CrossRef] [PubMed]

56. Prakash, N.; Simuni, T. Infusion Therapies for Parkinson's Disease. *Curr. Neurol. Neurosci. Rep.* **2020**, *20*, 44. [CrossRef] [PubMed]
57. Antonini, A.; Odin, P.; Pahwa, R.; Aldred, J.; Alobaidi, A.; Jalundhwala, Y.J.; Kukreja, P.; Bergmann, L.; Inguva, S.; Bao, Y.; et al. The Long-Term Impact of Levodopa/Carbidopa Intestinal Gel on 'Off'-time in Patients with Advanced Parkinson's Disease: A Systematic Review. *Adv. Ther.* **2021**. [CrossRef] [PubMed]
58. Honig, H.; Antonini, A.; Martinez-Martin, P.; Forgacs, I.; Faye, G.C.; Fox, T.; Fox, K.; Mancini, F.; Canesi, M.; Odin, P.; et al. Intrajejunal levodopa infusion in Parkinson's disease: A pilot multicenter study of effects on nonmotor symptoms and quality of life. *Mov. Disord.* **2009**, *24*, 1468–1474. [CrossRef] [PubMed]
59. Ray Chaudhuri, K.; Antonini, A.; Robieson, W.Z.; Sanchez-Soliño, O.; Bergmann, L.; Poewe, W. Burden of non-motor symptoms in Parkinson's disease patients predicts improvement in quality of life during treatment with levodopa-carbidopa intestinal gel. *Eur. J. Neurol.* **2019**, *26*, 581-e43. [CrossRef]
60. Katzenschlager, R.; Poewe, W.; Rascol, O.; Trenkwalder, C.; Deuschl, G.; Chaudhuri, K.R.; Henriksen, T.; van Laar, T.; Spivey, K.; Vel, S.; et al. Apomorphine subcutaneous infusion in patients with Parkinson's disease with persistent motor fluctuations (TOLEDO): A multicentre, double-blind, randomised, placebo-controlled trial. *Lancet Neurol.* **2018**, *17*, 749–759. [CrossRef]
61. Todorova, A.; Ray Chaudhuri, K. Subcutaneous apomorphine and non-motor symptoms in Parkinson's disease. *Parkinsonism Relat. Disord.* **2013**, *19*, 1073–1078. [CrossRef] [PubMed]
62. Rosa-Grilo, M.; Qamar, M.A.; Evans, A.; Chaudhuri, K.R. The efficacy of apomorphine—A non-motor perspective. *Parkinsonism Relat. Disord.* **2016**, *33* (Suppl. S1), S28–S35. [CrossRef] [PubMed]
63. Martinez-Martin, P.; Reddy, P.; Antonini, A.; Henriksen, T.; Katzenschlager, R.; Odin, P.; Todorova, A.; Naidu, Y.; Tluk, S.; Chandiramani, C.; et al. Chronic subcutaneous infusion therapy with apomorphine in advanced Parkinson's disease compared to conventional therapy: A real life study of non motor effect. *J. Parkinson's Dis.* **2011**, *1*, 197–203. [CrossRef]
64. Ellis, C.; Lemmens, G.; Parkes, J.D.; Abbott, R.J.; Pye, I.F.; Leigh, P.N.; Chaudhuri, K.R. Use of apomorphine in parkinsonian patients with neuropsychiatric complications to oral treatment. *Parkinsonism Relat. Disord.* **1997**, *3*, 103–107. [CrossRef]
65. Drapier, S.; Gillioz, A.S.; Leray, E.; Péron, J.; Rouaud, T.; Marchand, A.; Vérin, M. Apomorphine infusion in advanced Parkinson's patients with subthalamic stimulation contraindications. *Parkinsonism Relat. Disord.* **2012**, *18*, 40–44. [CrossRef] [PubMed]
66. Himeno, E.; Ohyagi, Y.; Ma, L.; Nakamura, N.; Miyoshi, K.; Sakae, N.; Motomura, K.; Soejima, N.; Yamasaki, R.; Hashimoto, T.; et al. Apomorphine treatment in Alzheimer mice promoting amyloid-β degradation. *Ann. Neurol.* **2011**, *69*, 248–256. [CrossRef] [PubMed]
67. Antonini, A.; Isaias, I.U.; Rodolfi, G.; Landi, A.; Natuzzi, F.; Siri, C.; Pezzoli, G. A 5-year prospective assessment of advanced Parkinson disease patients treated with subcutaneous apomorphine infusion or deep brain stimulation. *J. Neurol.* **2011**, *258*, 579–585. [CrossRef] [PubMed]
68. Bouwyn, J.P.; Derrey, S.; Lefaucheur, R.; Fetter, D.; Rouille, A.; Le Goff, F.; Maltête, D. Age Limits for Deep Brain Stimulation of Subthalamic Nuclei in Parkinson's Disease. *J. Parkinson's Dis.* **2016**, *6*, 393–400. [CrossRef]
69. Levi, V.; Carrabba, G.; Rampini, P.; Locatelli, M. Short term surgical complications after subthalamic deep brain stimulation for Parkinson's disease: Does old age matter? *BMC Geriatr.* **2015**, *15*, 116. [CrossRef]
70. Dryden, M.; Baguneid, M.; Eckmann, C.; Corman, S.; Stephens, J.; Solem, C.; Li, J.; Charbonneau, C.; Baillon-Plot, N.; Haider, S. Pathophysiology and burden of infection in patients with diabetes mellitus and peripheral vascular disease: Focus on skin and soft-tissue infections. *Clin. Microbiol. Infect. Off. Publ. Eur. Soc. Clin. Microbiol. Infect. Dis.* **2015**, *21* (Suppl. S2), S27–S32. [CrossRef]
71. Marshall, T.; Pugh, A.; Fairchild, A.; Hass, S. Patient Preferences for Device-Aided Treatments Indicated for Advanced Parkinson Disease. *Value Health J. Int. Soc. Pharm. Outcomes Res.* **2017**, *20*, 1383–1393. [CrossRef]
72. Sharma, J.C.; Lewis, A. Weight in Parkinson's Disease: Phenotypical Significance. *Int. Rev. Neurobiol.* **2017**, *134*, 891–919. [CrossRef] [PubMed]
73. Titova, N.; Ray Chaudhuri, K. Intrajejunal levodopa infusion therapy for Parkinson's disease: Practical and pragmatic tips for successful maintenance of therapy. *Expert Rev. Neurother.* **2017**, *17*, 529–537. [CrossRef] [PubMed]
74. Senek, M.; Nielsen, E.I.; Nyholm, D. Levodopa-entacapone-carbidopa intestinal gel in Parkinson's disease: A randomized crossover study. *Mov. Disord. Off. J. Mov. Disord. Soc.* **2017**, *32*, 283–286. [CrossRef] [PubMed]
75. Leta, V.; van Wamelen, D.J.; Sauerbier, A.; Jones, S.; Parry, M.; Rizos, A.; Chaudhuri, K.R. Opicapone and Levodopa-Carbidopa Intestinal Gel Infusion: The Way Forward Towards Cost Savings for Healthcare Systems? *J. Parkinson's Dis.* **2020**, *10*, 1535–1539. [CrossRef] [PubMed]

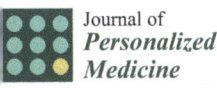

Article

Physiotherapy versus Consecutive Physiotherapy and Cognitive Treatment in People with Parkinson's Disease: A Pilot Randomized Cross-Over Study

Valentina Varalta [1,2], Paola Poiese [3], Serena Recchia [3], Barbara Montagnana [3], Cristina Fonte [1], Mirko Filippetti [1], Michele Tinazzi [4], Nicola Smania [1,2,*] and Alessandro Picelli [1,2]

[1] Neuromotor and Cognitive Rehabilitation Research Center, Section of Physical and Rehabilitation Medicine, Department of Neurosciences, Biomedicine and Movement Sciences, University of Verona, 37134 Verona, Italy; valentina.varalta@univr.it (V.V.); cristina.fonte@univr.it (C.F.); mirko.filippetti@univr.it (M.F.); alessandro.picelli@univr.it (A.P.)

[2] Neurorehabilitation Unit, University Hospital of Verona, 37126 Verona, Italy

[3] Centro Polifunzionale Don Calabria, 37138 Verona, Italy; paola.poiese@centrodoncalabria.it (P.P.); serena.recchia@centrodoncalabria.it (S.R.); barbara.montagnana@centrodoncalabria.it (B.M.)

[4] Neurology Unit, Movement Disorders Division, Department of Neurosciences, Biomedicine and Movement Sciences, University of Verona, 37134 Verona, Italy; michele.tinazzi@univr.it

* Correspondence: nicola.smania@univr.it; Tel.: +39-045-812-4573

Abstract: Background: Parkinson's disease (PD) is characterized by motor and cognitive dysfunctions that can usually be treated by physiotherapy or cognitive training, respectively. The effects of consecutive physiotherapy and cognitive rehabilitation programs on PD deficits are less investigated. Objective: We investigated the effects of 3 months of physiotherapy (physiotherapy treatment group) or consecutive physiotherapy and cognitive (physiotherapy and cognitive treatment group) rehabilitation programs on cognitive, motor, and psychological aspects in 20 PD patients. Methods: The two groups switched programs and continued rehabilitation for another 3 months. The outcomes were score improvement on cognitive (Montreal Cognitive Assessment, Frontal Assessment Battery, Trail Making Test, Verbal Phonemic Fluency, Digit Span, and Rey Auditory Verbal Learning), motor (Unified Parkinson's Disease Rating Scale-III, Berg Balance Scale, Two-Minute Walking Test, and Time Up and Go), and psychological (Beck Depression Inventory and State-Trait Anxiety Inventory) scales. Results: Between-group comparison revealed a significant difference in functional mobility between the two rehabilitation programs. Improvements in walking abilities were noted after both interventions, but only the patients treated with consecutive training showed better performance on functional mobility and memory tasks. Conclusion: Our findings support the hypothesis that consecutive physiotherapy plus cognitive rehabilitation may have a greater benefit than physiotherapy alone in patients with PD.

Keywords: rehabilitation; cognition; movement disorders

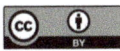

1. Introduction

Parkinson's disease (PD) is a neurodegenerative disorder characterized by motor and nonmotor symptoms [1]. Motor symptoms include bradykinesia, resting tremor, and postural instability [2], resulting in impaired gait and balance [3]. Common nonmotor manifestations are cognitive deficits in attention, memory, visuospatial, and executive functions [4], and mood disorders, particularly depression and anxiety [5].

While motor manifestations have long been investigated, nonmotor symptoms are now recognized as the main components that interfere with functionality in PD [6]. Cognitive deficits seem to be related to motor abilities [7,8]. Basal ganglia functional connectivity, which is compromised in PD by dopaminergic reduction, may have an important role in modulating both cognitive and motor functions [9].

These findings suggest the importance of evaluating and treating both motor and cognitive dysfunctions. Nonetheless, rehabilitation programs are often limited to physical training. While the effectiveness of physiotherapy in improving motor abilities is well documented [10–13], it is only in recent years that its effects on cognition have been better investigated [12,13]. Few studies to date have investigated cognitive outcomes before and after motor treatment [12,13]. The improvement in attention and executive functions after physical activity [12,13] suggested a relationship between cognitive and motor improvement in PD in which a common mechanism may underlie cognition and movement [13].

The effects of other rehabilitation interventions besides physiotherapy on motor and cognitive dysfunctions have been investigated in PD patients. An increase in motor and cognitive performance was found after combined (dual-tasking) [14] and consecutive training physiotherapy and cognitive treatment [14,15]. The studies concluded that the effectiveness of combined or consecutive treatment was comparable to motor treatment alone [14,15]. One study suggested that isolated cognitive training may reduce the severity of freezing of gait in PD patients [16].

Study findings suggest that physiotherapy [12,13], cognitive [17] combined [14] or consecutive physiotherapy, and cognitive training [14,15] can improve dysfunctions in PD patients. However, usually the studies measured changes in some functional features (motor, cognitive, psychological) but did not deeply assess cognitive or motor abilities.

The aim of the present study was to investigate the effects of physiotherapy alone versus consecutive physiotherapy and cognitive treatment on cognitive, motor, and psychological aspects in patients with mild to moderate PD.

2. Materials and Methods

2.1. Study Design

Block randomization for this pilot randomized cross-over trial was generated by a computer with a web tool (randomization.com; accessed on: 25 august 2016). The patients took part in two rehabilitation programs (PT or PCT); each program consisted of 3 months of treatment, and 8 sessions/month. The two groups switched to the PT and the PCT arm, respectively, after a 1-month wash out period (Figure 1).

2.2. Ethical Aspects

All participants were outpatients and gave their informed, written consent to participate. The study was carried out according to the Declaration of Helsinki and approved by the Centro Polifunzionale Don Calabria Review Board (no. 05/2016). The patients enrolled in this study are a subgroup involved in a clinical trial registered at http://clinicaltrials.gov (NCT03741959).

2.3. Subjects

The study population was composed of 20 patients with confirmed diagnosis of idiopathic PD, according to the Movement Disorder Society (MDS) PD diagnostic criteria [18], and with Hoehn and Yahr stage 3, determined in the "on" phase [19]. Hoehn and Yahr stage 3 was chosen in line with the physiotherapy program, which focused primarily on walking and balance (see Intervention and Procedures subsection for details) and with outcome measures that require sufficient walking ability (2-Minute Walking Test and Time Up and Go).

Exclusion criteria were severe unpredictable "on-off" fluctuations that could have compromised participation in the rehabilitation program, history of alcohol or drug abuse, psychotic disorders, vestibular disorders or paroxysmal vertigo, and other neurological or orthopedic conditions involving the lower limbs (e.g., musculoskeletal diseases, severe osteoarthritis, and peripheral neuropathy).

All patients received physiotherapy training (PT) or consecutive physiotherapy and cognitive training (PCT). Ten were allocated to the same training in reverse order (Figure 1).

Patients were monitored between September 2016 and May 2017. At the end of the study, PT and PCT included 20 patients in each group.

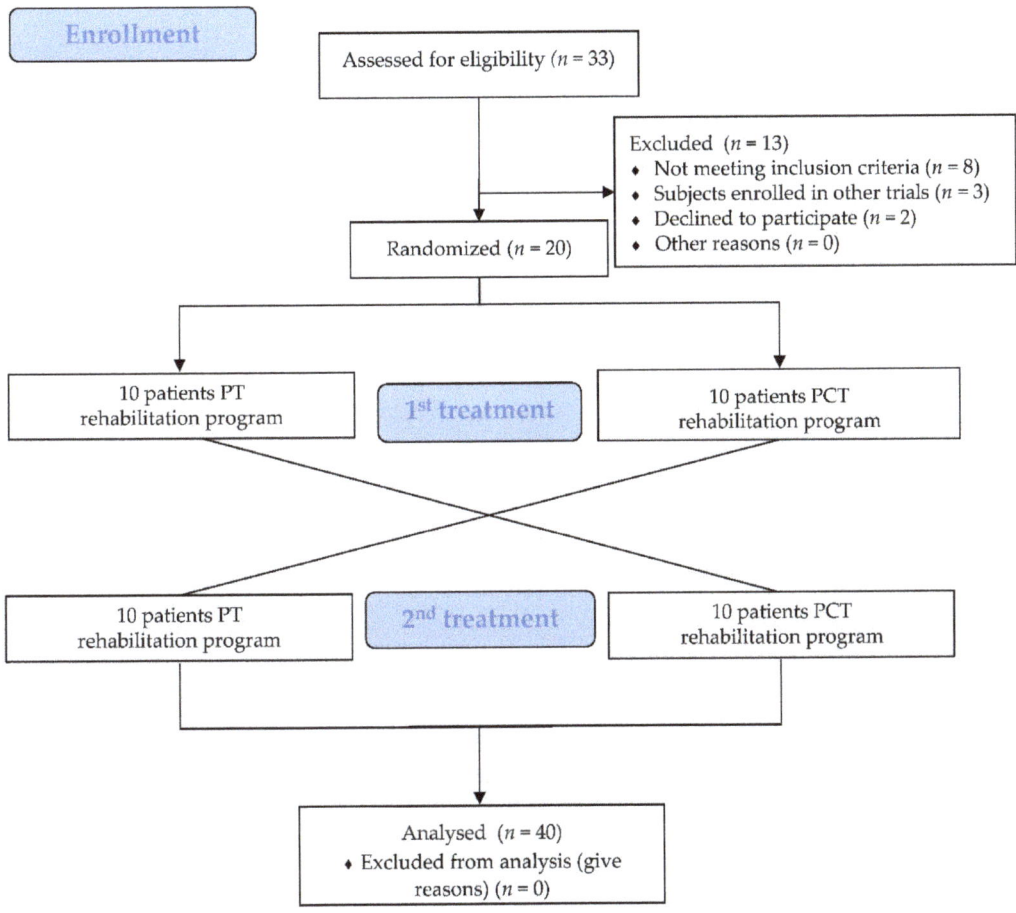

Figure 1. Study flow.

2.4. Intervention and Procedures

Patients received group treatment for 50 min/day, 2 days/week, for a total of 24 treatment sessions. Each group was composed of 10 patients with comparable motor and cognitive abilities. The PT program consisted of 24 physiotherapy sessions: one 50 min session/day, 2 days a week, for 12 consecutive weeks. The PCT program consisted of 12 physiotherapy sessions plus 12 cognitive sessions: a 50 min physiotherapy session one day/week and a 50 min cognitive session on another day during the same week for 12 consecutive weeks. Participation in other types of rehabilitation was not permitted during the study period.

The motor interventions were conducted in a well-lit and wide gym by two trained physiotherapists with experience in neuromotor rehabilitation. Each session consisted of three parts with a 5 min rest in between. In adherence to clinical practice guidelines for physical therapy in PD [20], the motor intervention focused on balance, gait, transfers, posture, and upper limb ability. Motor interventions primarily train gait and balance functions because these are usually impaired in PD and have an important impact on daily life activities.

First, patients performed active joint mobilization of the lower limbs (hip, knee, ankle) for 10 min. Lower limb mobilization was carried out with the patient supine (internal/external hip mobilization, active straight leg raise, knee flexion/extension, ankle mobilization) and prone (active hip extension) positions. During each training session, a total of five exercises were performed (four in supine and one in prone position).

Second, patients performed conventional gait and balance therapy for 20 min based on the proprioceptive neuromuscular facilitation concept and aimed at improving both feedforward and feedback postural reactions [21]. Two types of exercises were carried out. In the first of the exercises, patients performed voluntary motor actions in static or dynamic conditions (transferring body weight onto the tips of the toes and onto the heels; bouncing a ball during gait with the two hands alternating to the right and the left side). The second type of exercises trained coordination between leg and arm movement during walking and locomotor dexterity over an obstacle course. During each treatment session, a total of four exercises were performed (two from the first group and two from the second). Each single exercise was repeated three times in 5 min.

Finally, upper limb, lower limb, and trunk motor coordination exercises were executed for 10 min. Specifically a sequence of two exercises using single-leg stance and a sequence of two exercises associated with upper limb movement were conducted. Each single exercise was repeated two times in 2–3 min.

The physiotherapists assisted patients by demonstrating the exercises and providing verbal instructions.

The cognitive interventions were conducted in a well-lit room by a psychologist with experience in neuropsychological field and cognitive rehabilitation. The objective was to improve cognitive skills by acquiring restorative and compensatory techniques (e.g., memory strategies). Each session consisted of four parts with a 5 min rest in between. To start, the psychologist introduced the aim of the session, then oral and paper-pencil exercises of three cognitive functions were performed in each session. Each function was trained for 10 min followed by a 5 min rest. Memory, concentration, orientation, calculation, dual tasking, and cognitive flexibility were practiced. During the session, the patient stayed seated near a table.

The psychologist supported patients by providing verbal instructions and suggesting useful cognitive strategies.

The TIDieR (Template for Intervention Description and Replication) Checklist are present in the Supplementary File S1.

2.5. Data Collection and Assessment Procedures

During the study, patients took their regular PD medications. All underwent cognitive, motor, and psychological assessment during the "on" phase (1 to 2.5 h after having taken their morning dose). The same raters, blinded to the rehabilitation program, evaluated all patients (P.P. performed cognitive and psychological assessment; S.R. performed motor assessment) in an outpatient clinical setting. Motor, cognitive, and psychological assessments were conducted before and after the completion of each rehabilitation program.

2.6. Outcome Measures

2.6.1. Primary Outcome Measures

The primary outcome measures were the Montreal Cognitive Assessment (MoCA) [22] and Unified Parkinson's Disease Rating Scale Part III (UPDRS III) [23].

The MoCA was used to investigate a patient's global cognitive level. The total score is the sum of all trials, with a maximum score of 30 (best performance) [22]. To decrease possible learning effects between consecutive assessment timing, we used different versions of the MoCA (7.1, 7.2, 7.3) [24].

The UPDRS III was used to assess movement capacity. It consists of 14 items (each rated on a scale from 0 to 4 points) about tremor, slowness (bradykinesia), stiffness (rigidity), and balance. The total score is the sum of all items; the range is from 0 (best performance) to 56 (worst performance) [23].

2.6.2. Secondary Outcome Measures

The secondary outcome measures were other cognitive (Frontal Assessment Battery—FAB-it, Trail Making Test—TMT, F-A-S Verbal Phonemic Fluency Test—FAS, Digit Span Forward—DSF and Backward—DSB, and Rey Auditory Verbal Learning Test—RAVL), psychological (Beck Depression Inventory—BDI and State-Trait Anxiety Inventory—STAI), and motor (Berg Balance Scale—BBS, 2-Minute Walking Test—2MWT, and Time Up and Go—TUG) tests.

The FAB-it assesses executive functions (conceptualization, mental flexibility, programming, sensitivity interference, inhibitory control, and environmental autonomy). It consists of six tests, each of which is rated on a scale from 0 to 3 points. The total score is the sum of all items; the range is from 0 (worst performance) to 18 (best performance) [25].

Selective attention, psychomotor speed, and sequencing skills were evaluated with the TMT part A. The ability to switch attention between two rules and cognitive flexibility were assessed with the TMT part B. The time taken to complete the trials was recorded (longer = worse performance) [26].

The FAS assesses verbal fluency by determining the number of words beginning with a letter (F, A, or S) generated in 60 s. The total score is the average number of words produced (greater = better performance) [27].

Short-term memory was assessed with the DSF. Subjects are asked to repeat forward a list of single digit numbers in the correct order immediately after presentation. The maximum score is 9 (best performance) [28].

Working memory was assessed with the DSB. Subjects are asked to repeat backward a list of single-digit numbers in the correct order immediately after presentation. The maximum score is 8 (best performance) [28].

In order to assess learning and long-term verbal memory abilities, we used the RAVL. The test consists of two parts: immediate recall (RAVL-I) for learning and delayed recall (RAVL-D) for long-term memory. The maximum score for RAVL-I is 75 (best performance) and 15 (best performance) for RAVL-D [29].

The BDI consists of 21 items rated on a 4-point scale of severity of psychological aspects of depression. The total score is the sum of all items; the maximum score is 63 (worst mood) [30].

State anxiety level was assessed with the STAI-Y2, which consists of 20 questions, each rated on a 4-point Likert-like scale. Higher scores are positively correlated with higher levels of anxiety [31].

The BBS is a 14-item scale (each rated on a scale from 0 to 4 points) that evaluates balance abilities during sitting, standing, and positional changes. The total score is the sum of all items; the range is from 0 (worst performance) to 56 (best performance) [32].

The 2MWT measures self-paced walking ability. The total score is the distance (meters) covered in 2 min (greater = better performance) [33].

The TUG is a functional mobility test associated with balance problems and falls in older adults, in which a subject must stand up, walk 3 m, turn around, walk back, and sit down. The time (seconds) taken to complete the test is recorded (longer = worse performance) and it is correlated with the level of functional mobility [34]. Patients can perform the TUG also under two dual-task conditions, one in which they are asked to count backwards from a randomly selected number between 20 and 100 (TUG-COG) and one in which they try to hold a full cup of water steady while walking (TUG-MOT). The time (seconds) taken to complete the test is recorded (longer = worse performance) and is correlated with the level of functional mobility under the dual-task condition [35].

2.7. Statistical Analysis

Data were analyzed using IBM SPSS software version 26.0 for Macintosh (IBM Corp., Armonk, NY, USA). Normal distribution of data was determined using the Kolmogorov–Smirnov and Shapiro–Wilk tests, and the homogeneity of variance was assessed with the Levene test. The normal and homogeneous variables were analyzed with two-way mixed ANOVA with a between-individual factor "group" (PT and PCT) and a within-individual factor "time" (pre- and post-treatment). Post hoc comparisons were corrected with the LSD method.

The other variables were analyzed with the Mann–Whitney U-test to compare the effects of treatment between the two groups and with the Wilcoxon signed-rank test for within-group comparison. Descriptive analysis was used to evaluate the effect size measures between groups (Cohen's d calculation) and the 95% confidence intervals [36]. The alpha level for significance was set at $p < 0.05$.

3. Results

For this pilot study, the study population was 20 patients (12 females, 8 males; mean age 70.8 ± 5.09; mean years of schooling 10.15 ± 4.69) with idiopathic PD (mean disease duration 7 ± 3.83 years) recruited from among 33 outpatients consecutively admitted to the Centro Polifunzionale Don Calabria of Verona, Italy, between June and August 2016. No drop-outs or adverse events were recorded during the study. Figure 1 illustrates the study flow diagram.

3.1. Baseline

Among outcome measures, FAS, RAVL-I, RAVL-D, and BDI scores resulted as normally distributed (Kolmogorov–Smirnov and Shapiro–Wilk tests, $p > 0.05$) and homogeneous (Levene test, $p > 0.05$).

There were no statistically significant differences in primary (MoCA, $p=0.346$; UPDRS III, $p = 0.724$) and secondary outcome measures (FAB-it, $p = 0.955$; TMT-A, $p = 0.655$; TMT-B, $p = 0.891$; FAS, $p = 0.557$; DSF, $p = 0.319$; DSB, $p = 0.931$; RAVL-I, $p = 0.686$; RAVL-D, $p = 0.602$; BDI, $p = 0.666$; STAI, $p = 0.776$; BBS, $p = 0.924$; 2MWT, $p = 0.516$; TUG, $p = 0.482$; TUG-COG, $p = 0.402$; TUG-MOT, $p = 0.198$) between the PT and the PCT group before treatment.

3.2. Primary Outcomes

Analysis revealed no statistically significant differences between the PCT and the PT group after treatment (MoCA, $p = 0.257$, $z = -1.133$; UPDRS III, $p = 0.724$, $z = -0,352$). Within-group comparison showed significant changes in the UPDRS III scores pre-treatment versus post-treatment for both groups (PCT, $p = 0.002$, $z = -3,061$; PT, $p = 0.004$, $z = -2.892$).

3.3. Secondary Outcomes

For the outcome measures analyzed with non-parametric tests, the between-group comparison showed statistically significant differences in TUG ($p = 0.047$; $z = -1.988$) and TUG-MOT ($p = 0.023$; $z = -2.272$) between the PCT and the PT group after treatment. The within-group comparison showed significant changes in pre-treatment versus post-treatment scores for the PCT group in the 2MWT ($p = 0.006$; $z = -2.726$), TUG ($p = 0.033$; $z = -2.128$), and TUG-MOT ($p = 0.007$; $z = -2.700$) and for the PT group in 2MWT ($p = 0.011$; $z = -2.558$).

Table 1 presents the group data and results of the within-group comparison for outcome measures analyzed with non-parametric tests

Table 1. Within-group comparisons for outcome measures analyzed with non-parametric tests.

Outcome	Rehabilitation Program	Pre Treatment	Post Treatment	Within Group Comparison Post vs. Pre-Treatment p Value (95% CI)
MoCA (0–30)	PCT	26.5 (24.75; 28)	26 (24; 27.25)	0.099 (−1.41; 0.21)
median (IQR)	PT	26.5 (23; 27)	26 (24.5; 27.25)	0.536 (−1.01; 0.51)
UPDRS-III (0–56)	PCT	9.5 (5; 16.25)	13 (11; 21.5)	0.002 (1.64; 7.76) *
median (IQR)	PT	11 (7.5; 13)	13 (11; 17)	0.004 (1.19; 7.11) *
FABit (0–18)	PCT	16 (15; 18)	16 (13.5; 17)	0.243 (1.99; 0.59)
median (IQR)	PT	17 (14.75; 18)	17.5 (13.5; 18)	0.893 (−1.61; 1.01)
TMTa (seconds)	PCT	57.55 (24.37)	59.65 (37.21)	0.808 (−11.86; 16.06)
mean (SD)	PT	55.6 (25.37)	56.2 (27.77)	0.872 (−6.90; 8.10)
TMTb (seconds)	PCT	197.4 (93.54)	200.6 (92.96)	0.73 (−15.88; 22.28)
mean (SD)	PT	195.1 (94.27)	197.4 (94.07)	0.977 (−20.72; 25.32)
DSF (0–9)	PCT	6 (5; 6)	6 (5; 6)	0.564 (−0.47; 0.27)
median (IQR)	PT	5 (5; 6)	6 (5;6)	0.109 (−0.08; 0.68)
DSB (0–8)	PCT	4 (3; 4.25)	4 (4; 4)	0.571 (−0.40; 0.70)
median (IQR)	PT	4 (3; 4)	4 (3.75; 5)	0.35 (−0.35; 0.95)
BBS (0–56)	PCT	53.5 (50; 55)	54 (48; 55)	0.954 (2.37; 1.37)
median (IQR)	PT	52 (50.5; 55)	54 (50.75; 55)	0.652 (−3.62; 1.02)
2MWT (meters)	PCT	107.28 (30.54)	130.53 (38.32)	0.006 (7.63; 38.88) *
mean (SD)	PT	112.9 (48.48)	130.6 (39.07)	0.011 (5.13; 30.23) *
TUG (seconds)	PCT	11.96 (6.65)	10.89 (6.85)	0.033 (−2.37; 1.37) *
mean (SD)	PT	10.49 (4.46)	11.12 (6.73)	0.823 (−0.73; 1.98)
TUG-COG (seconds)	PCT	14.30 (6.99)	12.85 (6.96)	0.067 (−2.93; 0.05)
mean (SD)	PT	12.58 (5.19)	12.66 (7.37)	0.601 (−1.38; 1.54)
TUG-MOT (seconds)	PCT	13.37 (6.53)	9.36 (2.23)	0.007 (−9.05; -0.86) *
mean (SD)	PT	10.99 (4.98)	11.6 (6.94)	0.149 (−2.84; 5.11)
STAI-Y2 (0–80)	PCT	43 (38.75; 50)	43 (36; 48.25)	0.432 (−5.18; 3.18)
median (IQR)	PT	41 (36; 49)	40 (35; 50.25)	0.904 (−4.79; 6.79)

Abbreviations: IQR = interquartile range; SD = standard deviation; CI = confidence interval; MoCA = Montreal Cognitive Assessment; UPDRS-III = Unified Parkinson's Disease Rating Scale part III; FAB-it = Frontal Assessment Battery-Italian version; TMT = trail making test; DSF = digit Span Forward; DSB = Digit Span Backward; BBS = Berg Balance Scale; 2MWT = 2 min walking test; TUG = Time Up and Go; TUG-COG = cognitive; TUG-MOT = motor; STAI-Y2 = State-Trait Anxiety Inventory part Y2; * = statistically significant ($p < 0.05$).

For the outcome measures analyzed with parametric tests, ANOVA revealed a principal significant effect of "time" for RAVL-I ($F_{(1,38)}$ 9.459, $p = 0.004$, $\eta = 0.199$) and RAVL-D ($F_{(1,38)}$ 13.671, $p = 0.001$, $\eta = 0.265$). The RAVL-I score was significantly higher after treatment (mean score post-treatment RAVL-I 38.15 ± 9.102) compared to before treatment (mean score post-treatment RAVL-I 34.65 ± 8.438). The RAVL-D score was significantly higher after treatment than before treatment (mean score post-treatment RAVL-D 7.5 ± 3.138—mean score pre-treatment RAVL-D 5.85 ± 2.975). Post hoc comparisons revealed significantly higher scores at post-treatment with respect to pre-treatment for RAVL-I and RAVL-D only in the PCT group (mean RAVL-I pre-treatment 34.1 ± 6.813; mean RAVL-I post-treatment 39.4 ± 10.58; mean RAVL-D pre-treatment 5.6 ± 2.854; mean RAVL-D post-treatment 7.65 ± 3.297).

ANOVA showed no group effect of FAS ($F_{(1,38)}$ 0.042, $p = 0.838$, $\eta = 0.001$), RAVL-I ($F_{(1,38)}$ 0.075, $p = 0.785$, $\eta = 0.002$), RAVL-D ($F_{(1,38)}$ 0.013, $p = 0.909$, $\eta = 0$), and BDI ($F_{(1,37)}$ 0.001, $p = 0.969$, $\eta = 0$). Additionally, no effect of "timeXgroup" interaction was found for FAS ($F_{(1,38)}$ 0.092, $p = 0.343$, $\eta = 0.024$), RAVL-I ($F_{(1,38)}$ 2.502, $p = 0.122$, $\eta = 0.062$), RAVL-D ($F_{(1,38)}$ 0.803, $p = 0.376$, $\eta = 0.021$), and BDI ($F_{(1,37)}$ 0.8091, $p = 0.374$, $\eta = 0.21$).

Table 2 presents the group data and results for outcome measures analyzed with the parametric tests.

Table 2. Group data and results for outcome measures analyzed with parametric tests.

Outcome	Rehabilitation Program	Pre Treatment	Post Treatment	Repeated Measures ANOVA		Post Hoc Analysis
				Group Between-Subjects *p*	Time Whitin-Subjects *p*	Whitin-Group Post vs. Pre-Treatment *p* Value (95% CI) *p*
FAS (no. words) mean (SD)	PCT	11.65 (3.99)	13.02 (3.98)	0.838	0.075	/
	PT	12.39 (3.91)	12.82 (5.57)			/
RAVL-I (0–75) mean (SD)	PCT	34.1 (6.81)	39.4 (10.58)	0.785	0.004 *	0.002 (2.04; 8.56) *
	PT	35.2 (9.96)	36.9 (7.4)			0.297 (−1,56; 4.96)
RAVL-D (0–15) mean (SD)	PCT	5.6 (2.86)	7.65 (3.3)	0.909	0.001 *	0.002 (0.77; 3.33) *
	PT	6.1 (3.14)	7.35 (3.05)			0.055 (−0.03; 2.53)
BDI (0–63) mean (SD)	PCT	12.37 (7.03)	12 (7.61)	0.906	0.577	/
	PT	11.3 (8.23)	12.9 (7.52)			/

Abbreviations: SD = standard deviation; CI = confidence interval; FAS = fonemic verbal fluency; RAVL = Rey Auditory Verbal Learning I = immediate, D = delay; BDI = Beck Depression Inventory; * = statistically significant ($p < 0.05$).

4. Discussion

In this pilot randomized cross-over trial, we compared improvement in cognitive, motor, and psychological domain scores after physiotherapy training alone and after consecutive physiotherapy and cognitive treatment in patients with PD.

We observed a statistically significant difference in motor abilities between the two groups after treatment.

There was a change in functional mobility performance, as evaluated with the single- (TUG) and the dual-task condition (TUG-MOT) after PCT. Patients showed an improvement in gait velocity, especially in the dual-task condition (about 4 s faster). In line with a previous study involving other types of patients [37], we speculate that this change may translate into a clinically meaningful improvement for the patients. Our data are shared by the previous study, in which patients who received training with separated gait and cognitive exercises showed an improvement on dual-tasking abilities after treatment [14].

Since the published data suggest a significant correlation between functional mobility (single- or dual-task condition) and cognitive abilities [7], we assume that specific training including cognitive rehabilitation is necessary to also enhance functional mobility under the dual-task condition in PD patients. In our patients, this improvement did not seem possible with physiotherapy alone. We speculate that consecutive treatment provides for training attention and dual-task abilities. This view is shared by previous work that reported a relationship between functional capacity and mobility and severity of cognitive impairment in neurological patients [38].

Our findings for cognitive change indicate that consecutive physiotherapy and cognitive treatment, but not physiotherapy alone, may help to improve performance on delay recall memory ability (as measured with the RAVL-D). This observation is shared by previous studies that reported improvements after cognitive [17] and motor plus cognitive [14,15] training. Furthermore, our data indicate that only the PD patients who underwent this training showed significant improvement in verbal learning (as measured with the RAVL-I). This suggests that cognitive rehabilitation enables patients to improve their memory learning abilities. Specific memory training is needed to increase verbal learning in which correct memory strategies can be acquired.

No changes in cognitive performance were found after treatment in the PT group. Differently from previous studies [13,15,39,40], our data suggest that physiotherapy alone does not result in improved cognitive abilities in PD. We assumed that group treatment might reduce cognitive engagement during rehabilitation exercises. Furthermore, our physiotherapy program, unlike others [39,40], did not include aerobic exercises, which are suggested to induce improvement in brain functional connectivity in the frontal areas [41] that are essential for cognitive functionality in PD patients.

As expected, both training modalities had a positive effect on walking ability (as measured with the 2MWT). This is in line with previous studies that indicated an improvement in motor performance after motor rehabilitation [10,12,39]. However, differently from others [15,39], we found a decrease in global motor performance (as measured with UPDRS III) after both types of training. Unlike other study designs, cross-over studies have natural progression of the disease as a bias. The UPDRS motor score progressed over time, with an annual score increase of 3.3 points [42]. This is in line with the changes in scores in our sample (about 2 points on UPDRS III for both groups during the 8-month study period). However, the pre-post treatment change in score did not have a clinical impact on the PD patients [43]. Due to an unfortunate mistake in the first version of this study, we did not use the revised version of the UPDRS (MDS-UPDRS). Future study protocols will include this version to confirm our data for the UPDRS III.

We believe that the discordant results between the 2MWT and the UPDRS III could stem from the type of intervention. For this study, the focus of the physiotherapy training was primarily on walking and balance, whereas the UPDRS III is a global measure that investigates all movement dysfunctions in patients with PD.

Differently from other studies, ours examined the effects of consecutive physiotherapy and cognitive rehabilitation on different motor abilities (balance, walking, and functional mobility). Barboza et al. investigated motor performance with only one motor outcome (UPDRS III) [15] and Strowen at al.'s study [14] specifically assessed gait velocity under single- and dual-task conditions. By using different outcome measures, we were able to investigate the different motor dysfunctions more deeply.

It is difficult to compare our findings with published data because of the differences in our consecutive training protocol compared to previous studies [14,15]. In our protocol, cognitive and physical training sessions were performed on two separate days (not in the same session) and the patients underwent group (not individual) treatment.

Again, different from a previous study [39], we found stabilization of pre-post treatment of mood (as measured with the BDI), as reported in another study [40]. Summarizing, few studies on rehabilitation in PD include psychological outcome measures, and current knowledge in this field is scarce. A future area of focus is the effect of rehabilitation (cognitive, motor, or combined) on mood in PD patients.

The present study has some limitations. The sample size was small and no follow-up assessment was performed. These limitations reflect the rehabilitation context where the study was conducted. The medical center can accept few patients at one time for rehabilitation care, and following the inclusion criteria, we further reduced the number of patients potentially eligible for the study. Since the majority of the study subjects went on to participate in other training sessions at other clinics immediately after the end of the present study, we could not perform follow-up assessments and compare the effects of our treatment with those of a control group.

In addition, since the patients were not tested in "off" medication, no conclusions can be drawn about the unmedicated state. Another area of focus would be to investigate the effects of cognitive training alone on more than one motor dysfunction in patients with PD and to compare its effectiveness with other approaches (physiotherapy or physiotherapy and cognitive treatment). It might also be interesting to conduct a randomized trial with a non-cross-over design involving two separate patient groups.

Overall, our data indicate a statistical difference pre-post treatment for some outcome measures, suggesting the benefit of consecutive motor and cognitive treatment for functional mobility and long-term memory in PD patients. Nonetheless, we cannot be certain that such differences translate into a clinical change. Further studies are needed to confirm our preliminary results and better investigate the clinical impact of rehabilitation programs in PD patients.

5. Conclusions

Our findings suggest potential effects of consecutive motor and cognitive interventions in PD. Our findings may also serve as starting points to better investigate the effects of this rehabilitation program on cognitive, motor, and psychological symptoms in PD patients. Finally, the clinical implications are that the identification and treatment of cognitive deficits are important in patients with PD and that a benefit can be gained with rehabilitation programs that include both motor and cognitive training.

Supplementary Materials: The following are available online at https://www.mdpi.com/article/10.3390/jpm11080687/s1, File S1: The TIDieR (Template for Intervention Description and Replication) Checklist.

Author Contributions: Conceptualization, V.V. and P.P.; Methodology, A.P. and B.M.; Formal Analysis, V.V. and M.F.; Investigation, S.R. and C.F.; Data Curation, P.P. and M.F.; Writing—Original Draft Preparation, V.V.; Writing—Review and Editing, V.V. and A.P.; Supervision, N.S. and M.T.; Project Administration, V.V. and N.S. All authors have read and agreed to the published version of the manuscript.

Funding: This research received no external funding.

Institutional Review Board Statement: The study was conducted according to the guidelines of the Declaration of Helsinki and approved by the Institutional Review Board of Centro Polifunzionale Don Calabria (protocol code no. 05/2016, date of approval: 05/16/2016).

Informed Consent Statement: All participants were outpatients and gave their informed, written consent to participate.

Data Availability Statement: Data is contained within the article or Supplementary Materials.

Conflicts of Interest: The authors have no conflict of interest to declare.

References

1. Wang, Y.X.; Zhao, J.; Li, D.K.; Peng, F.; Wang, Y.; Yang, K.; Liu, Z.Y.; Liu, F.T.; Wu, J.J.; Wang, J. Associations between cognitive impairment and motor dysfunction in Parkinson's disease. *Brain Behav.* **2017**, *7*, e00719. [CrossRef]
2. Pothakos, K.; Kurz, M.J.; Lau, Y.S. Restorative effect of endurance exercise on behavioral deficits in the chronic mouse model of Parkinson's disease with severe neurodegeneration. *BMC Neurosci.* **2009**, *10*, 6. [CrossRef]
3. Picelli, A.; Camin, M.; Tinazzi, M.; Vangelista, A.; Cosentino, A.; Fiaschi, A.; Smania, N. Three-dimensional motion analysis of the effects of auditory cueing on gait pattern in patients with Parkinson's disease: A preliminary investigation. *Neurol. Sci.* **2010**, *31*, 423–430. [CrossRef]
4. Muslimović, D.; Post, B.; Speelman, J.D.; Schmand, B. Cognitive profile of patients with newly diagnosed Parkinson disease. *Neurology* **2005**, *65*, 1239–1245. [CrossRef]
5. Uekermann, J.; Daum, I.; Peters, S.; Wiebel, B.; Przuntek, H.; Müller, T. Depressed mood and executive dysfunction in early Parkinson's disease. *Acta Neurol. Scand.* **2003**, *107*, 341–348. [CrossRef] [PubMed]
6. Lawson, R.A.; Yarnall, A.J.; Duncan, G.W.; Khoo, T.K.; Breen, D.P.; Barker, R.A.; Collerton, D.; Taylor, J.P.; Burn, D.J. Severity of mild cognitive impairment in early Parkinson's disease contributes to poorer quality of life. *Parkinsonism Relat. Disord.* **2014**, *20*, 1071–1075. [CrossRef] [PubMed]
7. Varalta, V.; Picelli, A.; Fonte, C.; Amato, S.; Melotti, C.; Zatezalo, V.; Saltuari, L.; Smania, N. Relationship between cognitive performance and motor dysfunction in patients with Parkinson's disease: A pilot cross-sectional study. *Biomed. Res. Int.* **2015**, *2015*, 365959. [CrossRef]
8. Varalta, V.; Fonte, C.; Munari, D. The influence of cognitive factors on balance and gait. In *Advanced Technologies for the Rehabilitation of Gait and Balance Disorders*; Sandrini, G., Homberg, V., Saltuari, L., Smania, N., Pedrocchi, A., Eds.; Springer: Cham, Switzerland, 2018; Volume 19.
9. Nagano-Saito, A.; Martinu, K.; Monchi, O. Function of basal ganglia in bridging cognitive and motor modules to perform an action. *Front. Neurosci.* **2014**, *8*, 187. [CrossRef]
10. Tomlinson, C.L.; Patel, S.; Meek, C.; Herd, I.P.; Clarke, C.E.; Stowe, R.; Shah, L.; Sackley, C.; Deane, K.H.O.; Wheatley, K.; et al. Physiotherapy intervention in Parkinson's disease: Systematic review and meta-analysis. *BMJ* **2012**, *345*, e5004. [CrossRef] [PubMed]
11. Abbruzzese, G.; Marchese, R.; Avanzino, L.; Pelosin, E. Rehabilitation for Parkinson's disease: Current outlook and future challenges. *Parkinsonism Relat. Disord.* **2016**, *22* (Suppl. 1), S60–S64. [CrossRef]
12. Lauzé, M.; Daneault, J.F.; Duval, C. The Effects of Physical Activity in Parkinson's Disease: A Review. *J. Parkinsons Dis.* **2016**, *6*, 685–698. [CrossRef] [PubMed]

13. Intzandt, B.; Beck, E.N.; Silveira, C.R.A. The effects of exercise on cognition and gait in Parkinson's disease: A scoping review. *Neurosci. Biobehav. Rev.* **2018**, *95*, 136–169. [CrossRef] [PubMed]
14. Strouwen, C.; Molenaar, E.; Münks, L.; Keus, S.; Zijlmans, J.; Vandenberghe, W.; Bloem, B.R.; Nieuwboer, A. Training dual tasks together or apart in Parkinson's disease: Results from the DUALITY trial. *Mov. Disord.* **2017**, *32*, 1201–1210. [CrossRef] [PubMed]
15. Barboza, N.M.; Terra, M.B.; Brandão Bueno, M.E.; Christofoletti, G.; Smaili, S.M. Physiotherapy versus physiotherapy plus cognitive training on cognition and quality of life in Parkinson disease randomized clinical trial. *Am. J. Phys. Med. Rehabil.* **2019**, *98*, 460–468. [CrossRef] [PubMed]
16. Walton, C.C.; Mowszowski, L.; Gilat, M.; Hall, J.M.; O'Callaghan, C.; Muller, A.J.; Georgiades, M.; Szeto, J.; Ehgoetz Martens, K.A.; Shine, J.M.; et al. Cognitive training for freezing of gait in Parkinson's disease: A randomized controlled trial. *NPJ Parkinsons Dis.* **2018**, *4*, 15. [CrossRef]
17. Leung, I.H.; Walton, C.C.; Hallock, H.; Lewis, S.J.; Valenzuela, M.; Lampit, A. Cognitive training in Parkinson disease: A systematic review and meta-analysis. *Neurology* **2015**, *85*, 1843–1851. [CrossRef]
18. Postuma, R.B.; Berg, D.; Stern, M.; Poewe, W.; Olanow, C.W.; Oertel, W.; Obeso, J.; Marek, K.; Litvan, I.; Lang, A.E.; et al. MDS clinical diagnostic criteria for Parkinson's disease. *Mov. Disord.* **2015**, *30*, 1591–1601. [CrossRef]
19. Hoehn, M.M.; Yahr, M.D. Parkinsonism: Onset, progression and mortality. *Neurology* **1967**, *17*, 427–442. [CrossRef]
20. European Physiotherapy Guideline for Parkinson's Disease. 2014. Available online: https://www.parkinsonnet.nl/app/uploads/sites/3/2019/11/eu_guideline_parkinson_guideline_for_pt_s1.pdf (accessed on 12 July 2021).
21. Smania, N.; Corato, E.; Tinazzi, M.; Stanzani, C.; Fiaschi, A.; Girardi, P.; Gandolfi, M. Effect of balance training on postural instability in patients with idiopathic Parkinson's disease. *Neurorehabil. Neural Repair* **2010**, *24*, 826–834. [CrossRef] [PubMed]
22. Santangelo, G.; Siciliano, M.; Pedone, R.; Vitale, C.; Falco, F.; Bisogno, R.; Siano, P.; Barone, P.; Grossi, D.; Santangelo, F.; et al. Normative data for the Montreal Cognitive Assessment in an Italian population sample. *Neurol. Sci.* **2015**, *36*, 585–591. [CrossRef]
23. Song, J.; Fisher, B.E.; Petzinger, G.; Wu, A.; Gordon, J.; Salem, G.J. The relationships between the unified Parkinson's disease rating scale and lower extremity functional performance in persons with early-stage Parkinson's disease. *Neurorehabil. Neural Repair* **2009**, *23*, 657–661. [CrossRef] [PubMed]
24. Chertkow, H.; Nasreddine, Z.; Johns, E.; Phillips, N.; McHenry, C. P1-143: The Montreal cognitive assessment (MoCA): Validation of alternate forms and new recommendations for education corrections. *Alzheimer's Dement. J. Alzheimer's Assoc.* **2011**, *7*, S157. [CrossRef]
25. Appollonio, I.; Leone, M.; Isella, V.; Piamarta, F.; Consoli, T.; Villa, M.L.; Forapani, E.; Russo, A.; Nichelli, P. The frontal assessment battery (FAB): Normative values in an Italian population sample. *Neurol. Sci.* **2005**, *26*, 108–116. [CrossRef]
26. Giovagnoli, A.R.; Del Pesce, M.; Mascheroni, S.; Simoncelli, M.; Laiacona, M.; Capitani, E. Trail Making Test: Normative values from 287 normal adult controls. *Ital. J. Neurol. Sci.* **1996**, *17*, 305–309. [CrossRef] [PubMed]
27. Costa, A.; Bagoj, E.; Monaco, M.; Zabberoni, S.; De Rosa, S.; Papantonio, A.M.; Mundi, C.; Caltagirone, C.; Carlesimo, G.A. Standardization and normative data obtained in the Italian population for a new verbal fluency instrument, the phonemic/semantic alternate fluency test. *Neurol. Sci.* **2014**, *35*, 365–372. [CrossRef]
28. Monaco, M.; Costa, A.; Caltagirone, C.; Carlesimo, G.A. Forward and backward span for verbal and visuo-spatial data: Standardization and normative data from an Italian adult population. *Neurol. Sci.* **2013**, *34*, 749–754. [CrossRef]
29. Carlesimo, G.A.; Caltagirone, C.; Gainotti, G. The Mental Deterioration Battery: Normative data, diagnostic reliability and qualitative analyses of cognitive impairment. The Group for the Standardization of the Mental Deterioration Battery. *Eur. Neurol.* **1996**, *36*, 378–384. [CrossRef]
30. Beck, A.T.; Ward, C.H.; Mendelson, M.; Mock, J.; Erbaugh, J. An inventory for measuring depression. *Arch. General Psych.* **1961**, *4*, 561–571. [CrossRef] [PubMed]
31. Spielberger, C.D.; Gorsuch, R.L.; Lushene, R.; Vagg, P.R.; Jacobs, G.A. *Manual for the State-Trait Anxiety Inventory*; Consulting Psychologists Press: Palo Alto, CA, USA, 1983.
32. Berg, K.; Wood-Dauphinee, S.; Williams, J.I. The balance scale: Reliability assessment with elderly residents and patients with an acute stroke. *Scand. J. Rehab. Med.* **1995**, *27*, 27–36.
33. Light, K.E.; Behrman, A.L.; Thigpen, M.; Triggs, W.J. The 2-min walk test: A tool for evaluating walking endurance in clients with Parkinson's disease. *J. Neurol. Phys. Ther.* **1997**, *21*, 136.
34. Morris, S.; Morris, M.E.; Iansek, R. Reliability of measurements obtained with the Timed 'Up & Go' test in people with Parkinson disease. *Phys. Ther.* **2001**, *81*, 810–818.
35. Shumway-Cook, A.; Brauer, S.; Woollacott, M. Predicting the probability for falls in community-dwelling older adults using the timed up & go test. *Phys. Ther.* **2000**, *80*, 896–903.
36. Benjamini, Y.; Hochberg, Y. Controlling the false discovery rate: A practical and powerful approach to multiple testing. *J. R. Statist. Soc. B* **1995**, *57*, 289–300. [CrossRef]
37. Gautschi, O.P.; Stienen, M.N.; Corniola, M.V.; Joswig, H.; Schaller, K.; Hildebrandt, G.; Smoll, N.R. Assessment of the Minimum Clinically Important Difference in the Timed Up and Go Test After Surgery for Lumbar Degenerative Disc Disease. *Neurosurgery* **2017**, *80*, 380–385. [CrossRef] [PubMed]
38. Domenech-Cebrián, P.; Martinez-Martinez, M.; Cauli, O. Relationship between mobility and cognitive impairment in patients with Alzheimer's disease. *Clin. Neurol. Neurosurg* **2019**, *179*, 23–29. [CrossRef] [PubMed]

39. Picelli, A.; Varalta, V.; Melotti, C.; Zatezalo, V.; Fonte, C.; Amato, S.; Saltuari, L.; Santamato, A.; Fiore, P.; Smania, N. Effects of treadmill training on cognitive and motor features of patients with mild to moderate Parkinson's disease: A pilot, single-blind, randomized controlled trial. *Funct. Neurol.* **2016**, *31*, 25–31. [PubMed]
40. Altmann, L.J.P.; Stegemöller, E.; Hazamy, A.A.; Wilson, J.P.; Bowers, D.; Okun, M.S.; Hass, C.J. Aerobic exercise improves mood, cognition, and language function in parkinson's disease: Results of a controlled study. *J. Inter. Neuropsy. Soc.* **2016**, *22*, 878–889. [CrossRef] [PubMed]
41. Voss, M.W.; Prakash, R.S.; Erickson, K.I.; Basak, C.; Chaddock, L.; Kim, J.S.; Alves, H.; Heo, S.; Szabo, A.N.; White, S.M.; et al. Plasticity of brain networks in a randomized intervention trial of exercise training in older adults. *Front. Aging Neurosci.* **2010**, *2*, 32. [CrossRef] [PubMed]
42. Alves, G.; Wentzel-Larsen, T.; Aarsland, D.; Larsen, J.P. Progression of motor impairment and disability in Parkinson disease: A population-based study. *Neurology* **2005**, *65*, 1436–1441. [CrossRef]
43. Sánchez-Ferro, Á.; Matarazzo, M.; Martínez-Martín, P.; Martínez-Ávila, J.C.; Gómez de la Cámara, A.; Giancardo, L.; Arroyo Gallego, T.; Montero, P.; Puertas-Martín, V.; Obeso, I.; et al. Minimal Clinically Important Difference for UPDRS-III in Daily Practice. *Mov. Disord. Clin. Pract.* **2018**, *5*, 448–450. [CrossRef] [PubMed]

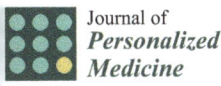

Review

Parkinson's Disease: Personalized Pathway of Care for Device-Aided Therapies (DAT) and the Role of Continuous Objective Monitoring (COM) Using Wearable Sensors

Vinod Metta [1,2,*], Lucia Batzu [1,2], Valentina Leta [1,2], Dhaval Trivedi [1,2], Aleksandra Powdleska [1], Kandadai Rukmini Mridula [3], Prashanth Kukle [4], Vinay Goyal [5], Rupam Borgohain [3], Guy Chung-Faye [1,2] and K. Ray Chaudhuri [1,2]

[1] Department of Neurosciences, Institute of Psychiatry, Psychology & Neuroscience, King's College London, London WC2R 2LS, UK; l.batzu@nhs.net (L.B.); Valentina.leta@nhs.net (V.L.); dhaval.trivedi1@nhs.net (D.T.); aleksandra.powdlewska@nhs.net (A.P.); Guy.chung-faye@nhs.net (G.C.-F.); Ray.chaudhuri@nhs.net (K.R.C.)
[2] Parkinson's Foundation Centre of Excellence, King's College Hospital, London SE5 9RS, UK
[3] Nizams Institute of Medical Sciences, Hyderabad 500082, India; rukminimridula@gmail.com (K.R.M.); b_rupam@hotmail.com (R.B.)
[4] Vikram Hospitals, Benguluru 560052, India; drprashanth.lk@gmail.com
[5] Medanta Institute of Neurosciences, New Delhi 122001, India; drvinaygoyal@gmail.com
* Correspondence: Vinod.metta@nhs.net

Abstract: Parkinson's disease (PD) is a chronic, progressive neurological disorder and the second most common neurodegenerative condition. Advanced PD is complicated by erratic gastric absorption, delayed gastric emptying in turn causing medication overload, and hence the emergence of motor and non-motor fluctuations and dyskinesia, which is initially predictable and then becomes unpredictable. As the patient progresses to the advanced stage, advanced Parkinson's disease (APD) is characterized by refractory motor and non motor fluctuations, unpredictable OFF periods, and troublesome dyskinesias. The management of APD is a complex affair. There is growing recognition that GI dysfunction is common in PD, with virtually the entire GI system (the upper and lower GI tracts) causing problems from dribbling to defecation. The management of PD should focus on personalized care addressing both motor and non-motor symptoms, ideally including not only dopamine replacement but also associated non-dopaminergic circuits, particularly focusing on noradrenergic, serotonergic, and cholinergic therapies bypassing the gastrointestinal tract (GIT) by infusion or device-aided therapies (DAT), including levodopa–carbidopa intestinal gel infusion, apomorphine subcutaneous infusion, and deep brain stimulation, which are available in many countries for the management of the advanced stage of Parkinson's disease (APD). The PKG (KinetiGrap) can be used as a continuous objective monitoring (COM) aid, as a screening tool to help to identify advanced PD (APD) patients suitable for DAT, and can thus improve clinical outcomes.

Keywords: advanced Parkinson's disease (APD); precision medicine; apomorphine subcutaneous infusion therapy; pain; intrajejunal; levodopa; motor and non-motor symptoms; PKG (KinetiGrap)

Citation: Metta, V.; Batzu, L.; Leta, V.; Trivedi, D.; Powdleska, A.; Mridula, K.R.; Kukle, P.; Goyal, V.; Borgohain, R.; Chung-Faye, G.; et al. Parkinson's Disease: Personalized Pathway of Care for Device-Aided Therapies (DAT) and the Role of Continuous Objective Monitoring (COM) Using Wearable Sensors. *J. Pers. Med.* **2021**, *11*, 680. https://doi.org/10.3390/jpm11070680

Academic Editor: David Alan Rizzieri

Received: 17 June 2021
Accepted: 14 July 2021
Published: 19 July 2021

Publisher's Note: MDPI stays neutral with regard to jurisdictional claims in published maps and institutional affiliations.

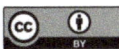

Copyright: © 2021 by the authors. Licensee MDPI, Basel, Switzerland. This article is an open access article distributed under the terms and conditions of the Creative Commons Attribution (CC BY) license (https://creativecommons.org/licenses/by/4.0/).

1. Introduction

Parkinson's disease is the second most common neurodegenerative disease, affecting 1–2% of the population over the age of 60 [1,2]. Advanced Parkinson's disease (APD) is associated with unmanageable, unpredictable motor and non-motor symptom fluctuations, which are refractory to standard oral/transdermal therapies, compromising quality of life (QOL) [3–6]. A recent consensus-based initiative based on a multi-country Delphi-panel (5-2-1) model, an approach to identifying functional indicators of advanced Parkinson's disease, was externally validated in the OBSERVE-PD study [7]. This led to the development of the 5-2-1 motor paradigm (>5 oral levodopa doses/day, >2 h of "off" symptoms/day, and >1 h of troublesome dyskinesia/day [8]) used in clinical practice to identify advanced Parkinson's patients and ensure timely referrals for device-aided treatments.

Managing advanced Parkinson's disease is a complex affair. There is growing recognition that GI dysfunction is common in PD, with almost the entire GI system (the upper and lower GI tracts) causing problems from dribbling to defecation [9]. As the disease progresses, over 80% of patients with PD develop dysphagia and life-threatening aspiration pneumonia. Lower GI dysfunction results in slowed colonic transit, a reduced frequency of bowel movements, constipation, etc. [10–13]. The initial years with oral pulsatile dopaminergic treatment are relatively easy and effective. As patients reach the advanced stage, APD is complicated by erratic gastric absorption, delayed gastric emptying (causing medication overload), and poor levodopa absorption, hence the emergence of motor and non-motor fluctuations and dyskinesia, which is initially predictable and then becomes unpredictable [3,14–16]. Once unpredictable fluctuations or refractory "offs" start, one should start looking at non-oral infusion therapies or device-aided therapies (DAT) [17].

2. Available Infusion Therapies or Device-Aided Therapies (DAT) and Patient Selection

In this situation, we should consider infusion or device-aided therapies, including levodopa–carbidopa intestinal gel infusion (LCIG), levodopa–entacapone–carbidopa intestinal gel infusion (LECIG), subcutaneous apomorphine infusion (APO), and deep brain stimulation (DBS). Many national guidelines have attempted to address the indications of these device-aided therapies (DAT) (Figure 1), and ideal patient selection remains somewhat of an unmet need [18].

If we look at the National Institute Centre of Excellence (Figure 2) indications for advanced device-aided therapies, the essential concept is based on offering the best medical therapy, which may start with subcutaneous apomorphine infusion (CSAI), or, if the symptoms are not adequately controlled, especially with severe dyskinesias, intrajejunal levodopa infusion (IJLI) or deep brain surgery (DBS) should be considered [19].

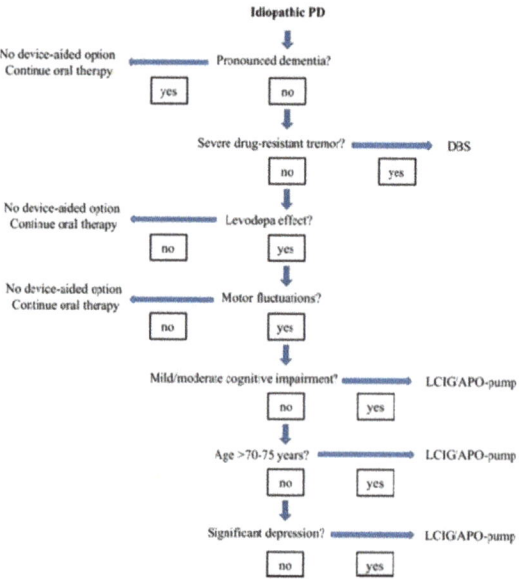

Figure 1. Patient selection for DAT therapies (Ref-Navigate PD) [18].

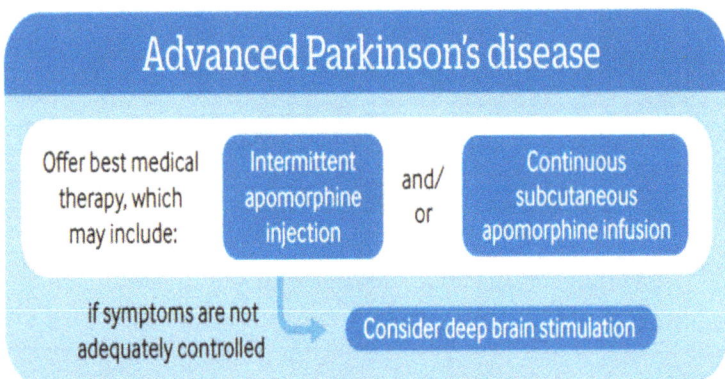

Figure 2. NICE guidelines 2017—Managing symptoms of Parkinson's disease.

2.1. Selection of the Ideal Patient

While therapeutic decisions and research on device-aided treatments have largely focused on the influence and effect on motor symptoms, we now know that Non Motor Symptoms (NMS) are an integral feature of PD and, therefore, should play a part (Figure 1) in the decision-making process for selecting the ideal patient [8,18].

2.2. Apomorphine: History and Molecular Structure

Apomorphine is considered one of the oldest antiparkinsonians. It is a drug found in water lilies that acts as an emetic, aphrodisiac, or hallucinogen [20]. In 1845, Adolf Edvard Arppe synthesized apomorphine from morphine and sulfuric acid [21]. In 1851, Thomas Anderson also synthesized apomorphine by heating codeine with sulfuric acid. It gained interest in medicine in 1868, when Matthiessen and Wright [22] heated morphine with concentrated hydrochloric acid and synthesized apomorphine hydrochloride. Figure 3 shows the history and evolution of apomorphine as a treatment for PD.

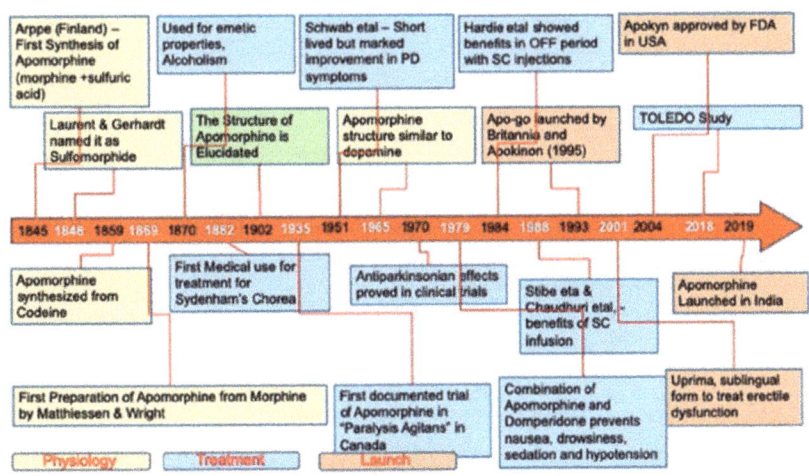

Figure 3. History and evolution of apomorphine as a treatment for PD.

Apomorphine ($C_{17}H_{17}NO_2$), a derivative of morphine, is a non-ergot dopamine agonist (DA) with high selectivity for D2, D3, D4, and D5 and, to a lesser extent, for D1 dopamine receptors. It activates serotonergic 5HT1A receptors but has antagonist effects on the serotonergic 5HT2A, 5HT2B, and 5HT2C receptors and adrenergic α2A, α2B, and α2C receptors [23].

While apomorphine has poor oral bioavailability (<4%), following its subcutaneous administration into the abdominal wall, 100% of it is rapidly absorbed. The time to peak plasma concentration is 10–60 min. Its concentration in the cerebrospinal fluid (CSF) peaks about 10–30 min later [23]. Its extremely lipophilic structure allows it to cross the blood–brain barrier. Its bioavailability after subcutaneous administration is similar to that after intravenous administration. It shows linear pharmacokinetics at 2–8 mg when a single subcutaneous injection is administered in the abdominal wall. Apomorphine is available in two presentations (Figure 4): A randomized double blinded study by Pfierffer et al. [24] looked at Continued efficacy and safety of subcutaneous apomorphine (Apo) in 62 patients with advanced Parkinson's disease (APD) who had previously received APO for 3 months and placebo showed Significantly greater improvement in mean Unified PD rating scale motor scores in treatment group with no overall adverse event incidence observed in both groups supporting the the long-term use of intermittent APO as effective acute therapy for off episodes in advanced PD patients (APD) [24].

Compared with a placebo, apomorphine resulted in significantly and rapidly improved mobility, as assessed by an improvement in mean UPDRS motor scores, within a few minutes of administration. Maximal results were observed 20 min after administration. This effect persisted for at least 40 min after dosing [24]. In another study by Isaacson SH et al. [25], patients achieved an "on" state 37 min sooner, on average, with apomorphine injection than with oral levodopa, helping with early-morning akinesia, with a 61% reduction in the time to "on" (TTO) [25].

The Expert Consensus Group (Trenkwalder C et al. [26]) proposed the following clinical practice recommendations regarding the use of apomorphine in PD (Tables 1 and 2).

Table 1. Expert Consensus Group report on the use of apomorphine in PD—clinical practice recommendations.

PEN (Figure 4)	PUMP (Figure 4)
Anticipated rescue when required during motor and non-motor "off" periods	Patient considers that rescue doses required too frequently
When absorption of oral levodopa is impaired or the patient has gastric emptying problems (gastroparesis)	Dyskinesias limit further therapy optimization
To treat delayed "on"	Simplify complex PD dosing regimens to improve convenience and compliance
To treat early-morning problems (akinesia and dystonia)	Alternative to surgical therapy or LCIG, if contraindicated, or due to patient preference
	Absorption or gastric emptying of oral levodopa is impaired

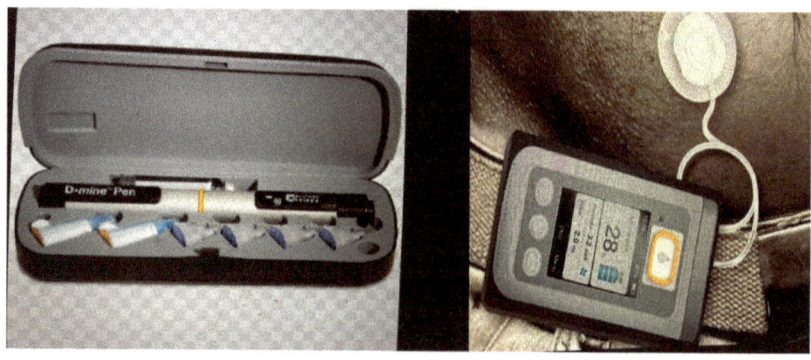

Figure 4. APO pen and pump.

Factors influencing supportive usage of APO.

Table 2. Navigate PD: Factors influencing the use of CSAI.

Symptoms That Support Use	Symptoms That Discourage Use
Dyskinesias	Marked ongoing hallucinations/psychosis
Maintenance insomnia	Impulse-control disorders
Pronounced therapy-refractory depression	Drug-related daytime somnolence
Non-motor fluctuations	Orthostatic hypotension
Dysarthria	Marked ongoing hallucinations/psychosis
Restless legs	

Another recent multicentre, double-blind, randomized, placebo-controlled study (TOLEDO) [27] demonstrated the long-term efficacy of apomorphine infusion for motor fluctuations in PD. The significant reduction in off and increase in on time without troublesome side effects also led to substantial reductions in oral PD medication [27].

Levodopa–carbidopa (LD–CD) intrajejunal infusion (LCIG Figure 5) is a treatment in which traditional gold-standard levodopa in gel form is administered continuously into the primary site of levodopa absorption, the proximal jejunum. This is achieved via a percutaneous endoscopic gastrojejunostomy tube connected to a portable infusion pump. This was first launched in Sweden in 2004, after pioneering work by Professor Aquilonius and colleagues in Uppsala University, and it has now been on the market for 17 years [28].

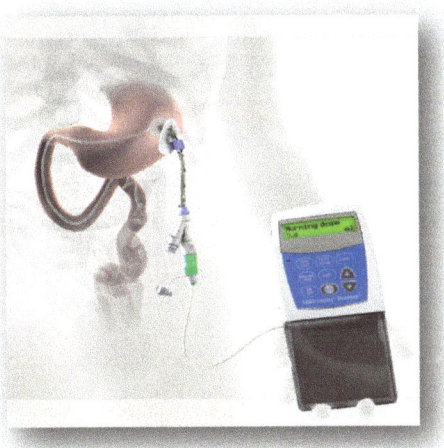

Figure 5. Intrajejunal levodopa infusion.

An observational study (DUOGLOBE study) [29] evaluating the long-term (24 months follow up) effectiveness of LCIG in advanced PD (APD) patients, in which 20% of patients met all of the 5-2-1 criteria, showed sustained improvements in motor and non-motor scores and in quality of life (QoL), with supporting real-world data on the effectiveness, safety profile, and caregiver burden in APD patients. LCIG is probably the device-aided treatment for which we have the most robust evidence on the effect on NMS. In 2015, a systematic review identified eight open-label studies confirming that LCIG improved the NMS burden after a follow-up period ranging from 6 to 25 months, with specific positive effects on sleep and autonomic dysfunction, particularly gastrointestinal issues [30]. This was further explored and consolidated by the GLORIA registry, whose 24-month follow-up data showed a remarkable beneficial effect of LCIG on sleep disturbances, apathy, and gastrointestinal dysfunction [31].

DBS (Figure 6) is a widely accepted, conventional, and effective surgical treatment for Parkinson's disease that involves implanting a device to stimulate targeted regions of the brain with electrical impulses generated by a battery-operated neurostimulator. DBS is thought to act by shifting the low-frequency (15–30 Hz) oscillatory activity observed in PD to a higher frequency, thus increasing the firing rate of the stimulated nucleus (commonly the sub-thalamic nucleus (STN), globus pallidus internus (GPi), or caudal zona incerta (cZi) [32]. Several randomized controlled trials (RCTs) comparing DBS (STN, GPi, or other) showed a superior efficacy and safety profile in patients with advanced Parkinson's compared with basic medical dopaminergic treatment (BMT) [33,34].

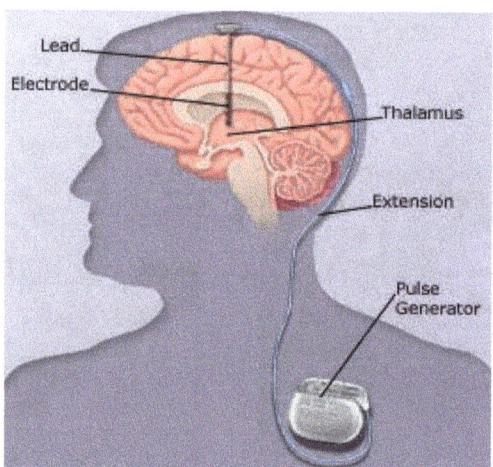

Figure 6. Deep brain surgery (DBS).

2.3. DAT Therapies: Evidence-Based Clinical Motor and Non-Motor Outcomes

Parkinson's disease (PD) is a progressive disorder. While the early motor phases of PD can be effectively managed by oral/transdermal dopaminergic therapy, as the disease progresses to advanced stages, it poses a challenge for neurologists to treat, complicated by the requirement to choose the ideal patients for device-aided therapies, including levodopa–carbidopa intestinal gel infusion (LCIG), levodopa–entacapone–carbidopa intestinal gel infusion (LECIG), subcutaneous apomorphine infusion (APO), and deep brain stimulation (DBS).

Personalizing treatment choices requires evidence and clinical-experience-based guidance for the device-aided management of PD, and it is paramount for better clinical outcomes. Several national guidelines and the Navigate PD program have attempted to address bespoke and ideal patient selection; the latter remains somewhat of an unmet need, as discussed above [18]. APO, LCIG, and bilateral STN-DBS have been available since early 2000 for the treatment of advanced Parkinson's disease (APD) in many countries. Although several individual studies of LCIG, STN-DBS, and APO supported beneficial motor and non-motor outcomes [25–31], head-to-head comparative studies are limited. An open-label, non-randomized comparative study [35] (the Euroinf study) showed that, in advanced Parkinson's patients, both IJLI and Apo infusion therapy appear to provide improvements in motor symptoms and quality of life, with IJLI resulting in better improvements in sleep/fatigue, gastrointestinal function, urinary domains, and sexual function compared to Apo [3].

Another prospective, multicentre, international, real-life cohort observation study of 173 PD patients, the Euroinf 2 study [36], the first and only study comparing all three device-aided treatments (APO, LCIG, and STN-DBS), was in agreement with previous studies [28–36]. It showed improvements in motor, non-motor, and quality-of-life outcomes [36]. However, interestingly, this study highlighted that each device-aided therapeutic option (DAT) showed biased outcomes in specific non-motor domains, with an overall reduction in non-motor burden. For instance, bilateral STN-DBS and LCIG appeared to benefit urogenital and gastrointestinal dysfunction, respectively, whereas APO showed supremacy in controlling attention/memory deficits. All three treatment options had a beneficial effect on depression and anxiety. Aspects of sleep dysfunction (insomnia, excessive daytime sleepiness, and restless leg syndrome) and fatigue improved with both LCIG and bilateral STN-DBS (Tables 3 and 4), compared with APO, which showed a beneficial effect on perceptual problems and hallucinations. All three (STN-DBS, APO, and LCIG) had beneficial effects on the miscellaneous domain of the NMS scale, which incorporates unexplained pain, olfaction, weight changes, etc. Overall, this study highlights (Figure 7) the importance of personalizing therapeutic options based on holistic assessments of motor and non-motor symptoms [36].

Factors influencing supportive usage of IJLI.

Table 3. Navigate PD: Factors influencing the use of LCIG.

Symptoms That Support Use	Symptoms That Discourage Use
Dyskinesias	No specific symptoms (like severe dementia) to discourage use; presence of some symptoms may require further investigation
Drug-related hallucinations and/or delusions in patient history	
Impulse-control disorders	
Maintenance insomnia	
Mild cognitive impairment	
Pronounced therapy-refractory depression	
Dysarthria	
Restless legs	

Factors influencing supportive usage of STN-DBS.

Table 4. Navigate PD: Factors influencing the use of STN-DBS.

Symptoms That Support Use	Symptoms That Discourage Use
Dyskinesias	Marked ongoing hallucinations
Drug-related hallucinations and/or delusions in patient history	Dementia
Impulse-control disorders	Pronounced therapy-refractory depression
Maintenance insomnia	Dysphagia
Non-motor fluctuations	Dysarthria
	L-dopa-unresponsive postural and gait problems, falls
	Marked ongoing hallucinations

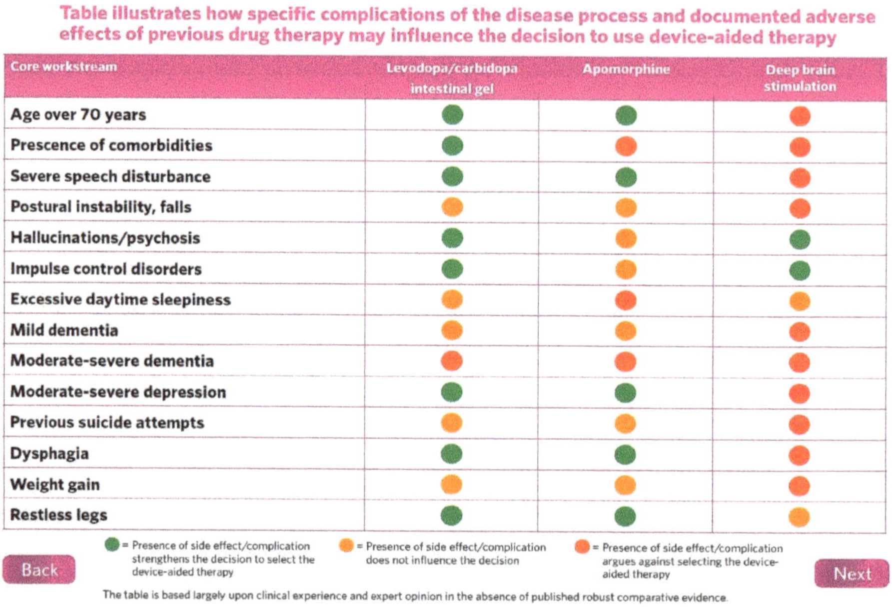

Core workstream	Levodopa/carbidopa intestinal gel	Apomorphine	Deep brain stimulation
Age over 70 years	🟢	🟢	🔴
Prescence of comorbidities	🟢	🔴	🔴
Severe speech disturbance	🟢	🟢	🔴
Postural instability, falls	🟠	🟠	🔴
Hallucinations/psychosis	🟢	🔴	🔴
Impulse control disorders	🟢	🔴	🟢
Excessive daytime sleepiness	🟠	🔴	🟠
Mild dementia	🟠	🟠	🔴
Moderate-severe dementia	🔴	🔴	🔴
Moderate-severe depression	🟢	🟢	🔴
Previous suicide attempts	🟠	🟠	🔴
Dysphagia	🟢	🟢	🔴
Weight gain	🟠	🟠	🔴
Restless legs	🟢	🟢	🔴

🟢 = Presence of side effect/complication strengthens the decision to select the device-aided therapy
🟠 = Presence of side effect/complication does not influence the decision
🔴 = Presence of side effect/complication argues against selecting the device-aided therapy

The table is based largely upon clinical experience and expert opinion in the absence of published robust comparative evidence.

Figure 7. Euroinf 2 Study [36] showing DAT vs. specification of NMS domains for (DAT therapies—overall table).

2.4. Objective Measurements of Patient Outcomes in Parkinson's Disease: Rating Scales

2.4.1. MDS-UPDRS Scale

This unified Parkinson's disease rating scale (UPDRS) is a tool for monitoring the course of Parkinson's and the degree of disability. The scale has three sections that evaluate key areas of disability, together with a fourth section that evaluates any complications of treatment [37,38].

Part I: Evaluation of mental activity, behaviour and mood, intellectual impairment, thought disorder motivation/initiative depression, sleep, pain, bladder and bowel problems, and fatigue. This subscale has scores from 0 to 4, with 4 representing the greatest level of dysfunction, and it can range from 0 (normal) to 16.

Part II: Self-evaluation of activities of daily living: speech, salivation, swallowing, handwriting, cutting food, dressing, hygiene, turning in bed, falling, freezing, walking, tremor, and sensory difficulties. This 14-item subscale ranges from 0 (normal) to 56.

Part III: Evaluation of motor function: speech, facial expression, tremor at rest, action tremor, rigidity, finger taps, hand movements, rotation of hands and forearms so palms face downward, rotation of hands and forearms so palms face upward, toe taps, leg agility, rising from chair, posture, gait, postural stability, and bradykinesia. This is the most commonly used subscale and has 14 different types of ratings, ranging from 0 to 4. The total score for subscale 3 ranges from 0 (normal) to 108, the sum of scores from 27 observations.

Part IV: Evaluation of complications of therapy; dyskinesia; early-morning "off" period deterioration, including the duration of "off" periods, predictability based on dosage, and whether onset is sudden or gradual; anorexia (including nausea and/or vomiting); and sleep disturbance. This subscale includes 11 questions, and the scores on this subscale range from 0 to 23.

2.4.2. Hoehn and Yahr Rating Scale

Hoehn and Yahr staging is probably the most widely known means for evaluating people with PD and was first described in 1967. It reflects motor manifestations of PD and is intended to reflect the degree of progression, combining features of motor impairment and disability, for scores of 0–5, with 0 = no signs of disease; 1 = unilateral disease (on one side); 1.5 = unilateral disease plus axial involvement; 2 = bilateral disease, without impairment of balance; 2.5 = bilateral disease, with recovery on the pull test; 3 = mild to moderate bilateral disease, needing assistance to prevent falling on the pull test, and physically independent; 4 = severe disability but still able to walk or stand unassisted; and 5 = wheelchair-bound or bedridden unless aided [39].

2.4.3. Short Parkinson's Evaluation Scale/Scales for Outcomes in Parkinson's Disease (SPES/SCOPA)

The SPES/SCOPA [40,41]. is a short, reliable, and valid scale used to evaluate the motor function of PD patients and includes three sections: A) Motor Evaluation (10 items, maximum of 42 points), B) Activities of Daily Living (7 items, 21 points), and C) Motor Complications (4 items, 12 points—with 2 items on motor fluctuations [6 points] and 2 on dyskinesias [6 points]). The response options for all the items range from 0 to 3.

2.4.4. Non-Motor Symptoms Scale (NMSS)

The Non-Motor Symptoms Scale (NMSS) [12] is a 30-item validated tool for assessing a wide range of non-motor symptoms in patients with Parkinson's disease (PD). The NMSS measures the severity and frequency of a range of non-motor symptoms across nine dimensions: cardiovascular, sleep/fatigue mood/cognition, perceptual problems, attention/memory, gastrointestinal, urinary, sexual function, and miscellany. The score for each item is based on a multiple of severity (from 0 to 3) and frequency scores (from 1 to 4), for total scores of 0 (none) to 360.

2.4.5. PDSS (Parkinson's Disease Sleep Scale)

The PDSS [42] is a simple bedside screening instrument for the evaluation of sleep disturbances in Parkinson's disease. The PDSS is a visual analogue scale addressing 15 commonly reported symptoms associated with sleep disturbance. The 15 items are the overall quality of a night's sleep (item 1), sleep onset and maintenance insomnia (items 2 and 3), nocturnal restlessness (items 4 and 5), nocturnal psychosis (items 6 and 7), nocturia (items 8 and 9), nocturnal motor symptoms (items 10–13), sleep refreshment (item 14), and daytime dozing (item 15). The severity of symptoms is reported by marking a cross along a 10 cm line (labelled from the worst to best state), and the scores for each item range from 0 (symptom severe and always experienced) to 10 (symptom-free). The maximum cumulative score for the PDSS is 150 (the patient is free of all symptoms).

2.4.6. King's Parkinson's Pain Scale (KPSS)

KPSS (King's PD Pain Scale) [43] seems to be a reliable and valid scale for grading various types of pain in PD. Its seven domains (musculoskeletal pain, chronic pain, fluctuation-related pain, nocturnal pain, orofacial pain, discoloration/oedema/swelling, and radicular pain) include 14 items, with each item scored by severity (0–3) multiplied by frequency (0–4), resulting in a subscore of 0 to 12, with the total possible scores ranging from 0 to 168.

2.4.7. Montreal Cognitive Assessment (MoCA)

The Montreal Cognitive Assessment (MoCA) [44] is a widely used screening assessment for detecting cognitive impairment. It helps to assess several domains including memory recall, which involves two learning trials with five nouns, and delayed recall after approximately five minutes (scores out of 5 points), as well as visuospatial abilities using a clock drawing task (3 points) and a three-dimensional cube copy (1 point). Multiple aspects of executive function are assessed, by the trail-making B task (1 point), a phonemic fluency task (1 point), and a two-item verbal abstraction task (2 points).

Orientation to time and place is evaluated by asking the subject for the date on which and the city in which the test is occurring (6 points). Abstract reasoning is assessed (2 points). One point each is given for attention, concentration, and working memory, which are evaluated using a sustained attention task (target detection using tapping; 1 point), and digits forward and backward, as well as 3 points for a serial subtraction task. The assessment of language using three-item naming (familiar animals such as lions, camels, rhinos, etc.) scores 3 points, and repetition of two complex sentences scores 2 points.

The MoCA test is a one-page 30-point test, assessing several cognitive domains, and the MoCA scores range between 0 and 30. A score of 26 or over is considered to be normal; people with mild cognitive impairment (MCI) score an average of 22.1; people with Alzheimer's disease score an average of 16.2.

2.4.8. Hospital Anxiety and Depression Scale (HADS)

HADS is a frequently used self-rating scale developed by Zigmond AS and Snaith RP for measuring anxiety and depression in non-psychiatric patients. The questionnaire comprises seven questions for anxiety (HADS Anxiety) and seven questions for depression (HADS Depression) [45]. The scoring for each item ranges from zero to three, with three denoting the highest level of anxiety or depression. A total subscale score of >8 points out of a possible 21 denotes considerable symptoms of anxiety or depression: 8–10 (mild), 11–14 (moderate), 15–21 (severe).

2.4.9. Parkinson's Disease Questionnaires (PDQ-8 and PDQ-39)

The Parkinson's Disease Questionnaire (PDQ-39) [46,47] is a validated disease-specific tool for measuring health-related quality of life in Parkinson's disease patients. It covers eight dimensions—mobility, activities of daily of living, emotional well-being, stigma, social support, cognition, communication, and bodily discomfort—and it contains 39 questions. Each question is scored 0–4 points, transformed to a score ranging from 0 (good health) to 100 (poor health). The total score is derived from the sum of 39 scale scores divided by eight (the number of scales), which yields a score between 0 and 100 (100 = more health problems). This is equivalent to expressing the sum of all 39 item responses as a percentage score.

2.4.10. Parkinson's Disease Questionnaire (PDQ-8)

The PDQ-8 is a shorter questionnaire derived from the PDQ-39. It is an eight-question instrument with a question taken from each domain of mobility, activities of daily of living, emotional well-being, stigma, social support, cognition, communication, and bodily discomfort. The questions are scored 0–4, and the sum is taken.

3. Continuous Objective Monitoring (COM) Using Wearable Sensors and Its Role in Identifying Potential Candidates for Device-Aided Therapies (DAT)

After 5 years of disease [48,49], approximately 50% of PwP can develop motor fluctuations (bradykinetic fluctuations) and dyskinesia. Motor fluctuations and dyskinesia are the motor manifestations of reduced or excess (respectively) dopamine transmission, which also cause significant non-motor fluctuations [50]. Dyskinesias can sometimes be confused with tremor, and bradykinesia can be attributed to tiredness rather than a decline in the effectiveness of dopaminergic treatment. Some patients with cognitive issues have problems with compliance with their treatment, and in routine clinical practice, patient diaries are impractical and not commonly used apart from in clinical trials [51]. Objective measurement by capturing data during activities of daily living in the home environment helps not only with compliance but also with career burden, and for clinicians, it can provide continuous objective information that helps to optimize treatment and patient outcomes.

3.1. About PKG

The Personal KinetiGraph® (PKG®) Movement Recording System (Figure 8) is a new COM technology that provides scores for bradykinesia, dyskinesia, motor fluctuations, and tremor, as well as immobility as a proxy for daytime sleepiness. The Personal KinetiGraph (PKG) is a commercially available wrist-worn data logger system approved by the FDA, providing a continuous, objective, motor and ambulatory assessment of bradykinesia, dyskinesia, and motor fluctuations in PD. The logger is a smartwatch that is worn on the most affected wrist, weighs 35 g, and contains a rechargeable battery and a 3-axis iMEMS accelerometer. It provides data points every two minutes and produces a series of graphs and scores in a clinically useful format known as the PKG [52]. The device is water resistant. The logger is programmed to remind patients to take their PD medications by delivering vibrations, and consumption is acknowledged by swiping the logger's smart screen. It also has sensors to detect whether the device is being worn.

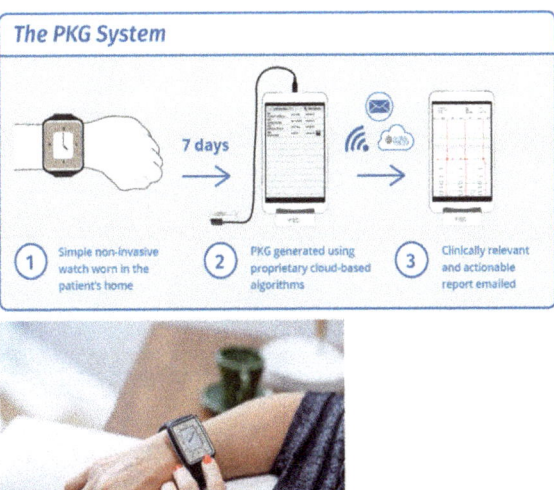

Figure 8. Monitoring Parkinson's disease: PKG.

The PKG is the graphical representation of the bradykinetic scores (BKS) and dyskinetic scores (DKS) collected every 2 min over an extended period of 6 days. It also provides sleep scores (as it is worn at night), daytime sleepiness scores, and inactivity [53], and also provides tremor scores [54]. The times at which medications are due and consumed are also shown, making it possible to assess whether there are dose-related variations in the BKS or DKS [55] (Figure 9).

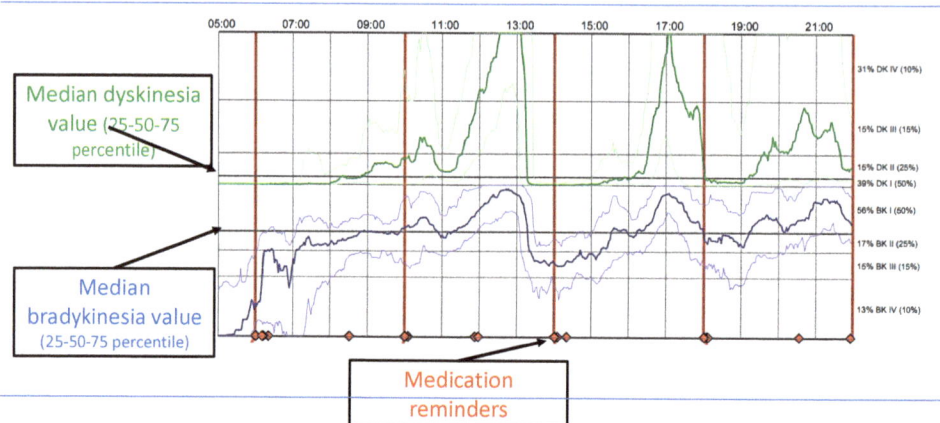

Figure 9. PKG: dyskinesia and bradykinesia.

The variables provided by the PKG are objective measures of these same factors that are considered clinically suitable candidates for DAT [18,56], which are recognized by the presence of increased "off" time and/or dyskinesia in subjects taking five or more doses/day [57]. Whilst there are many other factors taken into account before DAT is recommended, PKG is useful as a screening tool; for instance, the timing for deep brain stimulation (DBS) is important because there is a window of optimum benefit [58], and delay means that suitable candidates may have shorter benefit or lower benefit, or miss out on DBS entirely. Previous studies have shown [59,60] that 67% of patients referred for DBS are unsuitable for the procedure, yet only 1% of people with PD receive DBS [61], although as many as 20% may, in fact, be eligible [62].

One of the main reasons and indications for any DAT is motor fluctuations [63], which are frequently overlooked by both patients and clinicians [64]. The information from the PKG could be used to build a classifier (DAT classifier) that identifies patients eligible for DAT therapies with high sensitivity and specificity, correlating with the clinical criteria for DAT, and that can be used as a referral tool [65,66].

3.2. Glossary of PKG Terms

The PKG produces a graphical representation of the BKS and DKS collected every 2 min over an extended period (typically 6 days) [52–54,67,68].

- Median BKS. The median BKS was the 50th percentile of the BKS for all 6 days the PKG was worn (usually 6 days).
- The interquartile range of the BKS was a measure of the fluctuation of the BKS.
- The percent time in bradykinesia (PTB). Epochs whose BKS lay between 26.1 and 49.4 and whose 25th percentiles of the BKS were >18.5 and 90th percentiles, <80. Additionally, any epoch whose BKS was >49.9 but contained tremor was included.
- Median DKS: This is the 50th percentile for all the days that the PKG was worn. Brisk walking introducing resonant peaks may artificially increase the DKS. An algorithm was used to detect and remove epochs affected in this way.
- Interquartile range of DKS: calculates the median BKS and is a measure of the fluctuation of the DKS.
- Percent time in dyskinesia (PTD): Those DKS used to estimate the median DKS were passed through a median filter (most of the epochs in the filter period must be in the dyskinetic range (DKS > 7) for the centre to be classed as dyskinetic).
- Percent time with tremor (PTT): This was the percentage of 2 min epochs estimated over all the days that the PKG was worn that contained tremor. Tremor is likely to be present if the PTT score is >1%.

- The percent time immobile (PTI): This was the percentage of 2 min epochs with BKS > 80 from all the days that the PKG was worn. These scores were associated with daytime sleep.
- The doses of levodopa/day. These were calculated from the number of reminders programmed into the logger.

Bradykinesia was considered adequately treated if the BKS was <25, which relates to a Unified Parkinson's Disease Rating (UPDRS) score of ~40 [52–54,67,68], and inadequately treated if the BKS was >25 [8,19–23]. Dyskinesia was considered "controlled" if DKS < 9, which relates to an Abnormal Involuntary Movement Score (AIMS) of 10 [52–54,67,68]. The percent time immobile (PTI) was defined as the percentage of 2-min periods between 9 AM and 6 PM where the movement data recorded by the PKG device were very low and correlated with the daytime sleep measured by polysomnography (PSG) and the Epworth Sleepiness Scale Scores (ESS). The percent time with tremor (PTT) was defined as the percentage of 2-min periods between 9 AM and 6 PM that contained tremor [68]. Tremor is likely to be present if the PTT score is >1% [52–54,67,68]. The other scores include compliance with the reminders.

3.3. PKG Database and Associated Studies

Currently we have a 6-year database (January 2012 to August 2018) with 27,834 complete and de-identified PKGs from 21 countries where the device has received regulatory approval. Data from seven countries (Australia, the UK, the USA, Sweden, Germany, the Netherlands, and France) where more than 500 PKGs had been performed (referred to as the Top 7 countries) were analysed, and these constituted 94% (26,112/27,834) of the PKGs in the database [52–54,67,68].

The first sub-analysis was based on the median scores of only those PD patients with serial PKGs (i.e., more than one PKG). There were statistically significant differences in BKS from the 1st to 2nd through to the 6th PKG readings in this stratified population (all $p < 0.0001$). The average time between each PKG order ranged from 23 to 42 days for the first 6 PKG readings. While the BKS improved by 3.3 points (30.9 to 27.6 points), the DKS increased by 0.3 points (0.8 to 1.1 points), suggesting improvements in the BKS due to clinicians optimizing the treatment regime [52–54,67,68]. Interestingly, these changes in treatment plan/dose optimization did not adversely affect the DKS, suggesting no significant increase in side effects or any abnormal movements.

4. Conclusions

PKG can be used as a COM in daily clinical practice. It aids in clinical decision making and the identification and quantification of PD motor symptoms, can be useful as a screening tool to help to identify advanced PD (APD) patients suitable for DAT, and improves clinical outcomes.

4.1. Clinical Scenario 1

A 64-year-old Asian patient (British Indian), a retired GP diagnosed with Parkinson's disease 7 years ago, had an initial beneficial response to dopaminergic treatment and then presented with refractory motor (troublesome dyskinesias) and non-motor fluctuations (mild cognitive decline and non-intrusive perceptual issues, apathy, hallucinations, etc.). There were no obvious sleep-related issues or bowel/bladder complaints. Other problems included well-controlled type 2 diabetes treated with metformin monotherapy (1 g/day), and essential hypertension treated with captopril at 5 mg/day; there was no other significant past medical history, family history of dementia or history of allergies.

4.1.1. Current PD Medications

- Stalevo (l'dopa, 200 mg carbidopa, 50 mg; entacopone, 200 mg) QDS;
- Sinemet, controlled release, 250 mg (l'dopa, 200 mg; carbidopa, 50 mg) ON;

- Rotigotine, 8 mg (he responded very well initially and then started developing rashes, on rotigotine patches for 3 years);
- Previously tried a dopaminergic regime (selegiline, ropinorole, sinemet, etc.).

4.1.2. Current Ongoing Problems

- Troublesome dyskinesias;
- Unpredictable offs/freezing episodes;
- Attention/memory/cognitive problems;
- Apathy/hallucinations and non-intrusive perceptual issues.

4.2. Clinical Scenario 2

A 71-year-old Caucasian patient of Scottish heritage diagnosed with Parkinson's disease 11 years ago, who had problems with dopamine agonists in the past (developed dopamine dysregulation syndrome with pramipexole and severe somnolence issues with ropinirole). They showed a good initial beneficial response to levodopa treatment, but then presented with unpredictable wearing offs, troublesome dyskinesias, and non-motor fluctuations, predominantly in terms of cardiovascular, urinary, and gastrointestinal dysfunction, as well as severe sleep-related issues (excessive daytime sleepiness). Other problems included symptoms suggestive of restless legs (RLS), with well-controlled hypertension treated with amlodipine at 5 mg/day, and no other significant past medical history.

4.2.1. Current PD Medications

- Sinemet PLUS (l'dopa, 100 mg; carbidopa, 25 mg) at 7 am, 10 am, 1 pm, 4 pm, and 7 pm;
- Sinemet, controlled release, 250 mg (l'dopa, 200 mg; carbidopa, 50 mg) at 10 pm;
- Opicopone, 50 mg, 8 pm;
- Previously tried a dopaminergic regime (pramipexole, ropinorole, and entacopone).

4.2.2. Current Ongoing Problems

- Troublesome dyskinesias;
- Unpredictable offs/freezing episodes/falls;
- Cardiovascular, urinary, and gastrointestinal dysfunction;
- Severe sleep-related issues (excessive daytime sleepiness);
- Previous adverse reactions to dopamine agonists.

4.3. Discussion and Outcomes

Patient 1. Being a medical practitioner who is well-versed about his condition and the available options, he is personally not keen on STN-DBS (patient preference). On the basis of the motor and non-motor profiles according to Euroinf 2 data, APO may represent a good therapeutic choice, keeping in line with the patient's personal preference (not keen on surgery). He responded well to previous agonists (ropinorole/rotigotine). Based on the best medical therapy and available guidelines and evidence, APO (subcutaneous apomorphine infusion) was opted for, and the continuous, objective, motor, and ambulatory assessment of bradykinesia, dyskinesia, and motor fluctuations was performed to evaluate the efficacy of the device-aided therapy (apomorphine) with the wearable sensor monitor (COM) Personal KinetiGraph® (PKG®).

Patient 2. Elderly gentleman with a history of previous adverse events in response to dopamine agonists (DDS) and with motor and non-motor (mainly cardiovascular, gastrointestinal, and sleep-related) problems and falls. On the basis of motor and non-motor profiles according to Euroinf 2 data, intrajejunal levodopa infusion may represent a good therapeutic choice, in keeping with the patient's age and non-motor profiles. Surgery may not be a viable option, and due to a history of adverse events in response to dopamine agonists, APO is not indicated. Therefore, based on the best medical therapy and available guidelines and evidence, intrajejunal levodopa infusion (IJLI) was opted for, and the continuous, objective, motor, and ambulatory assessment of bradykinesia, dyskinesia, and motor fluctuations was performed to evaluate the efficacy of the device-aided therapy (IJLI) with the wearable sensor monitor (COM) Personal KinetiGraph® (PKG®).

Overall clinical assessments revealed that both patients had refractory motor and non-motor fluctuations, unpredictable offs, and refractory freezing episodes, and both were on multi/varied dosing, with a combination of oral dopaminergic and transdermal dopamine treatments, with no obvious therapeutic effects or benefits compared to traditional conventional treatment. This indeed complements the Delphi model (5-2-1) [8] and was confirmed on COM (PKG recordings indeed showed variable BKS/DKS scores before the usage of DAT therapies, and Patient 1's non-motor profile was dominated by mild cognitive decline, non-intrusive perceptual issues, apathy, hallucinations, etc.). Another factor to be considered for Patient 1 is how his personal preference was also implicated in the delivery of personalized advanced treatment. As he was not keen on surgery, according to available Euroinf 2 data, Apo (CSAI) [36] was considered the best option, and this was also the patient's choice. He was monitored using COM (PKG), and 6-day recording showed an improvement in overall BKS/DKS scores (for the 20th to 14th percentiles before and after Apo (Figures 10–12) respectively, and likewise for the bradykinesia scores).

Meanwhile, for our second patient, APO may not be suitable, as he has previously had problems with dopamine agonists, having developed dopamine dysregulation syndrome with pramipexole and severe somnolence issues with ropinirole. Other factors are also implicated, especially in this patient, in considering the delivery of personalized advanced treatment. His age, for instance, represents a key aspect in the assessment for DBS suitability; an age > 70 or 75 years is an exclusion criterion for DBS in many centres given the associated higher risk of complications as discussed previously [18,19]. Based on his current non-motor profile, LCIG was considered, as it showed superior efficacy in improving gastrointestinal, cardiovascular, and sleep-related problems and falls, and like our first patient, a 6-day PKG/COM recording was obtained (Figure 13) and showed an overall improvement in dyskinesias/fluctuating offs/bradykinesia scores.

Device-aided non-oral therapies are now considered and recommended worldwide for the management of advanced Parkinson's disease. Personalizing the pathway of care and the successful delivery of these therapies depend on patient selection, motor and non-motor profiles, and patient choices and preferences. Body weight has also emerged as an important aspect in the decision-making process [69]. The PKG can be used as a COM in daily clinical practice, since it aids in clinical decision making and the identification and quantification of PD motor symptoms, is useful as a screening tool to help to identify advanced PD (APD) patients suitable for DAT, and improves clinical outcomes.

PKG and Apomorphine at King's

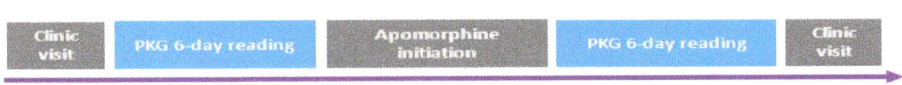

Figure 10. PKG and APO.

Pre-Apomorphine

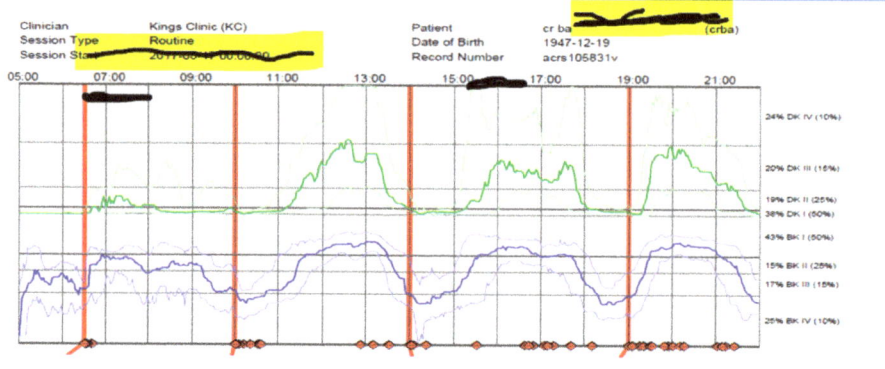

Figure 11. Pre APO.

Post-Apomorphine

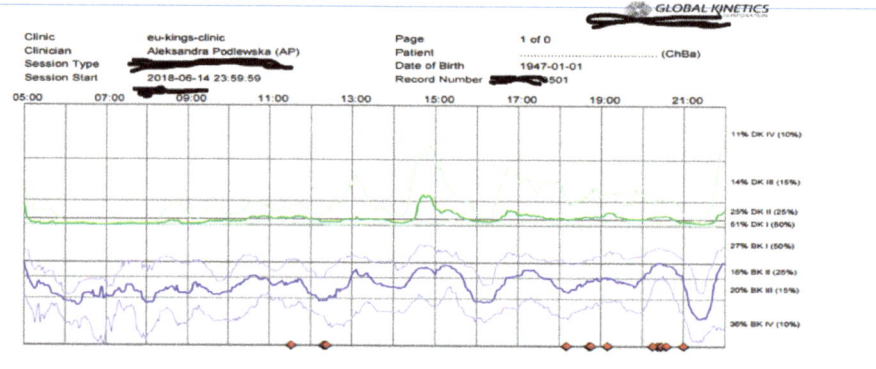

Figure 12. Post APO.

Monitoring Parkinson's disease: LCIG effect

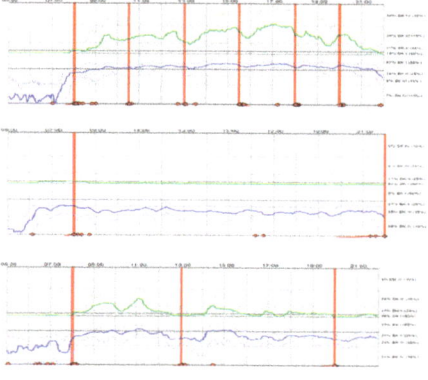

Figure 13. PRE and POST Duodopa.

Funding: This research received no external funding.

Institutional Review Board Statement: Not applicable.

Informed Consent Statement: This is a review article, clinical cases described and discussed in this review (patient names and details annoymised/blinded) however written informed consent has been obtained to publish their PKG reports in this paper.

Data Availability Statement: Not applicable.

Conflicts of Interest: The authors declare no conflict of interest.

References

1. Reeve, A.; Simcox, E.; Turnbull, D. Ageing and Parkinson's disease: Why is advancing age the biggest risk factor? *Ageing Res. Rev.* **2014**, *14*, 19–30. [CrossRef]
2. Parkinson's Foundation. Statistics. Available online: https://www.parkinson.org/Understanding-Parkinsons/Statistics (accessed on 25 October 2019).
3. Ray Chaudhuri, K.; Poewe, W.; Brooks, D. Motor and Nonmotor Complications of Levodopa: Phenomenology, Risk Factors, and Imaging Features. *Mov. Disord. Off. J. Mov. Disord. Soc.* **2018**, *33*, 909–919. [CrossRef] [PubMed]
4. Leta, V.; Jenner, P.; Chaudhuri, K.R.; Antonini, A. Can therapeutic strategies prevent and manage dyskinesia in Parkinson's disease? An update. *Expert Opin. Drug Saf.* **2019**, *18*, 1203–1218. [CrossRef] [PubMed]
5. Chapuis, S.; Ouchchane, L.; Metz, O.; Gerbaud, L.; Durif, F. Impact of the motor complications of Parkinson's disease on the quality of life. *Mov. Disord. Off. J. Mov. Disord. Soc.* **2005**, *20*, 224–230. [CrossRef] [PubMed]
6. Politis, M.; Wu, K.; Molloy, S.; Bain, P.G.; Chaudhuri, K.R.; Piccini, P. Parkinson's disease symptoms: The patient's perspective. *Mov. Disord. Off. J. Mov. Disord. Soc.* **2010**, *25*, 1646–1651. [CrossRef] [PubMed]
7. Fasano, A.; Fung, V.S.C.; Lopiano, L.; Elibol, B.; Smolentseva, I.G.; Seppi, K.; Takáts, A.; Onuk, K.; Parra, J.C.; Bergmann, L.; et al. Characterizing advanced Parkinson's disease: OBSERVE-PD observational study results of 2615 patients. *BMC Neurol.* **2019**, *19*, 1–11. [CrossRef] [PubMed]
8. Antonini, A.; Stoessl, A.J.; Kleinman, L.S.; Skalicky, A.M.; Marshall, T.S.; Sail, K.R.; Onuk, K.; Odin, P.L.A. Developing consensus among movement disorder specialists on clinical indicators for identification and management of advanced Parkinson's disease: A multi-country Delphi-panel approach. *Curr. Med. Res. Opin.* **2018**, *34*, 2063–2073. [CrossRef]
9. Cloud, L.J.; Greene, J.G. Gastrointestinal Features of Parkinson's Disease. *Curr. Neurol. Neurosci. Rep.* **2011**, *11*, 379–384. [CrossRef]
10. Dubow, J.S. Autonomic Dysfunction in Parkinson's Disease. *Dis. A Mon.* **2007**, *53*, 265–274. [CrossRef] [PubMed]
11. Stacy, M. Nonmotor symptoms in Parkinson's disease. *Int. J. Neurosci.* **2011**, *121* (Suppl. 2), 9–17. [CrossRef] [PubMed]
12. Chaudhuri, K.R.; Martinez-Martin, P.; Brown, R.G.; Sethi, K.; Stocchi, F.; Odin, P.; Ondo, W.; Abe, K.; MacPhee, G.; MacMahon, D.; et al. The metric properties of a novel non-motor symptoms scale for Parkinson's disease: Results from an international pilot study. *Mov. Disord.* **2007**, *22*, 1901–1911. [CrossRef] [PubMed]
13. Chaudhuri, K.R.; Schapira, A.H. Non-motor symptoms of Parkinson's disease: Dopaminergic pathophysiology and treatment. *Lancet Neurol.* **2009**, *8*, 464–474. [CrossRef]
14. Fahn, S. Adverse effects of levodopa. In *The Scientific Basis for the Treatment of Parkinson's Disease*; Olanow, C.W., Lieberman, A.N., Eds.; Parthenon Publishing Group: Carnforth, UK, 1992; pp. 89–112.
15. Fahn, S.; Bressman, S.B. Should Levodopa Therapy for Parkinsonism be Started Early or Late? Evidence against Early Treatment. *Can. J. Neurol. Sci. J. Can. Des. Sci. Neurol.* **1984**, *11* (Suppl. 1), 200–205. [CrossRef] [PubMed]
16. Fahn, S.; Elton, R.L.; Members of the UPDRS Development Committee. Unified Parkinson's disease rating scale. In *Recent Developments in Parkinson's Disease*; Fahn, S., Marsden, C.D., Calne, D.B., Goldstein, M., Eds.; MacMillan Healthcare Information: Florham Park, NJ, USA, 1987; Volume 2, pp. 153–163.
17. Timpka, J.; Nitu, B.; Datieva, V.; Odin, P. Antonini: ADevice-Aided Treatment Strategies in Advanced Parkinson's DiseaseInternational Review of Neurobiology. *Int. Rev. Neurobiol.* **2017**, *132*, 453–474.
18. Odin, P.; Chaudhuri, K.R.; Slevin, J.T.; Volkmann, J.; Dietrichs, E.; Martinez-Martin, P.; Krauss, J.K.; Henriksen, T.; Katzenschlager, R.; Antonini, A.; et al. Collective physician perspectives on non-oral medication approaches for the management of clinically relevant unresolved issues in Parkinson's disease: Consensus from an international survey and discussion program. *Park. Relat. Disord.* **2015**, *21*, 1133–1144. [CrossRef]
19. Nyholm, D. The rationale for continuous dopaminergic stimulation in advanced Parkinson's disease. *Park. Relat. Disord.* **2007**, *13*, S13–S17. [CrossRef] [PubMed]
20. Rätsch, C.; Hofmann, A. *The Encyclopedia of Psychoactive Plants*; Simon & Schuster: New York, NY, USA, 2005.
21. Arppe, A.E. UebereinemerkwürdigeVeränderung des MorphinsdurchSchwefelsäure. *Justus Liebigs Ann. Chem.* **1845**, *55*, 96–101. [CrossRef]
22. Matthiessen, A. Researches into the chemical constitution of the opium bases. Part I—On the action of hydrochloric. *Proc. R. Soc. Lond.* **1868**, *17*, 455–460.
23. Ribarič, S. The pharmacological properties and therapeutic use of apomorphine. *Molecules* **2012**, *17*, 5289–5309. [CrossRef]

24. Pfeiffer, R.F.; Gutmann, L.; Hull, K.L.; Bottini, P.B.; Sherry, J.H. Continued efficacy and safety of subcutaneous apomorphine in patients with advanced Parkinson's disease. *Park. Relat. Disord.* **2007**, *13*, 93–100. [CrossRef]
25. Isaacson, S.; Lew, M.; Ondo, W.; Hubble, J.; Clinch, T.; Pagan, F. Apomorphine subcutaneous injection for the management of morning akinesia in Parkinson's disease. *Mov. Disord. Clin. Pract.* **2017**, *4*, 78–83. [CrossRef] [PubMed]
26. Trenkwalder, C.; Chaudhuri, K.R.; Ruiz, P.J.G.; LeWitt, P.; Katzenschlager, R.; Sixel-Döring, F.; Henriksen, T.; Sesar, Á.; Poewe, W.; Baker, M.; et al. Expert Consensus Group for Use of Apomorphine in Parkinson's Disease. Expert consensus group report on the use of apomorphine in the treatment of Parkinson's disease—Clinical practice recommendations. *Park. Relat. Disord.* **2015**, *21*, 1023–1030. [CrossRef] [PubMed]
27. Katzenschlager, R.; Poewe, W.; Rascol, O.; Trenkwalder, C.; Deuschl, G.; Chaudhuri, K.R.; Henriksen, T.; Van Laar, T.; Spivey, K.; Vel, S.; et al. Apomorphine subcutaneous infusion in patients with Parkinson's disease with persistent motor fluctuations (TOLEDO): A multicentre, double-blind, randomised, placebo-controlled trial. *Lancet Neurol.* **2018**, *17*, 749–759. [CrossRef]
28. Nyholm, D. Duodopa®treatment for advanced Parkinson's disease: A review of efficacy and safety. *Park. Relat. Disord.* **2012**, *18*, 916–929. [CrossRef] [PubMed]
29. Aldred, J.; Kovacs, N.; Pontieri, F.; Standaert, D.; Bourgeois, P.; Davis, T.; Cubo, E.; Anca-Herschkovitsch, M.; Iansek, R.; Siddiqui, M.; et al. Abstract. Improvements in Dyskinesia with Levodopa-Carbidopa Intestinal Gel in Advanced Parkinson's Disease Patients in a 'Real-World' Study: Interim Results of the Multinational DUO GLOBE Study With up to 24 Months Follow-Up. *Neurology* **2020**, *94* (Suppl. 15), 1824.
30. Wirdefeldt, K.; Odin, P.; Nyholm, D. Levodopa–Carbidopa Intestinal Gel in Patients with Parkinson's Disease: A Systematic Review. *CNS Drugs* **2016**, *30*, 381–404. [CrossRef] [PubMed]
31. Antonini, A.; Poewe, W.; Chaudhuri, K.R.; Jech, R.; Pickut, B.; Pirtošek, Z.; Szasz, J.; Valldeoriola, F.; Winkler, C.; Bergmann, L.; et al. Levodopa-carbidopa intestinal gel in advanced Parkinson's: Final results of the GLORIA registry. *Park. Relat. Disord.* **2017**, *45*, 13–20. [CrossRef] [PubMed]
32. Xu, W.; Russo, G.S.; Hashimoto, T.; Zhang, J.; Vitek, J.L. Subthalamic Nucleus Stimulation Modulates Thalamic Neuronal Activity. *J. Neurosci.* **2008**, *28*, 11916–11924. [CrossRef] [PubMed]
33. Perestelo-Pérez, L.; Rivero-Santana, A.; Pérez-Ramos, J.; Serrano-Pérez, P.; Panetta, J.; Hilarión, P. Deep brain stimulation in Parkinson's disease: Meta-analysis of randomized controlled trials. *J. Neurol.* **2014**, *261*, 2051–2060. [CrossRef]
34. Xie, C.-L.; Shao, B.; Chen, J.; Zhou, Y.; Lin, S.-Y.; Wang, W.-W. Effects of neurostimulation for advanced Parkinson's disease patients on motor symptoms: A multiple-treatments meta-analysis of randomized controlled trials. *Sci. Rep.* **2016**, *6*, 1–11. [CrossRef] [PubMed]
35. Martinez-Martin, P.; Reddy, P.; Katzenschlager, R.; Antonini, A.; Todorova, A.; Odin, P.; Henriksen, T.; Martin, A.; Calandrella, D.; Rizos, A.; et al. EuroInf: A multicenter comparative observational study of apomorphine and levodopa infusion in Parkinson's disease. *Mov. Disord. Off. J. Mov. Disord. Soc.* **2015**, *30*, 510–516. [CrossRef]
36. Dafsari, H.S.; Martinez-Martin, P.; Rizos, A.; Trost, M.; dos Santos Ghilardi, M.G.; Reddy, P.; Sauerbier, A.; Petry-Schmelzer, J.N.; Kramberger, M.; Borgemeester, R.W.; et al. EuroInf 2: Subthalamic stimulation, apomorphine, and levodopa infusion in Parkinson's disease. *Mov. Disord. Off. J. Mov. Disord. Soc.* **2019**, *34*, 353–365. [CrossRef]
37. Goetz, C.G.; Fahn, S.; Martinez-Martin, P.; Poewe, W.; Sampaio, C.; Stebbins, G.T.; Stern, M.B.; Tilley, B.C.; Dodel, R.; Dubois, B.; et al. Movement Disorder Society-Sponsored Revision of the Unified Parkinson's Disease Rating Scale (MDS-UPDRS): Process, format, and clinimetric testing plan. *Mov. Disord.* **2007**, *22*, 41–47. [CrossRef] [PubMed]
38. Goetz, C.G.; Stebbins, G.T.; Chmura, T.A.; Fahn, S.; Poewe, W.; Tanner, C.M. Teaching program for the Movement Disorder Society-Sponsored Revision of the Unified Parkinson's Disease Rating Scale:(MDS-UPDRS). *Mov. Disord.* **2010**, *25*, 1190–1194. [CrossRef]
39. Hoehn, M.M.; Yahr, M.D. Parkinsonism: Onset, progression, and mortality. *Neurology* **1967**, *17*, 427–442. [CrossRef] [PubMed]
40. Verbaan, D.; van Rooden, S.; Benit, C.; van Zwet, E.; Marinus, J.; van Hilten, J. SPES/SCOPA and MDS-UPDRS: Formulas for converting scores of two motor scales in Parkinson's disease. *Park. Relat. Disord.* **2011**, *17*, 632–634. [CrossRef]
41. Martinez-Martin, P.; Benito-León, J.; Burguera, J.A.; Castro, A.; Linazasoro, G.; Martínez-Castrillo, J.C.; Valldeoriola, F.; Vázquez, A.; Vivancos, F.; del Val, J.; et al. The SCOPA–Motor Scale for assessment of Parkinson's disease is a consistent and valid measure. *J. Clin. Epidemiol* **2005**, *58*, 674–679. [CrossRef] [PubMed]
42. Chaudhuri, K.R.; Pal, S.; DiMarco, A.; Whately-Smith, C.; Bridgman, K.; Mathew, R.; Pezzela, F.R.; Forbes, A.; Högl, B.; Trenkwalder, C. The Parkinson's disease sleep scale: A new instrument for assessing sleep and nocturnal disability in Parkinson's disease. *J. Neurol. Neurosurg. Psychiatry* **2002**, *73*, 629–635. [CrossRef]
43. Chaudhuri, K.R.; Rizos, A.; Trenkwalder, C.; Rascol, O.; Pal, S.; Martino, D.; Carroll, C.; Paviour, D.; Falup-Pecurariu, C.; Kessel, B.; et al. King's Parkinson's disease pain scale, the first scale for pain in PD: An international validation. *Mov. Disord.* **2015**, *30*, 1623–1631. [CrossRef] [PubMed]
44. Nasreddine, Z.S.; Phillips, N.A.; Bedirian, V.; Charbonneau, S.; Whitehead, V.; Collin, I.; Cummings, J.L.; Chertkow, H. The Montreal Cognitive Assessment, MoCA: A Brief Screening Tool For Mild Cognitive Impairment. *J. Am. Geriatr. Soc.* **2005**, *53*, 695–699. [CrossRef]
45. Zigmond, A.S.; Snaith, R.P. The Hospital Anxiety and Depression Scale. *Acta Psychiatr. Scand.* **1983**, *67*, 361–370. [CrossRef]
46. Jenkinson, C.; Fitzpatrick, R.; Peto, V.; Greenhall, R.; Hyman, N. The PDQ-8: Development and validation of a short-form Parkinson's disease questionnaire. *Psychol. Health* **1997**, *12*, 805–814. [CrossRef]

47. Peto, V.; Jenkinson, C.; Fitzpatrick, R.; Greenhall, R. The development and validation of a short measure of functioning and well being for individuals with Parkinson's disease. *Qual. Life Res.* **1995**, *4*, 241–248. [CrossRef] [PubMed]
48. Tysnes, O.B.; Storstein, A. Epidemiology of Parkinson's disease. *J. Neural. Transm.* **2017**, *124*, 901–905. [CrossRef] [PubMed]
49. Ahlskog, J.E.; Muenter, M.D. Frequency of levodopa-related dyskinesias and motor fluctuations as estimated from the cumulative literature. *Mov. Disord.* **2001**, *16*, 448–458. [CrossRef] [PubMed]
50. Storch, A.; Schneider, C.B.; Wolz, M.; Stürwald, Y.; Nebe, A.; Odin, P.; Mahler, A.; Fuchs, G.; Jost, W.H.; Chaudhuri, K.R.; et al. Nonmotor fluctuations in Parkinson disease: Severity and correlation with motor complications. *Neurology* **2013**, *80*, 800–809. [CrossRef] [PubMed]
51. Papapetropoulos, S. (Spyros) Patient Diaries As a Clinical Endpoint in Parkinson's Disease Clinical Trials. *CNS Neurosci. Ther.* **2011**, *18*, 380–387. [CrossRef]
52. Griffiths, R.I.; Kotschet, K.; Arfon, S.; Xu, Z.M.; Johnson, W.; Drago, J.; Evans, A.; Kempster, P.; Raghav, S.; Horne, M.K. Automated Assessment of Bradykinesia and Dyskinesia in Parkinson's Disease. *J. Park. Dis.* **2012**, *2*, 47–55. [CrossRef]
53. Kotschet, K.; Johnson, W.; McGregor, S.; Kettlewell, J.; Kyoong, A.; O'Driscoll, D.M.; Turton, A.R.; Griffiths, R.I.; Horne, M.K. Daytime sleep in Parkinson's Disease measured by episodes of immobility. *Park. Relat. Disord.* **2014**, *20*, 578–583. [CrossRef]
54. Braybrook, M.; O'Connor, S.; Churchward, P.; Perera, T.; Farzanehfar, P.; Horne, M. An Ambulatory Tremor Score for Parkinson's Disease. *J. Park. Dis.* **2016**, *6*, 723–731. [CrossRef]
55. Farzanehfar, P.; Horne, M. Evaluation of the Parkinson's KinetiGraph in monitoring and managing Parkinson's disease. *Expert Rev. Med. Devices* **2017**, *14*, 583–591. [CrossRef]
56. Horne, M.; Volkmann, J.; Sannelli, S.; Luyet, P.-P.; Moro, E. An evaluation of the parkinson'skinetigraph (pkg) as a tool to support deep brain stimulation eligibility assessment in patients with parkinson's disease. *Mov. Disord.* **2017**, *32* (Suppl. 2).
57. Schuepbach, W.; Rau, J.; Knudsen, K.; Volkmann, J.; Krack, P.; Timmermann, L.; Hälbig, T.; Hesekamp, H.; Navarro, S.; Meier, N.; et al. Neurostimulation for Parkinson's Disease with Early Motor Complications. *N. Engl. J. Med.* **2013**, *368*, 610–622. [CrossRef] [PubMed]
58. Moro, E.; Allert, N.; Eleopra, R.; Houeto, J.-L.; Phan, T.-M.; Stoevelaar, H.; International Study Group onReferral Criteria for DBS. A decision tool to support appropriate referral for deep brain stimulation in Parkinson's disease. *J. Neurol.* **2009**, *256*, 83–88. [CrossRef] [PubMed]
59. Okun, M.; Fernandez, H.H.; Pedraza, O.; Misra, M.; Lyons, K.E.; Pahwa, R.; Tarsy, D.; Scollins, L.; Corapi, K.; Friehs, G.M.; et al. Development and initial validation of a screening tool for Parkinson disease surgical candidates. *Neurology* **2004**, *63*, 161–163. [CrossRef] [PubMed]
60. Willis, A.W.; Schootman, M.; Kung, N.; Wang, X.-Y.; Perlmutter, J.S.; Racette, B.A. Disparities in deep brain stimulation surgery among insured elders with Parkinson disease. *Neurology* **2014**, *82*, 163–171. [CrossRef]
61. Lim, S.-Y.; O'Sullivan, S.S.; Kotschet, K.; Gallagher, D.A.; Lacey, C.; Lawrence, A.D.; Lees, A.J.; O'Sullivan, D.J.; Peppard, R.F.; Rodrigues, J.P.; et al. Dopamine dysregulation syndrome, impulse control disorders and punding after deep brain stimulation surgery for Parkinson's disease. *J. Clin. Neurosci.* **2009**, *16*, 1148–1152. [CrossRef]
62. Jenner, P. Wearing Off, Dyskinesia, and the Use of Continuous Drug Delivery in Parkinson's Disease. *Neurol. Clin.* **2013**, *31*, S17–S35. [CrossRef]
63. Stacy, M.; Hauser, R.; Oertel, W.; Schapira, A.; Sethi, K.; Stocchi, F.; Tolosa, E. End-of-dose wearing off in parkinson disease: A 9-question survey assessment. *Clin. Neuropharmacol.* **2006**, *29*, 312–321. [CrossRef]
64. Stocchi, F.; Antonini, A.; Barone, P.; Tinazzi, M.; Zappia, M.; Onofrj, M.; Ruggieri, S.; Morgante, L.; Bonuccelli, U.; Lopiano, L.; et al. Early DEtection of wEaring off in Parkinson disease: The DEEP study. *Park. Relat. Disord.* **2014**, *20*, 204–211. [CrossRef]
65. Florkowski, C.M. Sensitivity, Specificity, Receiver-Operating Characteristic (ROC) Curves and Likelihood Ratios: Communicating the Performance of Diagnostic Tests. *Clin. Biochem. Rev.* **2008**, *29* (Suppl. 1), S83–S87.
66. Khodakarami, H.; Farzanehfar, P.; Horne, M. The Use of Data from the Parkinson's KinetiGraph to Identify Potential Candidates for Device Assisted Therapies. *Sensors* **2019**, *19*, 2241. [CrossRef]
67. Odin, P.; Chaudhuri, K.R.; Volkmann, J.; Antonini, A.; Storch, A.; Dietrichs, E.; Pirtošek, Z.; Henriksen, T.; Horne, M.; Devos, D.; et al. Viewpoint and practical recommendations from a movement disorder specialist panel on objective measurement in the clinical management of Parkinson's disease. *NPJ Park. Dis.* **2018**, *4*, 1–7. [CrossRef] [PubMed]
68. Pahwa, R.; Isaacson, S.H.; Torres-Russotto, D.; Nahab, F.B.; Lynch, P.M.; Kotschet, K.E. Role of the Personal KinetiGraph in the routine clinical assessment of Parkinson's disease: Recommendations from an expert panel. *Expert Rev. Neurother.* **2018**, *18*, 669–680. [CrossRef] [PubMed]
69. Sharma, J.C.; Lewis, A. Weight in Parkinson's Disease: Phenotypic Significance. *Int. Rev. Neurobiol.* **2017**, *134*, 891–919. [PubMed]

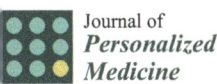

Review

Personalized Medicine in Parkinson's Disease: New Options for Advanced Treatments

Takayasu Mishima [1], Shinsuke Fujioka [1], Takashi Morishita [2], Tooru Inoue [2] and Yoshio Tsuboi [1,*]

[1] Department of Neurology, School of Medicine, Fukuoka University, 7-45-1, Nanakuma, Johnan-ku, Fukuoka 814-0180, Japan; mishima1006@fukuoka-u.ac.jp (T.M.); shinsuke@cis.fukuoka-u.ac.jp (S.F.)
[2] Department of Neurosurgery, School of Medicine, Fukuoka University, Fukuoka 814-0180, Japan; tmorishita@fukuoka-u.ac.jp (T.M.); toinoue@fukuoka-u.ac.jp (T.I.)
* Correspondence: tsuboi@cis.fukuoka-u.ac.jp; Tel.: +81-92-801-1011; Fax: +81-92-865-7900

Abstract: Parkinson's disease (PD) presents varying motor and non-motor features in each patient owing to their different backgrounds, such as age, gender, genetics, and environmental factors. Furthermore, in the advanced stages, troublesome symptoms vary between patients due to motor and non-motor complications. The treatment of PD has made great progress over recent decades and has directly contributed to an improvement in patients' quality of life, especially through the progression of advanced treatment. Deep brain stimulation, radiofrequency, MR–guided focused ultrasound, gamma knife, levodopa-carbidopa intestinal gel, and apomorphine are now used in the clinical setting for this disease. With multiple treatment options currently available for all stages of PD, we here discuss the most recent options for advanced treatment, including cell therapy in advanced PD, from the perspective of personalized medicine.

Keywords: Parkinson's disease; deep brain stimulation; levodopa-carbidopa intestinal gel; apomorphine; radiofrequency; focused ultrasound; induced pluripotent stem cells; cell therapy; gene therapy; personalized medicine

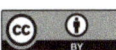

1. Introduction

Personalized medicine is an emerging field that seeks to tailor the treatment of individual patients based on their clinical characteristics, biomarkers, genetics, and other factors [1,2]. Other factors include specific comorbidities, complications, and patient background. To date, personalized medicine in Parkinson's disease (PD) has not been fully realized due to barriers such as cost and genetic counseling although personalized medicine is used in PD patients in clinical settings when treatments are tailored based on motor and non-motor features [3–7].

PD is a heterogeneous disorder in which motor and non-motor features of varying types and degrees may appear quite separately in individuals [1,8]. Indeed, the etiology and pathogenesis of PD include a mixture of factors without any diagnostically reliable biomarkers; therefore, the diagnosis of PD is still based on a clinical assessment [9,10]. It is known that the prognosis of PD differs between clinical types, with tremor-dominant types progressing slower than postural instability gait difficulty (PIGD) types [11]. The Parkinson's Progression Markers Initiative (PPMI) clinical study has revealed more detailed subtypes of PD [12]. The authors classified PD into mild motor-predominant, intermediate, and diffuse malignant types [12]. Several studies have been undertaken to address and detect possible biomarkers, which may predict the progression of individual PD patients [13].

Historically, the first PD treatments involved a surgical approach. In 1952, Narabayashi et al. performed the world's first pallidotomy for PD patients and described its positive effect [14]. In the early 1960s, L-dopa therapy was initiated, but initially, low doses failed to show efficacy in many PD patients; Cotzias then initiated the use of high-dose therapy, and the modern regimen for L-dopa therapy was established [15]. L-dopa is still the gold standard, and its combination with dopamine agonist, monoamine oxidase type B inhibitor, catechol-O-methyltransferase inhibitor and/or non-dopaminergic medication has been used to treat L-dopa related motor and non-motor complications for many years. However, in the advanced stage, despite adjustments to these medications, it is impossible to manage these complications, and finally surgical intervention is required in some patients. The use of stereotactic neurosurgery declined with the introduction of the drug L-dopa as an effective oral medication; but stereotactic neurosurgery was revived when it was shown to be effective in treating motor complications including wearing-off and dyskinesia [16,17]. Later, deep brain stimulation (DBS) was introduced, and became the gold standard of treatment for advanced PD motor features [18]. Today, various advanced treatments such as DBS, radiofrequency, MR–guided focused ultrasound (MRgFUS), gamma knife, levodopa-carbidopa intestinal gel (LCIG), and apomorphine are available, although the availability of treatments varies depending on country and region. Clinical practice guidelines for early treatment of PD have been published in various countries and are often recommended by experts [19–21]. Standard pharmacological and non-pharmacological treatments are required during treatment, and the need for personalized medicine becomes more obvious when aiming to achieve an appropriate symptomatic and disease-modifying treatment with the right dose, right time, and minimum side effects in a specific patient. On the other hand, guidelines for the treatment of advanced PD have not been established, and in particular, the indication criteria and exclusion criteria for device-aided therapy have not been clarified. DBS and LCIG are the most established treatments for advanced stage PD in recent years, apomorphine subcutaneous infusion and MRgFUS have also become available, and efforts to incorporate them into personalized medicine will become important in the future. This review focuses on the advanced treatment of PD including cell therapy and gene therapy. Furthermore, we discuss aspects of personalized medicine that are currently available for the advanced treatment of PD.

2. Advanced Treatments

In this review, we use the term "advanced treatments" when refering to DBS, LCIG, apomorphine injection, MRgFUS, and other non-medication approaches.

Although the aim of advanced treatment in PD is to improve motor features, this treatment has also been shown to be effective for certain non-motor features [22]. The timing of the introduction of advanced treatments such as DBS or LCIG varies from patient to patient, but, as suggested by Antonini et al. [23], the presence of off-symptoms for more than 2 h a day, troublesome dyskinesia for more than 1 h a day, and levodopa administration of more than 5 times a day may be indicators for advanced PD. The authors described the indications for advanced treatments in PD patients as follows. Patients with good L-dopa response, good cognition, and <70 years of age were considered as good candidates for DBS, LCIG, and apomorphine subcutaneous infusion. More specifically, patients with troublesome dyskinesia can be treated with DBS or LCIG. Patients with L-dopa-resistant tremor were considered good targets for DBS. Previous authors also propose an indicator of which device–aided therapy is appropriate, based on each patient's background, motor and non-motor features, and activities of daily living by using the Delphi approach [23]. However, with the emergence of new options, it may be necessary to further refine the criteria for personalized treatment. In addition, we should be mindful of whether these advanced treatments are suitable or unsuitable for individual patients on an evidence basis; this currently remains ambiguous.

Currently, or in the near future, the advanced treatment options for PD motor features include/will include DBS, LCIG, apomorphine, MRgFUS, cell therapy, and gene therapy (Figure 1). For medication-resistant tremor associated with PD, the main treatment options are DBS, MRgFUS, radiofrequency, and gamma knife. The characteristics of each treatment for tremor are shown in Supplementary Table S1. Below, we focus on and briefly describe the motor features of PD and outline each relevant advanced treatment. Table 1 briefly shows indication, advantages, disadvantages, and adverse effects for DBS, LCIG, and apomorphine, which are currently established advanced treatments for PD.

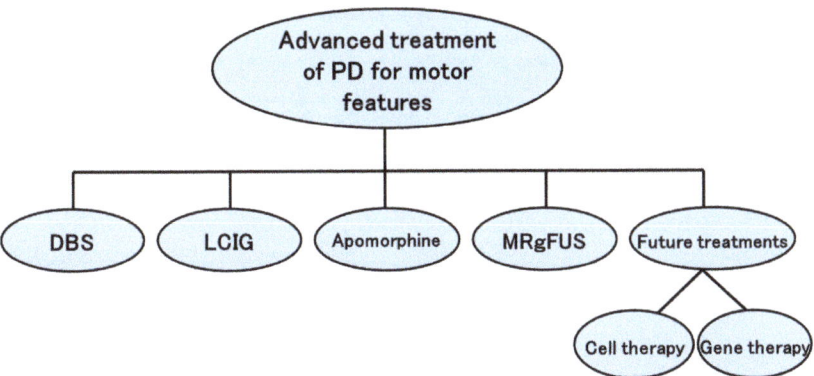

Figure 1. Advanced treatment for motor features of Parkinson's disease. PD: Parkinson's disease; DBS: deep brain stimulation; LCIG: Levodopa-carbidopa intestinal gel; MRgFUS: MR–guided focused ultrasound.

Table 1. Comparison of different advanced treatments.

	DBS	LCIG	Apomorphine
Indication	Motor complications (especially dyskinesia)	Motor complications	Motor complications (especially motor fluctuations)
Advantages	Dopaminergic medication reduction	No age limit	Minimally invasive procedures
Disadvantages	Invasive procedures	Requires caregivers to handle devices	Requires caregivers to handle devices
Adverse effects	Psychiatric and cognitive changes	Tube trouble	Skin reaction or trouble

DBS: deep brain stimulation; LCIG: Levodopa-carbidopa intestinal gel.

2.1. Deep Brain Stimulation (DBS)

Today, DBS has become one of the most successful surgical treatments in the advanced stages of PD and has been performed in many patients worldwide. During DBS, electrodes are implanted deep in the brain, a pulse generator is implanted in the chest wall, and an electric current is passed through a connected lead wire to stimulate the targeted deep brain tissue (Figure 2). In addition to the selection of the DBS target and the stimulation parameters, new technologies have enabled a personalized approach to PD.

Regarding the brain targets, the subthalamic nucleus (STN) and globus pallidus internus (GPi) are commonly used as targets for DBS in PD. Both targets have their own strengths, and previous studies have compared the therapeutic effects of DBS on motor and non-motor features in both targets. However, as yet, there are no clear criteria for the choice of DBS target for PD patients and this is often determined by the physician's preference. Negida et al. reviewed the selection between STN and GPi [24]. They report that STN-DBS is preferable from a cost point-of-view, as it allows a greater reduction in anti-Parkinson medication and less battery consumption, while GPi-DBS is better for patients who have problems with mood, speech, or cognition [24].

Other targets are the ventralis intermedius (Vim) and pedunculopontine nucleus (PPN) [25]. Vim-DBS is less effective for bradykinesia and rigidity, but very effective for tremor, and is therefore indicated for PD patients with tremor predominance and minimal motor features other than tremor. Meanwhile, PPN-DBS is effective for postural instability and gait disturbance, and has been suggested to reduce the incidence of falls; however, reported effects are variable [25,26]. In Supplementary Table S2, we show the effects of DBS on individual symptoms for each target (STN, GPi, Vim, and PPN). Although there are currently only a few reports, the effects of targeting the post-subthalamic area, or caudal zona incerta (PSA/cZi) are also expected to be positive [27]. Motor features of PD are bilateral in most cases and often have a right/left side dominance. The effectiveness of unilateral STN and GPi-DBS has also been reported [28,29], indicating that unilateral DBS may be an option, especially in cases with a strong left/right dominance. Furthermore, stepped GPi and STN-DBS, which is initially unilateral and then contralateral, or combined unilateral STN and contralateral GPi DBS may offer an effective resolution for certain PD patients [30,31]. It is also noteworthy that the connectomic approach has addressed the identification of stimulation targets in individual cases [32,33], and this technological advancement may also contribute to personalized DBS.

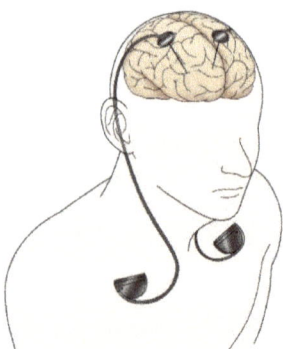

Figure 2. Deep brain stimulation (DBS).

In recent years, with the advancement of DBS technology, directional leads [34–40] and adaptive DBS (aDBS) [41] have been developed and made clinically available. There are many reports showing the usefulness of directional leads not only in PD but also in essential tremor (ET) [34–40]. Directional leads can be particularly useful in optimizing STN-DBS stimulation to expand therapeutic windows and avoid stimulation-induced side effects [34]. Krüger et al. showed that tremor was significantly improved after exchange from standard to directional DBS in ET patients. This is the first publication to date that showed a clinical superiority of directional DBS. Thus, directional DBS may have high potential for patients with advanced symptoms [40]. aDBS is a technique that was developed to enable analysis of local field potentials from leads in STN and/or GPi, revealing that beta oscillations are associated with motor features of PD [41]. Conventional DBS conveys sustained stimulation under conditions of constant stimulus, although a change in stimulus is possible. In contrast, aDBS, which uses beta oscillations as an index for control, may have higher therapeutic effects and lower battery consumption than conventional DBS [42]. Research in regulating the stimulation of DBS has also progressed, for example, low-frequency stimulation has been reported to have beneficial effects in patients with "freezing of gait" (FOG) [27]. In addition, recent studies have shown the efficacy of variable stimulation patterns for FOG [43] and cycling mode stimulation for tremor refractory to conventional continuous stimulation patterns [44]. With these new techniques and stimulus adjustments, further improvement of motor and non-motor features in PD patients is expected. Therefore, it is important for clinicians to understand the advantages of devices made by different manufacturers.

Thus, DBS may be the advanced treatment that is most suited to personalized medicine. Clinical teams should be aware that selection of the optimal brain target(s), device, and the stimulation parameters are all critically important. It is necessary to decide the optimal indication for surgical treatment according to the timing of treatment and an individual's unmet needs. In addition, most patients on whom surgery is performed are in an advanced stage of PD; therefore, support such as medical management, exercise therapy, and a suitable living environment are required even after DBS treatment. Motor complications are also indications for DBS. The advantage is that it does not require a caregiver, as shown in Table 1 above; however, the disadvantage is the possibility of psychiatric and cognitive changes. Multidisciplinary team medical care is a major driver behind solving these problems. This will be described in detail later.

We discuss potential treatments at the end of this section. Optogenetics is technology to control the functions of neurons by using genetically coded, light-gated ion channels or pumps, and light. This biological technique has contributed to our understanding of nervous system function. Although the application of optogenetics to non-human primates is limited, Watanabe et al. shows that neural activity and behavior in non-human primates can be manipulated optogenetically [45]. These studies may also lead to applications for DBS. In addition, the evolving technologies of magnetogenetics, which manipulating neurons with magnetic stimuli, and sonogenetics, which focuses on the genetic modulation of ultrasound-sensitive neurons and their specific responses to ultrasound, could contribute to the advanced treatment of PD for the possibility of being minimally invasive [46,47].

2.2. Levodopa-Carbidopa Intestinal Gel (LCIG)

Continuous dopaminergic delivery is required to resolve motor complications that are problematic in advanced PD patients. In addressing this situation, the mechanism of LCIG is ideal: it involves continuous infusion of levodopa directly into the jejunum (Figure 3), where it is absorbed via a transgastrostomal jejunal tube that maintains a constant blood levodopa concentration, thereby reducing motor complications [48]. The effect on motor complications such as reduction in off-time per day can be maintained for a lengthy period [49]. It is also effective in the treatment of cases of FOG that are resistant to pharmacological treatment [50]. LCIG is reported to improve non-motor features such as anxiety, sleep disorders, depression, hallucinations, impulse control disorders, and cognition [49,51,52]; however, there is less evidence than for its effects on motor features, so more research is needed in the future. The frequency of complications with LCIG is high [53]. Surgery-related complications include pain, gastrointestinal symptoms, and device failure, most of which decrease in frequency by two weeks post-surgery [53]. In addition to device failure, weight loss, cholecystitis, and neuropathy are complications of the long-term course [54–56]. It is necessary to check each patient's background before introducing an LCIG device, as, if the patient has difficulty with its use, a caregiver may be needed. The optimal indication for LCIG also needs to be determined. A multi-disciplinary medical team can be very helpful in advancing this treatment.

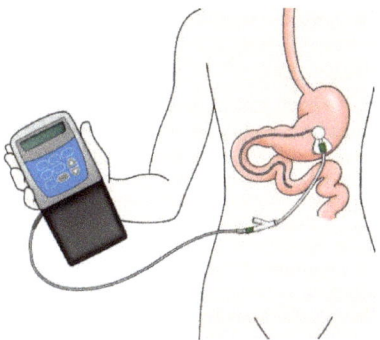

Figure 3. Levodopa-carbidopa intestinal gel (LCIG).

2.3. Apomorphine

Apomorphine, a dopamine agonist, is administered through subcutaneous rescue injection or subcutaneous infusion. Rescue injection is an established rescue therapy for patients with PD associated with motor fluctuations [57,58]. Katzenschlager et al. describes the efficacy of apomorphine subcutaneous infusion in patients with PD with motor fluctuations through the presentation of a multicenter, double-blind, randomized, placebo-controlled trial in 2018 [59]. This has now become one of the advanced treatment options for PD, along with DBS and LCIG. The indications for apomorphine are motor complications; this is a minimally invasive procedure compared to DBS and LCIG, as shown in Table 1 above; however, if the patient is unable to operate the device, a caregiver may be required. In Japan, rescue injection is available, but subcutaneous infusion is not, so further expansion of the treatment is expected in the near future.

2.4. Ablative Surgery

2.4.1. Radiofrequency Lesioning

Radiofrequency is the oldest surgical treatment for PD and was a cornerstone of the development of DBS. Radiofrequency thalamotomy is an established treatment for tremor. Tasker compares the efficacy and complications of radiofrequency thalamotomy and DBS for symptoms of tremor [60]. This study shows that DBS is more costly and requires more management, but DBS has fewer complications than radiofrequency thalamotomy because of the need to adjust stimulation parameters in DBS [60]. More recently, DBS has become the preferred choice over radiofrequency for tremor. Complications of both radiofrequency and DBS include cerebral hemorrhage. Radiofrequency thalamotomy can be repeated in cases of tremor recurrence, and additional DBS may be an option [60]. Schreglmann et al. reviews functional neurosurgery for tremor [61]. The authors indicate that when comparing the size of lesions following treatment with radiofrequency or MRgFUS, at 12 months after surgery, the size of lesions undergoing radiofrequency may be greater than that of FUS [61]. A study examining the recurrence rate of MRgFUS in patients with essential tremor shows that the recurrence rate decreases with increased lesion size [62]. Thus, at this time, radiofrequency may be less likely to result in recurrence than MRgFUS. For PD patients who are against the use of an implanted device for cosmetic reasons, thalamotomy is an alternative treatment option for tremor.

2.4.2. Gamma Knife

Similar to MRgFUS, gamma knife does not require burr hole craniotomy and is considered as a minimally invasive treatment; however, it does not allow the intraoperative observation of symptoms. In addition, physicians should be cautious that this therapy may result in late cyst formation and/or radiation necrosis in some cases as a high level of radiation is required for the treatment. Unilateral gamma knife thalamotomy has been shown to be effective in treating tremor in PD [63]. In addition, studies on the motor features of PD following the use of gamma knife pallidotomy and subthalamic gamma knife radiosurgery have been investigated [64,65]. Unilateral gamma knife thalamotomy is a potential alternative to DBS and radiofrequency thalamotomy for tremor in PD patients with contraindications for surgery [63]; however, due to the success and increased use of MRgFUS, the latter treatment may replace gamma knife in the future when MRgFUS overcomes the current technical issues because of the possibility of secondary neoplasia due to radiation exposure and difficulty in detecting complications during the procedure, due to the time for the treatment to take effect.

2.4.3. MR–Guided Focused Ultrasound (MRgFUS)

MRgFUS is a treatment that has recently received tremendous attention. FUS was originally difficult to apply for intracranial diseases due to the attenuation and scattering of ultrasound in the skull, but advances in technology have overcome these problems. MRgFUS can be repositioned, or treatment discontinued depending on the neurological condition of the patient being treated. It does require the total shaving of the patient's head, but it does not require the burr hole craniotomy that is needed for DBS or radiofrequency. Thus, MRgFUS is considered a minimally invasive therapy (Supplementary Table S1). However, physicians should be cautious that the incidence of permanent complications of MRgFUS may be higher than DBS due to the nature of lesioning [66]. For example, a recent randomized trial of MRgFUS subthalamotomy reveals a complication rate as high as 25%, including gait and speech disturbance as well as new onset of dyskinesia [67]. The complications reported in the same study are consistent with conventional radiofrequency subthalamotomy, despite the fact that subthalamotomy is performed unilaterally [68], so clinicians should be aware that any form of subthalamotomy may result in similar problems.

Bond et al. report the suppression of tremor following the application of unilateral MRgFUS thalamotomy in patients with PD [69]. Regarding other targets, MRgFUS subthalamotomy and pallidothalamic tractotomy for PD lead to the improvement of MDS UPDRS or UPDRS Part Three scores [67,70]. Based on these studies it is hoped that, in the not too distant future, this treatment will have an effect not only on tremor but also on other motor features. Furthermore, research into the relationship between lesion size and clinical outcome will help establish more optimal treatment methods. Because of concerns regarding complications of bilateral treatment of MRgFUS, it is a good indication for patients with prominent unilateral symptoms or tremor, and it is therefore thought to have the advantage over DBS therapy at this stage in patients who need improvement in unilateral symptoms [66,71].

2.5. Comparison of DBS and LCIG

A meta-analysis was performed based on comparisons between STN-DBS and LCIG [72]. In this study, no significant differences were noted between STN-DBS and LCIG on UPDRS Part Three and adverse events [72]. Furthermore, the results show no significant difference in motor features in the overall therapeutic effect of each surgical treatment. Moreover, EUROPAR and the International Parkinson and Movement Disorders Society Non-Motor Parkinson's Disease Study Group examined motor and non-motor features in STN-DBS, LCIG, and apomorphine [73]. The latter study, based on an eight-item Parkinson's disease questionnaire (PDQ-8), UPDRS Part Four, and NMSScale, reveals that total scores were improved significantly in all groups. The authors highlight the importance of holistic assessments to personalize treatment choices [73]. We show the advantages and disadvantages of DBS and LCIG from a perspective of holistic assessments in Supplementary Table S3.

2.6. Combination Therapy

In their study, Elkouzi et al. report a case series of advanced PD patients treated with DBS and LCIG [74]. Six patients were treated with DBS (bilateral STN DBS, bilateral GPi DBS, and unilateral GPi DBS) who subsequently received rescue LCIG therapy. Following this treatment, an improvement in the 39-item Parkinson's disease questionnaire (PDQ-39) was noted for four patients. The authors went on to propose an algorithm for the potential use of rescue LCIG therapy in PD-DBS patients. Therefore, PD-DBS patients with persistent or recurrent motor fluctuations who have difficulty with further DBS interventions may be candidates for additional LCIG treatment [74]. In addition to dual DBS and LCIG therapy, other surgical treatment combinations may be useful in selected cases, but cost does need to be considered.

2.7. Future Surgical Treatments

2.7.1. Cell Therapy

Since the 1980s, fetal dopaminergic transplantation has been performed in patients with PD and studies report an improvement in motor features following this treatment [75,76]. However, fetal dopaminergic transplantation encountered problems with ethical issues, including difficulty in obtaining sufficient amounts of fetal brain tissue, and contamination of serotonin neurons with associated dyskinesia. These problems have been solved following the introduction of induced pluripotent stem cell (iPSC) technology. Indeed, a primate study shows significant improvement two years after transplantation of human iPSCs into a primate PD model [77]. Human transplantation into PD patients was first practiced in Japan [78], where allogeneic transplantation is now performed [78]. In contrast, Schweitzer et al. performed autologous transplantations [79]; they report no significant change in MDS-UPDRS Part Three scores; however, they noted an improvement in PDQ-39 [79]. In autologous transplantation, if the patient has genetic variants, iPSCs are genome edited and differentiated into midbrain dopaminergic progenitor cells, which can then be transplanted (Figure 4). On the other hand, allogeneic transplantation requires immunosuppressive drugs; it is also advisable to check that the donated cells do not have genetic variants. Figure 4 shows the process of cell therapy in patients with PD using iPSCs. Drug treatment and rehabilitation are still needed in cases of cell therapy [80], and the collection of data from a greater series of cases is necessary to truly reflect the effectiveness of cell therapy using iPSCs.

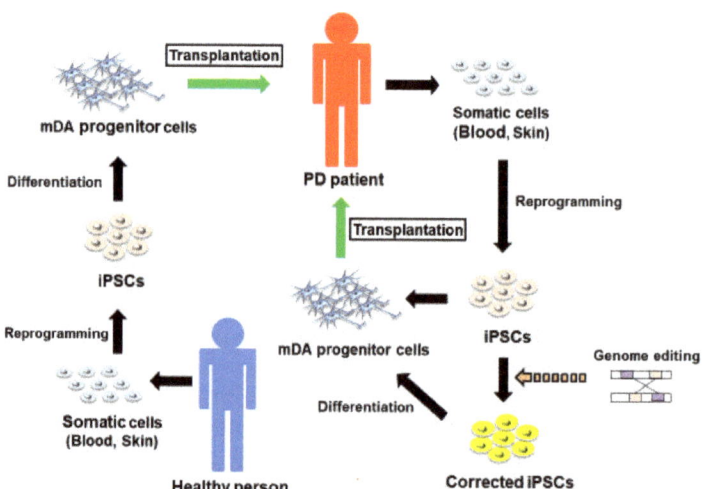

Figure 4. A schema showing cell therapy in patients with Parkinson's disease using induced pluripotent stem cells (iPSCs). PD: Parkinson's disease; mDA: midbrain dopaminergic.

2.7.2. Gene Therapy

Dopamine deficiency in the putamen causes motor features in PD. Therefore, gene therapy has been adopted to replenish dopamine by introducing genes of enzymes necessary for dopamine synthesis into neurons in the putamen [81]. An adeno-associated virus (AAV) vector has been the most commonly used gene therapy for PD patients in clinical trials, although an equine infectious anemia virus (EIAV) has also been used [81–86]. Muramatsu et al. [81] and Christine et al. [82] report that AAV vectors expressing aromatic-amino acid decarboxylase (AADC) were administered to the putamen of PD patients, and the patients subsequently showed improved UPDRS Part Three scores. Christine et al. further administered higher doses of AAV vectors to PD patients and showed increasing on-time in PD patients [83]. Gene therapy, implemented by injecting EIAV vectors carrying the three genes (tyrosine hydroxylase, AADC, and GTP-cyclohydrolase 1) into the putamen of PD patients, has also been performed [84]. Furthermore, gene therapy employing transfer of the trophic factor neurturin into the putamen [85] and glutamic acid decarboxylase into the STN [86] via an AAV vector have been conducted. The huge benefit of gene therapy is that it does not require immunosuppressive drugs, which are necessary for allogeneic cell transplantation using iPSCs; in addition, the mass production of vectors is possible.

Further research is needed to determine targets, dose, and which genes to introduce for the practical application of treatment in PD patients.

3. Evaluation of the Efficacy of Advanced Treatment

Since there are no disease-modifying treatments for PD, the current goal of PD treatment is to improve patient and caregiver satisfaction. Physicians may tend to focus on the improvement rate of MDS UPDRS Part Three scores when evaluating the effectiveness of advanced treatment. However, the possibility of a gap between physician evaluation of surgical treatment effectiveness and patient and caregiver satisfaction should be noted; despite this, few studies have examined patient satisfaction with advanced treatment for PD [87]. A large multicenter study of PD patients showed that MDS UPDRS Parts One and Two affect their quality of life (QOL) [88]. Although the short-form PDQ-8 and the PDQ-39 have been used in many studies [88–90], MDS UPDRS Parts One and Two, the patient reported outcome (PRO)-based assessments of patients' activities of daily living (ADL), is also useful in the assessment of advanced treatment. Regarding non-motor features, the Non-Motor Symptoms Scale for Parkinson's Disease (NMSS), the Non-Motor Symptoms Questionnaire (NMSQ), and MDS Non-Motor Rating Scale (MDS-NMS) may be useful for evaluating end points of advanced treatment. Furthermore, it is expected that outcomes assessed by caregivers [91] will also be used to judge the effectiveness of advanced treatment of PD.

4. Team Approach

Organization of multidisciplinary clinical care teams is recommended in PD treatment [92], and a team approach is essential for the realization of personalized medicine for advanced treatment in PD patients. An example of a team approach to advanced treatment of PD, particularly LCIG and stereotactic neurosurgery, is presented in Figure 5. Neurologists take a lead in determining treatment plans, but neurosurgeons are responsible for stereotactic neurosurgery, and gastroenterologists and colorectal surgeons are responsible for LCIG. Furthermore, psychiatrists are important in the evaluation and treatment of psychiatric symptoms, and dentists are needed to evaluate and care for dysphagia which is frequently seen in PD. Therapists play an important role in sustained rehabilitation, and assessment of ADL requires cooperation with therapists. The presence of a nurse is important for assessment of the patient's background, and PD nurses [92] are indispensable during the long process of advanced treatment. Caregivers as well as patients require nursing care. Pharmacist medication guidance is also important for the continuous treatment of various drugs. Higuchi et al. reveals that screening through the use of a team approach may be useful for more than just patient selection of DBS [93]. Supplementary Table S4 (DBS) and Table S5 (LCIG) show concerns from a multidisciplinary perspective in determining indications for advanced treatment of PD patients. Since any advanced treatment is invasive, patients may expect notable effects of such treatment in return, which may lead to reduced patient satisfaction [94]. Multidisciplinary informed consent is needed from patients and caregivers when advanced treatment is indicated. The above-mentioned improvement in QOL following cell therapy using iPSCs [79] may also benefit patient satisfaction with a team approach. Moreover, a team approach will be increasingly necessary in the implementation of cell therapy and gene therapy, which are expected to become more widespread in the near future.

A team approach also enables a tailored treatment plan for each patient based on patient-specific risks versus benefit analyses, accessibility to the center, supportive care circumstances, and cultural background. For example, surgical procedures requiring general anesthesia are contraindicated in patients with severe cardiopulmonary risks. Living in a remote area or poor supportive care circumstances may jeopardize LCIG, which requires daily medication renewal. Concerning cultural background, some patients may have a stigma against the use of devices, and in such cases lesion therapy and/or cell therapy may be a suitable option. Additionally, select patients may benefit from a combination of multiple treatment modalities (e.g., unilateral DBS and contralateral RF lesioning). We consider that a team approach at an experienced center would maximize the benefit of tailor-made treatment effects in the application of surgical procedures.

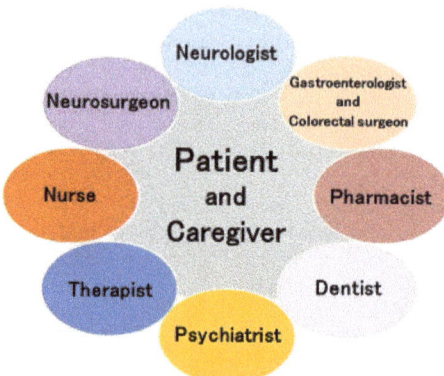

Figure 5. Team approach of advanced treatment for Parkinson's disease.

COVID-19 has led to major changes in medical systems globally [95]. It affects PD patients and particularly those that may have lost healthcare resources during the period of the pandemic [96]. During this period, the use of telemedicine, which is recommended in PD treatment, has been useful for outpatient care and may be continued into the future [97]. We conducted a questionnaire survey regarding telemedicine among PD patients in Japan [98]. The results revealed that a majority of patients were aware of the availability of this means of healthcare. Smartphone users, credit card users, and those who lived in regions distant from a hospital tend to prefer the convenience of this facility [98]. Although individual situations vary between countries and regions, telemedicine may be useful for continuing outpatient treatment of PD patients who have undergone advanced treatment. Indeed, the usefulness of telemedicine has been reported in DBS and LCIG even before the COVID-19 pandemic [99,100]. The spread of telemedicine may have a great impact on the choice of advanced treatment for PD.

5. Conclusions

Here, we have discussed various advanced treatments for advanced PD. In the future, there may be additional advanced treatment options, including cell therapy and gene therapy. In addition, the development of optogenetics, magnetogenetics, and sonogenetics is expected. Therefore, it is important to consider the individual symptoms, patient background, and cost of these options when deciding on advanced treatment.

Supplementary Materials: The following are available online at https://www.mdpi.com/article/10.3390/jpm11070650/s1, Table S1: comparison of DBS and LCIG; Table S2: effect of DBS on individual symptoms for each target; Table S3: comparison of DBS, MRgFUS, radiofrequency, and gamma knife; Table S4: a list of concerns to check when considering DBS; Table S5: a list of concerns to check when considering LCIG.

Author Contributions: T.M. (Takayasu Mishima): execution of the project; writing of the first draft; S.F.: review and critique; T.M. (Takashi Morishita): review and critique; T.I.: execution of the revision of the manuscript; Y.T.: conception and organization of the project; editing of the manuscript. All authors have read and agreed to the published version of the manuscript.

Funding: This research received no external funding.

Institutional Review Board Statement: Ethical review and approval was not required for this study because it is an analysis based on previously published studies.

Informed Consent Statement: Not applicable.

Data Availability Statement: All relevant data are included in the study and supplementary information.

Acknowledgments: This work was supported by AMED (20gm1010002h0305). The authors would also like to acknowledge Mai Takahashi for assembling the figures.

Conflicts of Interest: The authors declare no conflict of interest.

References

1. Titova, N.; Chaudhuri, K.R. Personalized medicine in Parkinson's disease: Time to be precise. *Mov. Disord.* **2017**, *32*, 1147–1154. [CrossRef] [PubMed]
2. Jameson, J.L.; Longo, D.L. Precision medicine—Personalized, problematic, and promising. *N. Engl. J. Med.* **2015**, *372*, 2229–2234. [CrossRef]
3. Schneider, S.A.; Alcalay, R.N. Precision medicine in Parkinson's disease: Emerging treatments for genetic Parkinson's disease. *J. Neurol.* **2020**, *267*, 860–869. [CrossRef] [PubMed]
4. Juengst, E.; McGowan, M.L.; Fishman, J.R.; Settersten, R.A., Jr. From "Personalized" to "Precision" Medicine: The Ethical and Social Implications of Rhetorical Reform in Genomic Medicine. *Hastings Cent. Rep.* **2016**, *46*, 21–33. [CrossRef] [PubMed]
5. Park, A.; Chang, H.; Lee, K.J. Action Research on Development and Application of Internet of Things Services in Hospital. *Healthc. Inform. Res.* **2017**, *23*, 25–34. [CrossRef] [PubMed]
6. Bandres-Ciga, S.; Diez-Fairen, M.; Kim, J.J.; Singleton, A.B. Genetics of Parkinson's disease: An introspection of its journey towards precision medicine. *Neurobiol. Dis.* **2020**, *137*, 104782. [CrossRef] [PubMed]
7. Gulilat, M.; Lamb, T.; Teft, W.A.; Wang, J.; Dron, J.S.; Robinson, J.F.; Tirona, R.G.; Hegele, R.A.; Kim, R.B.; Schwarz, U.I. Targeted next generation sequencing as a tool for precision medicine. *BMC Med. Genom.* **2019**, *12*, 81. [CrossRef]
8. Titova, N.; Padmakumar, C.; Lewis, S.J.G.; Chaudhuri, K.R. Parkinson's: A syndrome rather than a disease? *J. Neural Transm.* **2017**, *124*, 907–914. [CrossRef]
9. Gibb, W.R.; Lees, A.J. The relevance of the Lewy body to the pathogenesis of idiopathic Parkinson's disease. *J. Neurol. Neurosurg. Psychiatry* **1988**, *51*, 745–752. [CrossRef]
10. Postuma, R.B.; Berg, D.; Stern, M.; Poewe, W.; Olanow, C.W.; Oertel, W.; Obeso, J.; Marek, K.; Litvan, I.; Lang, A.E.; et al. MDS clinical diagnostic criteria for Parkinson's disease. *Mov. Disord.* **2015**, *30*, 1591–1601. [CrossRef]
11. Jankovic, J.; Kapadia, A.S. Functional decline in Parkinson disease. *Arch. Neurol.* **2001**, *58*, 1611–1615. [CrossRef] [PubMed]
12. Fereshtehnejad, S.M.; Zeighami, Y.; Dagher, A.; Postuma, R.B. Clinical criteria for subtyping Parkinson's disease: Biomarkers and longitudinal progression. *Brain* **2017**, *140*, 1959–1976. [CrossRef] [PubMed]
13. Bloem, B.R.; Marks, W.J., Jr.; Silva de Lima, A.L.; Kuijf, M.L.; van Laar, T.; Jacobs, B.P.F.; Verbeek, M.M.; Helmich, R.C.; van de Warrenburg, B.P.; Evers, L.J.W.; et al. The Personalized Parkinson Project: Examining disease progression through broad biomarkers in early Parkinson's disease. *BMC Neurol.* **2019**, *19*, 160. [CrossRef] [PubMed]
14. Narabayashi, H.; Okuma, T.; Shikiba, S. Procaine oil blocking of the globus pallidus. *AMA Arch. Neurol. Psychiatry* **1956**, *75*, 36–48. [CrossRef] [PubMed]
15. Fahn, S. The medical treatment of Parkinson disease from James Parkinson to George Cotzias. *Mov. Disord.* **2015**, *30*, 4–18. [CrossRef] [PubMed]
16. Laitinen, L.V. Brain targets in surgery for Parkinson's disease. Results of a survey of neurosurgeons. *J Neurosurg.* **1985**, *62*, 349–351. [CrossRef]
17. Laitinen, L.V.; Bergenheim, A.T.; Hariz, M.I. Leksell's posteroventral pallidotomy in the treatment of Parkinson's disease. *J. Neurosurg.* **1992**, *76*, 53–61. [CrossRef]
18. Schuepbach, W.M.; Rau, J.; Knudsen, K.; Volkmann, J.; Krack, P.; Timmermann, L.; Hälbig, T.D.; Hesekamp, H.; Navarro, S.M.; Meier, N.; et al. Neurostimulation for Parkinson's disease with early motor complications. *N. Engl. J. Med.* **2013**, *368*, 610–622. [CrossRef]
19. Fox, S.H.; Katzenschlager, R.; Lim, S.Y.; Barton, B.; de Bie, R.M.A.; Seppi, K.; Coelho, M.; Sampaio, C. Movement Disorder Society. Evidence-Based Medicine Committee. International Parkinson and movement disorder society evidence-based medicine review: Update on treatments for the motor symptoms of Parkinson's disease. *Mov. Disord.* **2018**, *33*, 248–1266. [CrossRef]
20. Ferreira, J.J.; Katzenschlager, R.; Bloem, B.R.; Bonuccelli, U.; Burn, D.; Deuschl, G.; Dietrichs, E.; Fabbrini, G.; Friedman, A.; Kanovsky, P.; et al. Summary of the recommendations of the EFNS/MDS-ES review on therapeutic management of Parkinson's disease. *Eur. J. Neurol.* **2013**, *20*, 5–15. [CrossRef]
21. National Institute for Health and Care Excellence. Parkinson's Disease in Adults. NICE Guideline [NG71]. July 2017. Available online: www.nice.org.uk/guidance/ng71 (accessed on 19 July 2017).
22. Jost, S.T.; Sauerbier, A.; Visser-Vandewalle, V.; Ashkan, K.; Silverdale, M.; Evans, J.; Loehrer, P.A.; Rizos, A.; Petry-Schmelzer, J.N.; Reker, P.; et al. A prospective, controlled study of non-motor effects of subthalamic stimulation in Parkinson's disease: Results at the 36-month follow-up. *J. Neurol. Neurosurg. Psychiatry* **2020**, *91*, 687–694. [CrossRef]
23. Antonini, A.; Stoessl, A.J.; Kleinman, L.S.; Skalicky, A.M.; Marshall, T.S.; Sail, K.R.; Onuk, K.; Odin, P.L.A. Developing consensus among movement disorder specialists on clinical indicators for identification and management of advanced Parkinson's disease: A multi-country Delphi-panel approach. *Curr. Med. Res. Opin.* **2018**, *12*, 2063–2073. [CrossRef]

24. Negida, A.; Elminawy, M.; El Ashal, G.; Essam, A.; Eysa, A.; Abd Elalem Aziz, M. Subthalamic and Pallidal Deep Brain Stimulation for Parkinson's Disease. *Cureus* **2018**, *10*, e2232. [CrossRef] [PubMed]
25. Mao, Z.; Ling, Z.; Pan, L.; Xu, X.; Cui, Z.; Liang, S.; Yu, X. Comparison of Efficacy of Deep Brain Stimulation of Different Targets in Parkinson's Disease: A Network Meta-Analysis. *Front. Aging Neurosci.* **2019**, *11*, 23. [CrossRef] [PubMed]
26. Wang, J.W.; Zhang, Y.Q.; Zhang, X.H.; Wang, Y.P.; Li, J.P.; Li, Y.J. Deep Brain Stimulation of Pedunculopontine Nucleus for Postural Instability and Gait Disorder After Parkinson Disease: A Meta-Analysis of Individual Patient Data. *World Neurosurg.* **2017**, *102*, 72–78. [CrossRef] [PubMed]
27. Yu, H.; Takahashi, K.; Bloom, L.; Quaynor, S.D.; Xie, T. Effect of Deep Brain Stimulation on Swallowing Function: A Systematic Review. *Front. Neurol.* **2020**, *11*, 547. [CrossRef]
28. Walker, H.C.; Watts, R.L.; Guthrie, S.; Wang, D.; Guthrie, B.L. Bilateral effects of unilateral subthalamic deep brain stimulation on Parkinson's disease at 1 year. *Neurosurgery* **2009**, *2*, 302–309. [CrossRef]
29. Okun, M.S.; Wu, S.S.; Fayad, S.; Ward, H.; Bowers, D.; Rosado, C.; Bowen, L.; Jacobson, C.; Butson, C.; Foote, K.D. Acute and Chronic Mood and Apathy Outcomes from a randomized study of unilateral STN and GPi DBS. *PLoS ONE* **2014**, *12*, e114140. [CrossRef] [PubMed]
30. Cernera, S.; Eisinger, R.S.; Wong, J.K.; Ho, K.W.D.; Lopes, J.L.; To, K.; Carbunaru, S.; Ramirez-Zamora, A.; Almeida, L.; Foote, K.D.; et al. Long-term Parkinson's disease quality of life after staged DBS: STN vs GPi and first vs second lead. *NPJ. Parkinsons Dis.* **2020**, *6*, 13. [CrossRef]
31. Zhang, C.; Wang, L.; Hu, W.; Wang, T.; Zhao, Y.; Pan, Y.; Almeida, L.; Ramirez-Zamora, A.; Sun, B.; Li, D. Combined Unilateral Subthalamic Nucleus and Contralateral Globus Pallidus Interna Deep Brain Stimulation for Treatment of Parkinson Disease: A Pilot Study of Symptom-Tailored Stimulation. *Neurosurgery* **2020**, *87*, 1139–1147.
32. Morishita, T.; Higuchi, M.A.; Kobayashi, H.; Abe, H.; Higashi, T.; Inoue, T. A retrospective evaluation of thalamic targeting for tremor deep brain stimulation using high-resolution anatomical imaging with supplementary fiber tractography. *J. Neurol. Sci.* **2019**, *398*, 148–156. [CrossRef] [PubMed]
33. Horn, A.; Reich, M.; Vorwerk, J.; Li, N.; Wenzel, G.; Fang, Q.; Schmitz-Hübsch, T.; Nickl, R.; Kupsch, A.; Volkmann, J.; et al. Connectivity Predicts deep brain stimulation outcome in Parkinson disease. *Ann. Neurol.* **2017**, *82*, 67–78. [CrossRef]
34. Eleopra, R.; Rinaldo, S.; Devigili, G.; Lettieri, C.; Mondani, M.; D'Auria, S.; Piacentino, M.; Pilleri, M. Brain impedance variation of directional leads implanted in subthalamic nuclei of Parkinsonian patients. *Clin. Neurophysiol.* **2019**, *130*, 1562–1569. [CrossRef]
35. Shao, M.M.; Liss, A.; Park, Y.L.; DiMarzio, M.; Prusik, J.; Hobson, E.; Adam, O.; Durphy, J.; Sukul, V.; Danisi, F.; et al. Early Experience With New Generation Deep Brain Stimulation Leads in Parkinson's Disease and Essential Tremor Patients. *Neuromodulation* **2020**, *23*, 537–542. [CrossRef]
36. Pollo, C.; Kaelin-Lang, A.; Oertel, M.F.; Stieglitz, L.; Taub, E.; Fuhr, P.; Lozano, A.M.; Raabe, A.; Schüpbach, M. Directional deep brain stimulation: An intraoperative double-blind pilot study. *Brain* **2014**, *137*, 2015–2026. [CrossRef] [PubMed]
37. Contarino, M.F.; Bour, L.J.; Verhagen, R.; Lourens, M.A.; de Bie, R.M.; van den Munckhof, P.; Schuurman, P.R. Directional steering: A novel approach to deep brain stimulation. *Neurology* **2014**, *83*, 1163–1169. [CrossRef] [PubMed]
38. Steigerwald, F.; Müller, L.; Johannes, S.; Matthies, C.; Volkmann, J. Directional deep brain stimulation of the subthalamic nucleus: A pilot study using a novel neurostimulation device. *Mov. Disord.* **2016**, *31*, 1240–1243. [CrossRef]
39. Dembek, T.A.; Reker, P.; Visser-Vandewalle, V.; Wirths, J.; Treuer, H.; Klehr, M.; Roediger, J.; Dafsari, H.S.; Barbe, M.T.; Timmermann, L. Directional DBS increases side-effect thresholds-A prospective, double-blind trial. *Mov. Disord.* **2017**, *32*, 1380–1388. [CrossRef] [PubMed]
40. Krüger, M.T.; Avecillas-Chasin, J.M.; Tamber, M.S.; Heran, M.K.S.; Sandhu, M.K.; Polyhronopoulos, N.E.; Sarai, N.; Honey, C.R. Tremor and Quality of Life in Patients With Advanced Essential Tremor Before and After Replacing Their Standard Deep Brain Stimulation With a Directional System. *Neuromodulation* **2021**, *24*, 353–360. [CrossRef]
41. Meidahl, A.C.; Tinkhauser, G.; Herz, D.M.; Cagnan, H.; Debarros, J.; Brown, P. Adaptive Deep Brain Stimulation for Movement Disorders: The Long Road to Clinical Therapy. *Mov. Disord.* **2017**, *32*, 810–819. [CrossRef]
42. Little, S.; Pogosyan, A.; Neal, S.; Zavala, B.; Zrinzo, L.; Hariz, M.; Foltynie, T.; Limousin, P.; Ashkan, K.; FitzGerald, J.; et al. Adaptive deep brain stimulation in advanced Parkinson disease. *Ann. Neurol.* **2013**, *74*, 449–457. [CrossRef]
43. Jia, F.; Wagle Shukla, A.; Hu, W.; Almeida, L.; Holanda, V.; Zhang, J.; Meng, F.; Okun, M.S.; Li, L. Deep Brain Stimulation at Variable Frequency to Improve Motor Outcomes in Parkinson's Disease. *Mov. Disord. Clin. Pract.* **2018**, *5*, 538–541. [CrossRef]
44. Enatsu, R.; Kitagawa, M.; Morishita, T.; Sasagawa, A.; Kuribara, T.; Hirano, T.; Arihara, M.; Mikami, T.; Mikuni, N. Effect of Cycling Thalamosubthalamic Stimulation on Tremor Habituation and Rebound in Parkinson Disease. *World Neurosurg.* **2020**, *144*, 64–67. [CrossRef]
45. Watanabe, H.; Sano, H.; Chiken, S.; Kobayashi, K.; Fukata, Y.; Fukata, M.; Mushiake, H.; Nambu, A. Forelimb movements evoked by optogenetic stimulation of the macaque motor cortex. *Nat. Commun.* **2020**, *11*, 3253. [CrossRef]
46. Nimpf, S.; Keays, D.A. Is magnetogenetics the new optogenetics? *EMBO J.* **2017**, *36*, 1643–1646. [CrossRef] [PubMed]
47. Wang, S.; Meng, W.; Ren, Z.; Li, B.; Zhu, T.; Chen, H.; Wang, Z.; He, B.; Zhao, D.; Jiang, H. Ultrasonic Neuromodulation and Sonogenetics: A New Era for Neural Modulation. *Front. Physiol.* **2020**, *11*, 787. [CrossRef] [PubMed]
48. Politis, M.; Sauerbier, A.; Loane, C.; Pavese, N.; Martin, A.; Corcoran, B.; Brooks, D.J.; Ray-Chaudhuri, K.; Piccini, P. Sustained striatal dopamine levels following intestinal levodopa infusions in Parkinson's disease patients. *Mov. Disord.* **2017**, *32*, 235–240. [CrossRef]

49. Antonini, A.; Poewe, W.; Chaudhuri, K.R.; Jech, R.; Pickut, B.; Pirtošek, Z.; Szasz, J.; Valldeoriola, F.; Winkler, C.; Bergmann, L.; et al. Levodopa-carbidopa intestinal gel in advanced Parkinson's: Final results of the GLORIA registry. *Parkinsonism Relat. Disord.* **2017**, *45*, 13–20. [CrossRef]
50. Zibetti, M.; Angrisano, S.; Dematteis, F.; Artusi, C.A.; Romagnolo, A.; Merola, A.; Lopiano, L. Effects of intestinal Levodopa infusion on freezing of gait in Parkinson disease. *J. Neurol. Sci.* **2018**, *385*, 105–108. [CrossRef] [PubMed]
51. Valldeoriola, F.; Santacruz, P.; Ríos, J.; Compta, Y.; Rumià, J.; Muñoz, J.E.; Martí, M.J.; Tolosa, E. l-Dopa/carbidopa intestinal gel and subthalamic nucleus stimulation: Effects on cognition and behavior. *Brain Behav.* **2017**, *7*, e00848. [CrossRef]
52. Catalan, M.J.; Molina-Arjona, J.A.; Mir, P.; Cubo, E.; Arbelo, J.M.; Martinez-Martin, P.; EDIS Study Group. Improvement of impulse control disorders associated with levodopa-carbidopa intestinal gel treatment in advanced Parkinson's disease. *J. Neurol.* **2018**, *265*, 1279–1287. [CrossRef] [PubMed]
53. Olanow, C.W.; Kieburtz, K.; Odin, P.; Espay, A.J.; Standaert, D.G.; Fernandez, H.H.; Vanagunas, A.; Othman, A.A.; Widnell, K.L.; Robieson, W.Z.; et al. Continuous intrajejunal infusion of levodopa-carbidopa intestinal gel for patients with advanced Parkinson's disease: A randomised, controlled, double-blind, double-dummy study. *Lancet Neurol.* **2014**, *13*, 141–149. [CrossRef]
54. Fabbri, M.; Zibetti, M.; Beccaria, L.; Merola, A.; Romagnolo, A.; Montanaro, E.; Ferreira, J.J.; Palermo, S.; Lopiano, L. Levodopa/carbidopa intestinal gel infusion and weight loss in Parkinson's disease. *Eur. J. Neurol.* **2019**, *26*, 490–496. [CrossRef] [PubMed]
55. Nose, K.; Fujioka, S.; Umemoto, G.; Yamashita, K.; Shiwaku, H.; Hayashi, Y.; Mishima, T.; Fukae, J.; Hasegawa, S.; Tsuboi, Y. Acute cholecystitis induced by surgery for levodopa-carbidopa intestinal gel therapy: Possible relationship to pre-existing gallstones. *Parkinsonism Relat. Disord.* **2018**, *54*, 107–109. [CrossRef]
56. Merola, A.; Romagnolo, A.; Zibetti, M.; Bernardini, A.; Cocito, D.; Lopiano, L. Peripheral neuropathy associated with levodopa-carbidopa intestinal infusion: A long-term prospective assessment. *Eur. J. Neurol.* **2016**, *23*, 501–509. [CrossRef]
57. Pessoa, R.R.; Moro, A.; Munhoz, R.P.; Teive, H.A.G.; Lees, A.J. Apomorphine in the treatment of Parkinson's disease: A review. *Arq. Neuropsiquiatr.* **2018**, *76*, 840–848. [CrossRef]
58. Ray Chaudhuri, K.; Qamar, M.A.; Rajah, T.; Loehrer, P.; Sauerbier, A.; Odin, P.; Jenner, P. Non-oral dopaminergic therapies for Parkinson's disease: Current treatments and the future. *NPJ. Parkinsons Dis.* **2016**, *2*, 16023. [CrossRef]
59. Katzenschlager, R.; Poewe, W.; Rascol, O.; Trenkwalder, C.; Deuschl, G.; Chaudhuri, K.R.; Henriksen, T.; van Laar, T.; Spivey, K.; Vel, S.; et al. Apomorphine subcutaneous infusion in patients with Parkinson's disease with persistent motor fluctuations (TOLEDO): A multicentre, double-blind, randomised, placebo-controlled trial. *Lancet Neurol.* **2018**, *17*, 749–759. [CrossRef]
60. Tasker, R.R. Deep brain stimulation is preferable to thalamotomy for tremor suppression. *Surg. Neurol.* **1998**, *49*, 145–153. [CrossRef]
61. Schreglmann, S.R.; Krauss, J.K.; Chang, J.W.; Martin, E.; Werner, B.; Bauer, R.; Hägele-Link, S.; Bhatia, K.P.; Kägi, G. Functional lesional neurosurgery for tremor: back to the future? *J. Neurol. Neurosurg. Psychiatry* **2018**, *89*, 727–735. [CrossRef] [PubMed]
62. Kapadia, A.N.; Elias, G.J.B.; Boutet, A.; Germann, J.; Pancholi, A.; Chu, P.; Zhong, J.; Fasano, A.; Munhoz, R.; Chow, C.; et al. Multimodal MRI for MRgFUS in essential tremor: Post-treatment radiological markers of clinical outcome. *J. Neurol. Neurosurg. Psychiatry* **2020**, *91*, 921–927. [CrossRef] [PubMed]
63. Higuchi, Y.; Matsuda, S.; Serizawa, T. Gamma knife radiosurgery in movement disorders: Indications and limitations. *Mov. Disord.* **2017**, *32*, 28–35. [CrossRef] [PubMed]
64. Cahan, L.D.; Young, R.F.; Li, F. Radiosurgical Pallidotomy for Parkinson's Disease. *Prog. Neurol. Surg.* **2018**, *33*, 149–157. [PubMed]
65. Drummond, P.S.; Pourfar, M.H.; Hill, T.C.; Mogilner, A.Y.; Kondziolka, D.S. Subthalamic Gamma Knife Radiosurgery in Parkinson's Disease: A Cautionary Tale. *Stereotact. Funct. Neurosurg.* **2020**, *98*, 110–117. [CrossRef] [PubMed]
66. Giordano, M.; Caccavella, V.M.; Zaed, I.; Foglia Manzillo, L.; Montano, N.; Olivi, A.; Polli, F.M. Comparison between deep brain stimulation and magnetic resonance-guided focused ultrasound in the treatment of essential tremor: A systematic review and pooled analysis of functional outcomes. *J. Neurol. Neurosurg. Psychiatry* **2020**, *91*, 1270–1278. [CrossRef] [PubMed]
67. Martínez-Fernández, R.; Máñez-Miró, J.U.; Rodríguez-Rojas, R.; Del Álamo, M.; Shah, B.B.; Hernández-Fernández, F.; Pineda-Pardo, J.A.; Monje, M.H.G.; Fernández-Rodríguez, B.; Sperling, S.A.; et al. Randomized Trial of Focused Ultrasound Subthalamotomy for Parkinson's Disease. *N. Engl. J. Med.* **2020**, *383*, 2501–2513. [CrossRef]
68. Alvarez, L.; Macias, R.; Guridi, J.; Lopez, G.; Alvarez, E.; Maragoto, C.; Teijeiro, J.; Torres, A.; Pavon, N.; Rodriguez-Oroz, M.C.; et al. Dorsal subthalamotomy for Parkinson's disease. *Mov. Disord.* **2001**, *16*, 72–78. [CrossRef]
69. Bond, A.E.; Shah, B.B.; Huss, D.S.; Dallapiazza, R.F.; Warren, A.; Harrison, M.B.; Sperling, S.A.; Wang, X.Q.; Gwinn, R.; Witt, J.; et al. Safety and Efficacy of Focused Ultrasound Thalamotomy for Patients With Medication-Refractory, Tremor-Dominant Parkinson Disease A Randomized Clinical Trial. *JAMA Neurol.* **2017**, *74*, 1412–1418. [CrossRef]
70. Gallay, M.N.; Moser, D.; Rossi, F.; Magara, A.E.; Strasser, M.; Bühler, R.; Kowalski, M.; Pourtehrani, P.; Dragalina, C.; Federau, C.; et al. MRgFUS Pallidothalamic Tractotomy for Chronic Therapy-Resistant Parkinson's Disease in 51 Consecutive Patients: Single Center Experience. *Front. Surg.* **2020**, *6*, 76. [CrossRef]
71. Mahajan, U.V.; Ravikumar, V.K.; Kumar, K.K.; Ku, S.; Ojukwu, D.I.; Kilbane, C.; Ghanouni, P.; Rosenow, J.M.; Stein, S.C.; Halpern, C.H. Bilateral deep brain stimulation is the procedure to beat for advanced Parkinson Disease: A meta-analytic, cost-effective threshold analysis for focused ultra-sound. *Neurosurgery* **2021**, *88*, 487–496. [CrossRef]

72. Liu, X.D.; Bao, Y.; Liu, G.J. Comparison Between Levodopa-Carbidopa Intestinal Gel Infusion and Subthalamic Nucleus Deep-Brain Stimulation for Advanced Parkinson's Disease: A Systematic Review and Meta-Analysis. *Front. Neurol.* **2019**, *10*, 934. [CrossRef] [PubMed]
73. Dafsari, H.S.; Martinez-Martin, P.; Rizos, A.; Trost, M.; Dos Santos Ghilardi, M.G.; Reddy, P.; Sauerbier, A.; Petry-Schmelzer, J.N.; Kramberger, M.; Borgemeester, R.W.K.; et al. EuroInf 2: Subthalamic stimulation, apomorphine, and levodopa infusion in Parkinson's disease. *Mov. Disord.* **2019**, *34*, 353–365. [CrossRef]
74. Elkouzi, A.; Ramirez-Zamora, A.; Zeilman, P.; Barabas, M.; Eisinger, R.S.; Malaty, I.A.; Okun, M.S.; Almeida, L. Rescue levodopa-carbidopa intestinal gel (LCIG) therapy in Parkinson's disease patients with suboptimal response to deep brain stimulation. *Ann. Clin. Transl. Neurol.* **2019**, *10*, 1989–1995. [CrossRef] [PubMed]
75. Barker, R.A.; Barrett, J.; Mason, S.L.; Björklund, A.F. Fetal dopaminergic transplantation trials and the future of neural grafting in Parkinson's disease. *Lancet Neurol.* **2013**, *12*, 84–91. [CrossRef]
76. Barker, R.A.; Drouin-Ouellet, J.; Parmar, M. Cell–based therapies for Parkinson disease—Past insights and future potential. *Nat. Rev. Neurol.* **2015**, *11*, 492–503. [CrossRef]
77. Kikuchi, T.; Morizane, A.; Doi, D.; Magotani, H.; Onoe, H.; Hayashi, T.; Mizuma, H.; Takara, S.; Takahashi, R.; Inoue, H.; et al. Human iPS cell-derived dopaminergic neurons function in a primate Parkinson's disease model. *Nature* **2017**, *548*, 592–596. [CrossRef]
78. UMIN. Kyoto Trial to Evaluate the Safety and Efficacy of iPSC-Derived Dopaminergic Progenitors in the Treatment of Parkinson's Disease. Available online: https://upload.umin.ac.jp/cgi-open-bin/ctr_e/ctr_view.cgi?recptno=R000038278 (accessed on 21 December 2018).
79. Schweitzer, J.S.; Song, B.; Herrington, T.M.; Park, T.Y.; Lee, N.; Ko, S.; Jeon, J.; Cha, Y.; Kim, K.; Li, Q.; et al. Personalized iPSC-Derived Dopamine Progenitor Cells for Parkinson's Disease. *N. Engl. J. Med.* **2020**, *382*, 1926–1932. [CrossRef]
80. Torikoshi, S.; Morizane, A.; Shimogawa, T.; Samata, B.; Miyamoto, S.; Takahashi, J. Exercise Promotes Neurite Extensions from Grafted Dopaminergic Neurons in the Direction of the Dorsolateral Striatum in Parkinson's Disease Model Rats. *J. Parkinsons Dis.* **2020**, *10*, 511–521. [CrossRef]
81. Muramatsu, S.; Fujimoto, K.; Kato, S.; Mizukami, H.; Asari, S.; Ikeguchi, K.; Kawakami, T.; Urabe, M.; Kume, A.; Sato, T.; et al. A phase I study of aromatic L-amino acid decarboxylase gene therapy for Parkinson's disease. *Mol. Ther.* **2010**, *18*, 1731–1735. [CrossRef]
82. Christine, C.W.; Starr, P.A.; Larson, P.S.; Eberling, J.L.; Jagust, W.J.; Hawkins, R.A.; VanBrocklin, H.F.; Wright, J.F.; Bankiewicz, K.S.; Aminoff, M.J. Safety and tolerability of putaminal AADC gene therapy for Parkinson disease. *Neurology* **2009**, *73*, 1662–1669. [CrossRef]
83. Christine, C.W.; Bankiewicz, K.S.; Van Laar, A.D.; Richardson, R.M.; Ravina, B.; Kells, A.P.; Boot, B.; Martin, A.J.; Nutt, J.; Thompson, M.E.; et al. Magnetic resonance imaging-guided phase 1 trial of putaminal AADC gene therapy for Parkinson's disease. *Ann. Neurol.* **2019**, *85*, 704–714. [CrossRef]
84. Palfi, S.; Gurruchaga, J.M.; Lepetit, H.; Howard, K.; Ralph, G.S.; Mason, S.; Gouello, G.; Domenech, P.; Buttery, P.C.; Hantraye, P.; et al. Long-Term Follow-Up of a Phase I/II Study of ProSavin, a Lentiviral Vector Gene Therapy for Parkinson's Disease. *Hum. Gene Ther. Clin. Dev.* **2018**, *29*, 148–155. [CrossRef]
85. Marks, W.J., Jr.; Bartus, R.T.; Siffert, J.; Davis, C.S.; Lozano, A.; Boulis, N.; Vitek, J.; Stacy, M.; Turner, D.; Verhagen, L.; et al. Gene delivery of AAV2-neurturin for Parkinson's disease: A double-blind, randomised, controlled trial. *Lancet Neurol.* **2010**, *9*, 1164–1172. [CrossRef]
86. Niethammer, M.; Tang, C.C.; LeWitt, P.A.; Rezai, A.R.; Leehey, M.A.; Ojemann, S.G.; Flaherty, A.W.; Eskandar, E.N.; Kostyk, S.K.; Sarkar, A.; et al. Long-term follow-up of a randomized AAV2- GAD gene therapy trial for Parkinson's disease. *JCI Insight* **2017**, *2*, e90133. [CrossRef]
87. Elsayed, G.A.; Menendez, J.Y.; Tabibian, B.E.; Chagoya, G.; Omar, N.B.; Zeiger, E.; Walters, B.C.; Walker, H.; Guthrie, B.L. Patient Satisfaction in Surgery for Parkinson's Disease: A Systematic Review of the Literature. *Cureus* **2019**, *11*, e4316. [CrossRef] [PubMed]
88. Skorvanek, M.; Martinez-Martin, P.; Kovacs, N.; Zezula, I.; Rodriguez-Violante, M.; Corvol, J.C.; Taba, P.; Seppi, K.; Levin, O.; Schrag, A.; et al. Relationship between the MDS-UPDRS and Quality of Life: A large multicenter study of 3206 patients. *Parkinsonism Relat. Disord.* **2018**, *52*, 83–89. [CrossRef] [PubMed]
89. Neff, C.; Wang, M.C.; Martel, H. Using the PDQ-39 in routine care for Parkinson's disease. *Parkinsonism Relat. Disord.* **2018**, *53*, 105–107. [CrossRef] [PubMed]
90. Kurihara, K.; Nakagawa, R.; Ishido, M.; Yoshinaga, Y.; Watanabe, J.; Hayashi, Y.; Mishima, T.; Fujioka, S.; Tsuboi, Y. Impact of motor and nonmotor symptoms in Parkinson disease for the quality of life: The Japanese Quality-of-Life Survey of Parkinson Disease (JAQPAD) study. *J. Neurol. Sci.* **2020**, *419*, 117172. [CrossRef] [PubMed]
91. Onozawa, R.; Tsugawa, J.; Tsuboi, Y.; Fukae, J.; Mishima, T.; Fujioka, S. The impact of early morning off in Parkinson's disease on patient quality of life and caregiver burden. *J. Neurol. Sci.* **2016**, *364*, 1–5. [CrossRef]
92. Radder, D.L.M.; Nonnekes, J.; van Nimwegen, M.; Eggers, C.; Abbruzzese, G.; Alves, G.; Browner, N.; Chaudhuri, K.R.; Ebersbach, G.; Ferreira, J.J.; et al. Recommendations for the Organization of Multidisciplinary Clinical Care Teams in Parkinson's Disease. *J. Parkinsons Dis.* **2020**, *10*, 1087–1098. [CrossRef]

93. Higuchi, M.A.; Martinez-Ramirez, D.; Morita, H.; Topiol, D.; Bowers, D.; Ward, H.; Warren, L.; DeFranco, M.; Hicks, J.A.; Hegland, K.W.; et al. Interdisciplinary Parkinson's Disease Deep Brain Stimulation Screening and the Relationship to Unintended Hospitalizations and Quality of Life. *PLoS ONE* **2016**, *11*, e0153785. [CrossRef] [PubMed]
94. Timpka, J.; Nitu, B.; Datieva, V.; Odin, P.; Antonini, A. Device-Aided Treatment Strategies in Advanced Parkinson's Disease. *Int. Rev. Neurobiol.* **2017**, *132*, 453–474. [PubMed]
95. Bhidayasiri, R.; Virameteekul, S.; Kim, J.M.; Pal, P.K.; Chung, S.J. COVID-19: An Early Review of Its Global Impact and Considerations for Parkinson's Disease Patient Care. *J. Mov. Disord.* **2020**, *13*, 105–114. [CrossRef]
96. Fasano, A.; Antonini, A.; Katzenschlager, R.; Krack, P.; Odin, P.; Evans, A.H.; Foltynie, T.; Volkmann, J.; Merello, M. Management of Advanced Therapies in Parkinson's Disease Patients in Times of Humanitarian Crisis: The COVID-19 Experience. *Mov. Disord. Clin. Pract.* **2020**, *7*, 361–372. [CrossRef] [PubMed]
97. Papa, S.M.; Brundin, P.; Fung, V.S.C.; Kang, U.J.; Burn, D.J.; Colosimo, C.; Chiang, H.L.; Alcalay, R.N.; Trenkwalder, C.; MDS-Scientific Issues Committee. Impact of the COVID-19 Pandemic on Parkinson's Disease and Movement Disorders. *Mov. Disord.* **2020**, *35*, 711–715. [CrossRef] [PubMed]
98. Kurihara, K.; Nakagawa, K.; Inoue, K.; Yamamoto, S.; Mishima, T.; Fujioka, S.; Ouma, S.; Tsuboi, Y. Attitudes toward telemedicine of patients with Parkinson's disease during the COVID-19 pandemic. *Neurol. Clin. Neurosci.* **2021**, *9*, 77–82. [CrossRef]
99. Jitkritsadakul, O.; Rajalingam, R.; Toenjes, C.; Munhoz, R.P.; Fasano, A. Tele-health for patients with deep brain stimulation: The experience of the Ontario Telemedicine Network. *Mov. Disord.* **2018**, *33*, 491–492. [CrossRef]
100. Willows, T.; Dizdar, N.; Nyholm, D.; Widner, H.; Grenholm, P.; Schmiauke, U.; Urbom, A.; Growth, K.; Larsson, J.; Permert, J.; et al. Initiation of Levodopa-Carbidopa Intestinal Gel Infusion Using Telemedicine (Video Communication System) Facilitates Efficient and Well-Accepted Home Titration in Patients with Advanced Parkinson's Disease. *J. Parkinsons Dis.* **2017**, *7*, 719–728. [CrossRef]

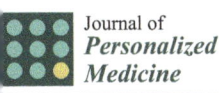

Article

Effectiveness of Cognitive Rehabilitation in Parkinson's Disease: A Systematic Review and Meta-Analysis

Itsasne Sanchez-Luengos, Yolanda Balboa-Bandeira, Olaia Lucas-Jiménez, Natalia Ojeda, Javier Peña and Naroa Ibarretxe-Bilbao *

Department of Methods and Experimental Psychology, Faculty of Psychology and Education, University of Deusto, 48007 Bilbao, Spain; itsasnesanchez@deusto.es (I.S.-L.); yolandabalboa@deusto.es (Y.B.-B.); olaia.lucas@deusto.es (O.L.-J.); nojeda@deusto.es (N.O.); javier.pena@deusto.es (J.P.)
* Correspondence: naroa.ibarretxe@deusto.es

Abstract: Cognitive deficits influence the quality of life of Parkinson's disease (PD) patients. In order to reduce the impact of cognitive impairment in PD, cognitive rehabilitation programs have been developed. This study presents a systematic review and meta-analysis regarding the effectiveness of cognitive rehabilitation in non-demented PD patients. Twelve articles were selected according to PRISMA guidelines. The systematic review showed that attention, working memory, verbal memory, executive functions and processing speed were the most frequently improved domains. Meta-analysis results showed moderate effects on global cognitive status ($g = 0.55$) and working memory ($g = 0.50$); small significant effects on verbal memory ($g = 0.41$), overall cognitive functions ($g = 0.39$) and executive functions ($g = 0.30$); small non-significant effects on attention ($g = 0.36$), visual memory ($g = 0.29$), verbal fluency ($g = 0.27$) and processing speed ($g = 0.24$); and no effect on visuospatial and visuoconstructive abilities ($g = 0.17$). Depressive symptoms showed small effect ($g = 0.24$) and quality of life showed no effect ($g = -0.07$). A meta-regression was performed to examine moderating variables of overall cognitive function effects, although moderators did not explain the heterogeneity of the improvement after cognitive rehabilitation. The findings suggest that cognitive rehabilitation may be beneficial in improving cognition in non-demented PD patients, although further studies are needed to obtain more robust effects.

Keywords: Parkinson's disease (PD); cognitive rehabilitation; intervention; cognition

1. Introduction

Parkinson's disease (PD) is the second most common neurodegenerative disease after Alzheimer's disease [1]. PD is associated with motor (bradykinesia, rigidity and tremor) and non-motor symptoms such as cognitive impairment, neuropsychiatric symptoms, sensory abnormalities, sleep disorders and autonomic disturbances [1,2].

Cognitive deficits are usually associated with PD [3], with 40% of PD patients developing mild cognitive impairment (MCI) during the course of the disease [4], and with attention, executive functions, visuospatial abilities and memory being the most affected domains [5,6]. In turn, the risk of dementia increases with the deterioration of cognitive deficits and disease progression [7], with 83% of PD patients with cognitive impairment presenting dementia after 20 years [8].

Non-pharmacological interventions have been developed [9] with the aim of intervening on the cognitive and functional impairment of PD, with cognitive rehabilitation being one of the strategies suggested for personalized medicine [10]. Several systematic reviews [11–16] and meta-analyses [17–19] have reviewed and analyzed the effect of cognitive rehabilitation in PD, suggesting that this intervention may be potentially beneficial in increasing cognitive performance or maintaining cognitive levels over time, especially when treatment is applied before dementia has set in [12]. As far as the authors are aware, there have only been three meta-analyses that analyze the effectiveness of cognitive rehabilitation in PD to date. Specifically, Leung and colleagues conducted the first meta-analysis published in 2015 [18], focused on the analysis of seven randomized controlled trials (RCTs), in which they showed improvements in working memory, executive functions and processing speed. Later, in 2017, Lawrence and colleagues [17] examined the effectiveness of cognitive rehabilitation along with non-invasive brain stimulation interventions, and found improvements in attention/working memory, memory and executive functions. Orgeta and colleagues [19] published the latest meta-analysis in 2020, which covered the effects of cognitive rehabilitation from seven RCTs in PD patients with MCI or dementia (excluding PD patients without MCI or dementia), and found no evidence of cognitive improvement after cognitive rehabilitation [19].

It is important to emphasize that there is an increasing number of studies that examine the effects of cognitive rehabilitation in PD patients without dementia. Therefore, it is essential to conduct an updated review of the literature to include and analyze the effect sizes that have been published to date. In addition, variables related to the characteristics and progression of the disease could interfere on the benefit of rehabilitation in people with PD [20]. The possible influence of rehabilitation characteristics (modality (paper/pencil or computer-based exercises), the duration of the entire program, and the frequency and duration of the sessions) should also be investigated. However, none of the meta-analyses published in PD performed moderator analyses to analyze the existence of possible factors that may influence the cognitive rehabilitation process. Therefore, the aim of this systematic review and meta-analysis was to conduct a critical review of the effectiveness of cognitive rehabilitation in PD and to analyze whether cognitive rehabilitation improves cognition, functionality, depressive symptoms and quality of life in people with PD. In addition, we analyzed the influence of age and years of education, variables related to intervention, baseline global cognitive scores and PD patient-related features on the effectiveness of cognitive rehabilitation in PD.

2. Materials and Methods

2.1. Search Strategy

A systematic review and meta-analysis of published research papers that focus on cognitive rehabilitation in PD patients was conducted according to the guidelines of "Preferred Information Elements for Systematic Reviews and Meta-Analysis" (PRISMA) [21]. This systematic review protocol was registered in the International Prospective Register of Systematic Reviews, PROSPERO (CRD42021243716). The bibliographic search was conducted in December 2020 and April 2021. PubMed database was used and the specific terms used for searching, identifying and selecting studies were: (1) Parkinson's disease and Parkinson disease; (2) cognitive rehabilitation/training/remediation/stimulation; (3) attention; (4) working memory; (5) memory; (6) executive functions and (7) rehabilitation/training/remediation/stimulation. The terms were combined in order to conduct a more comprehensive search: (1) + (2); (1) + (3) + (7); (1) + (4) + (7); (1) + (5) + (7); and (1) + (6) + (7). The search was filtered by title or abstract. In addition, we performed a citation search of the reference lists from the meta-analyses [17–19] of cognitive rehabilitation in PD published to date. For a detailed description of the search strategy applied and the number of results obtained, see Supplementary Material Table S1.

2.2. Eligibility Criteria

The inclusion criteria for studies were: (1) patients with a diagnosis of idiopathic PD, (2) PD patients receiving structured cognitive rehabilitation, (3) analysis of the effects on cognition and (if included in the studies) on functionality, depression and quality of life, (4) study design (parallel controlled trials), (5) studies that compared structured cognitive intervention with a control group receiving no specific cognitive intervention or unstructured cognitive intervention and (6) studies assessing outcomes immediately after the intervention period. As for the exclusion criteria, these were: (1) review papers, (2) single case studies, (3) conference abstract or presentation, (4) PD patients diagnosed with dementia, (5) brain stimulation studies, (6) only neuroimaging data, (7) lack of available data for effect size estimation, (8) lack of PD control group and (9) article language, as those written in any language other than English were excluded.

2.3. Quality Assessment and Risk of Bias in the Included Studies

The risk of bias in the included studies was assessed using the Cochrane Manual for Systematic Reviews of Interventions for RCTs (RoB 2 tool) [22] and non-randomized trials (ROBINS-I tool) [23]. This tool evaluated different aspects of the trial design, conduct and report, in order to obtain information about the characteristics of the trial relevant to the risk of bias [24]. Moreover, the methodological quality of the randomized studies was assessed using the Physiotherapy Evidence Database (PEDro-P) Rating Scale [25], comprising 11 items. For this purpose, the evaluation of the quality and risk of bias of the studies was evaluated independently by two reviewers (I.S.-L. and Y.B.-B.), obtaining an inter-rater reliability of 83.56%. The risk of bias was classified as low, unclear or high (See Table S2).

2.4. Data Extraction

Specific information was extracted for the systematic review from the studies selected, which included: (1) first author and year of publication; (2) sample size of the study; (3) characteristics of the sample; (4) characteristics of the disease; (5) type of intervention; (6) format of the intervention; (7) duration of the intervention; (8) cognitive domains trained and (9) variables in which improvements have been obtained after cognitive rehabilitation. In the meta-analysis, all effect sizes were calculated from the means and standard deviations, and/or F scores. Effect sizes were calculated for overall cognitive functions, global cognitive status and eight specific cognitive subdomains: attention, working memory, verbal memory, visual memory, verbal fluency, executive functions, visuospatial and visuoconstructive abilities, and processing speed. The effect sizes of the overall cognitive functions were calculated based on the mean of the global cognitive status and cognitive subdomains obtained from this meta-analysis. For this purpose, studies included in this meta-analysis that had reported at least two cognitive domains were selected. Moreover, the effect sizes of depressive symptoms and quality of life were also calculated. The tests included were classified according to the domain assessed by the test itself (See Table S3). For the moderator or meta-regression analyses, the following were selected: specific scores of the age and years of education, variables related to intervention time, the modality of delivering the cognitive training (pencil and paper or computer), baseline global cognitive scores and PD patient-related features (disease duration, the Unified Parkinson's Disease Rating Scale (UPDRS) part III [26] and the Hoehn and Yahr scale (H&Y) [27]).

2.5. Statistical Analysis

In this meta-analysis, we estimated the effect sizes of 12 articles in order to analyze the differences in the effects of cognitive rehabilitation programs on PD patients compared to control groups. We calculated the standardized mean difference (SMD), using Cohen's d formula [28] first, to estimate all the different outcomes. SMD values were calculated with a 95% confidence interval (CI) from the means and standard deviations, and the F scores provided by the studies, and were corrected using Hedges' g small sample size bias adjustment formula [29]. For those studies that provided the necessary data, the change score to estimate the effects sizes was calculated based on the assumption that the correlation between measures at pretest and posttest times is zero. This is a conservative approach that was previously used in Orgeta and colleagues' meta-analysis [19]. A random-effects model was used to perform all meta-analysis estimations. We did not detect or remove any effect size as an outlier. Effect sizes were considered small ≥ 0.20, moderate ≥ 0.50, or large ≥ 0.80. Heterogeneity across the studies was estimated using Cochrane's Q test (Q) and I^2 indexes, where the I^2 index can indicate low (25%), medium (50%), or high (75%) heterogeneity [30].

We examined the possible influence of different predictor variables on the effect sizes obtained in overall cognitive functions, using multiple meta-regression analyses with the rma function and the dmetar package available in RStudio [31]. These moderator analyses were conducted using the mixed-effects model [32].

Publication bias refers to the tendency to submit or accept articles for publication based only on the positive findings [33], and is a concern in meta-analyses as it can influence the validity of the analyses conducted [34]. Therefore, publication bias was assessed for the different studies using funnel plots and the Egger regression test [35]. Finally, sensitivity analyses were conducted to assess possible changes in the previously obtained results, with only RCTs included.

All the effect size calculations and analyses were conducted using the Practical Meta-Analysis Effect Size Calculator, Review Manager (RevMan, Version 5.4, Cochrane, London, UK), and the meta and metafor packages in RStudio (Version 1.3.1093, RStudio, PBC, Boston, MA, USA).

3. Results

3.1. Study Selection

Initially, 1472 articles were identified in PubMed database. Four hundred and fifty-two articles were excluded because they were duplicates. From the remaining 1020 articles, 994 were removed following initial screening based on their title and abstract. Twenty-six articles were assessed for eligibility and 15 of those studies were excluded due to the inclusion and exclusion criteria. Additionally, three studies were selected by citation searching, of which two were excluded. Finally, 12 articles were selected for the systematic review and the meta-analysis (see Figure 1).

3.2. Study Characteristics

Twelve studies with a total of 512 participants with PD were included in the systematic review and meta-analysis. Selected studies were published between 2004 and 2020, with the number of participants involved in the studies ranging from 15 to 75. Eleven of the 12 studies found no differences at baseline in demographic variables, whereas one study showed significant differences in age, sex, and years of disease progression, so the subsequent analyses were adjusted. The disease stage score assessed by H&Y was between 1 and 3 in most studies. The frequency of the interventions ranged from twice a week to five times a week, with a maximum duration of 90 min, over a period of time that varied from three weeks to six months. Two different methods of intervention were used; four studies conducted cognitive rehabilitation activities using a pencil and paper format, and five studies with a computer-based format. Three studies also used both methods (pencil and paper and computer-based activities) in their cognitive rehabilitation sessions. Six studies conducted the intervention in a group format, while another study conducted the intervention individually. Most of the research focused on cognitive outcomes and reported improvements, although there was diversity in the number of cognitive domains showing improvement, ranging from a single domain to six. A summary of the studies included in cognitive rehabilitation for PD is shown in Table 1.

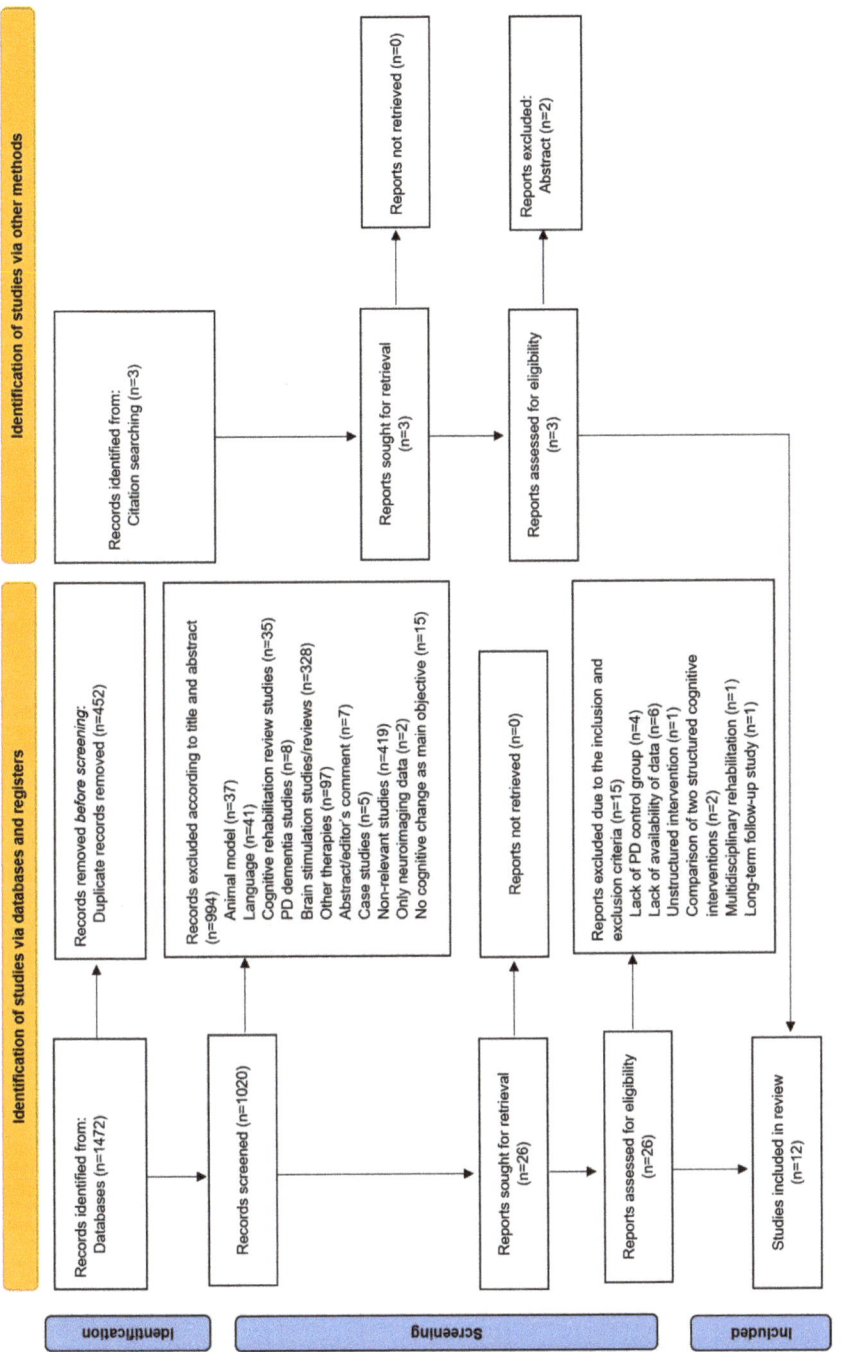

Figure 1. PRISMA summary of identified studies included in the review.

Table 1. Summary of cognitive rehabilitation studies for PD.

Authors	Sample	Characteristics of the Sample	H&Y Stages	Intervention	Format	Duration	Domains Trained	Outcomes
Sammer et al., 2006 [36]	26 PD 12 PD-CR 14 PD-ACG	Age: 70.8 PD-CR 68.5 PD-ACG Years of education: -	2–3	CR: Executive Function Training (Paper) ACG: Standard Treatment (Occupational Therapy, Physical Therapy and Treatment) (Paper)	Group	10 sessions 30 min/session	-Working memory -Executive functions	Improvements in PD-CR: -Executive functions
Paris et al., 2011 [37]	28 PD 12 PD-CR 16 PD-CG	Age: 64.7 PD-CR 65.4 PD-CG Years of education: 9.8 PD-CR 9.5 PD-CG	1–3	"SmartBrain Tool" (Paper + Computer)	Group + home	12 sessions 3 times/week 4 weeks 45 min/session	-Attention -Memory -Psychomotor speed -Executive functions -Visuospatial abilities -Language -Calculation abilities	Improvements in PD-CR: -Attention -Processing speed -Visual memory -Visuoconstructive abilities -Semantic fluency -Executive functions
Edwards et al., 2013 [38]	74 PD 32 PD-CR 42 PD-CG	Age: 69.4 PD-CR 68.2 PD-CG Years of education: 14.8 PD-CR 15.4 PD-CG	1–3	"Insight Software" (Computer)	Home	36 sessions 3 times/week 3 months 60 min/session	-Processing speed	Improvements in PD-CR: -Processing speed
Naismith et al., 2013 [39]	50 PD 35 PD-CR 15 PD-CG	Age: 68.5 PD-CR 64.9 PD-CG Years of education: 14.9 PD-CR 14.0 PD-CG	1–3	Cognitive training (Neuropsychological Educational Approach to Remediation (NEAR)) + Psychoeducation (Computer)	Group	14 sessions 2 times/week 7 weeks 60 min of CR 60 min psycho-education	-Memory -Psychomotor speed -Mental flexibility -Verbal fluency	Improvements in PD-CR: -Verbal memory
Cerasa et al., 2014 [40]	15 PD 8 PD-CR 7 PD-CG	Age: 61.1 PD-CR 58.3 PD-CG Years of education: 8 PD-CR 8 PD-CG	1–3	CR: "Rehacom" CG: Simple visuomotor coordination tapping task (Computer)	Group (CR) + Individual (CG)	6 weeks 2 times/week 60 min/session	-Attention -Information processing task	Improvements in PD-CR: -Attention/Processing speed -Working memory Increased functional brain activity: -Left dorsolateral prefrontal cortex -Superior left parietal cortex

Table 1. Cont.

Authors	Sample	Characteristics of the Sample	H&Y Stages	Intervention	Format	Duration	Domains Trained	Outcomes
Costa et al., 2014 [41]	17 PD-MCI 9 PD-CR 8 PD-CG	Age: 66.1 PD-CR 70.9 PD-CG Years of education: 11.2 PD-CR 10.6 PD-CG	1–3	CR: Cognitive change training CG: Breathing training (Paper)	–	4 weeks 3 times/week 45 min/session	-Shifting abilities (Verbal fluency and Trail Making Test)	Improvements in PD-CR: -Verbal fluency -Trail Making Test -Prospective memory procedures
Peña et al., 2014 [42]	42 PD 20 PD-CR 22 PD-ACG	Age: 67.7 PD-CR 68.1 PD-ACG Years of education: 10.5 PD-CR 10.2 PD-ACG	1–3	CR: "REHACOP" ACG: Occupational activities (Paper)	Group	39 sessions 13 weeks 2 times/week 60 min/session	-Attention -Memory -Language -Executive functions -Social cognition -Processing speed	Improvements in PD-CR: -Processing speed -Visual memory -Social cognition -Functional disability
Petrelli et al., 2014 [43]	65 PD 22 PD-NV 22 PD-MF 21 PD-CG	Age: 69.2 PD-NV 68.8 PD-MF 69.1 PD-CG Years of education: 13.1 PD-NV 13.6 PD-MF 12.8 PD-CG	1–3	NV: "NEUROvitalis" (Computer) MF: "Mentally fit" (Paper)	Group + Individual	12 sessions 6 weeks 2 times/week 90 min/session	NV -Attention -Verbal memory -Visual memory -Executive functions MF -Attention -Memory -Creativity	Improvements in PD-NV versus PD-CG: -Working memory -Verbal memory Improvements in PD-MF versus PD-CG: -Depressive symptoms Improvements in PD-NV versus PD-MF: -Working memory
Angelucci et al., 2015 [44]	15 PD-MCI 7 PD-CR 8 PD-CG	Age: 67.6 PD-CR 71.9 PD-CG Years of education: 11.7 PD-CR 10.6 PD-CG	–	CR: Cognitive change training CG: Simple cognitive tests (Paper)	–	12 sessions 4 weeks 3 times/week 45 min/session	-Executive functions	Improvements in PD-CR: -Executive functions
Fellman et al., 2018 [45]	52 PD 26 PD-CR 26 PD-ACG	Age: 64.8 PD-CR 65.5 PD-ACG Years of education: 5.3 PD-CR 5.5 PD-ACG	–	CR: Working memory ACG: Online quiz task "Älypää" (Computer)	Home	3 weeks 3 times/week 30 min/session	-Working memory	Improvements in PD-CR: -Working memory -Depressive symptoms

Table 1. *Cont.*

Authors	Sample	Characteristics of the Sample	H&Y Stages	Intervention	Format	Duration	Domains Trained	Outcomes
Bernini et al., 2020 [46]	53 PD 18 PD-CCT 12 PD-PCT 18 PD-CG	Age: 74.6 PD-CCT 69.8 PD-PCT 69.3 PD-CG Years of education: 9.5 PD-CCT 8.0 PD-PCT 7.6 PD-CG	≤3	CCT: "CoRe" (Computer) PCT: "CoRe" (Paper) CG: Unstructured activities	Group	3 weeks 4 times/week 45 min/session	-Logical executive functions - Attention/processing speed -Working memory -Episodic long-term memory	Improvements in PD-CCT versus PD-PCT: -Global cognition Improvements in PD-CCT versus CG: -Global cognition -Attention/processing speed
Ophey et al., 2020 [47]	75 PD 37 PD-CR 38 PD-CG	Age: 64.0 PD-CR 63.8 PD-CG Years of education: 15.0 PD-CR 15.5 PD-CG	2–3	CR: "NeuroNation" (Computer)	Individual + home	5 weeks 5 times/week 30 min/session	-Working memory	Improvements in PD-CR: -No improvements Assesment after 3 months: -Verbal working memory -Visuoconstructive abilities

PD = Parkinson's disease; CR = cognitive rehabilitation; ACG = active control group; CCT = computer cognitive training; PCT = paper-pencil cognitive training; CG = control group; H&Y = Hoehn and Yahr scale; MCI = Mild cognitive impairment

3.3. Effectiveness of Cognitive Rehabilitation

3.3.1. Overall Cognitive Functions

The effect size of overall cognitive functions was based on the mean of global cognitive status and cognitive subdomains from 10 studies reporting at least two cognitive variables. The random-effects model showed a small and statistically significant effect size ($g = 0.39$, $p = 0.01$) with a 95% CI (0.23 to 0.55). The heterogeneity test showed low levels of heterogeneity across the studies ($Q = 4.04$, $p = 0.91$; $I^2 = 0\%$) (Figure 2).

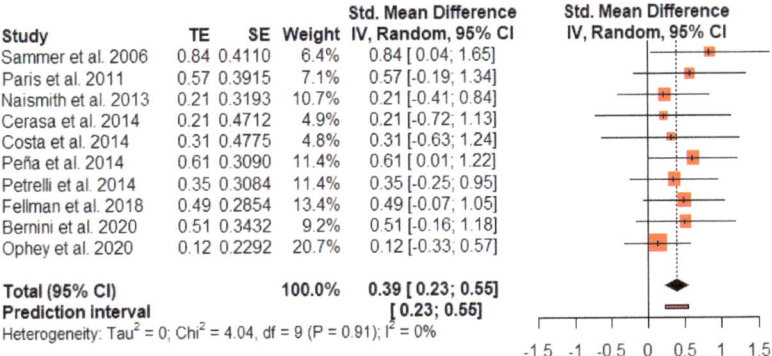

Figure 2. Effectiveness of cognitive rehabilitation in overall cognitive functions.

3.3.2. Global Cognitive Status

Four studies analyzed changes in global cognitive status after cognitive rehabilitation using global cognitive screening tests. The random-effects model showed a moderate and not significant effect size ($g = 0.55$, $p = 0.12$) with a 95% CI (-0.26 to 1.36). The heterogeneity test showed moderate levels of heterogeneity ($Q = 5.89$, $p = 0.12$; $I^2 = 49\%$) (Figure 3).

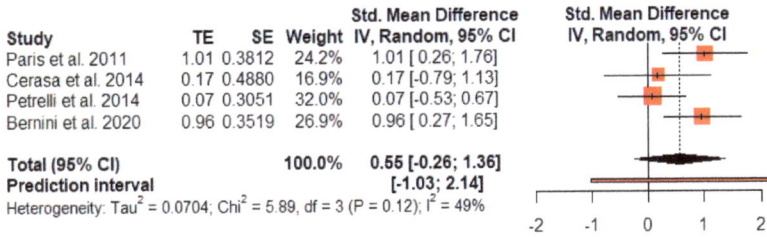

Figure 3. Effectiveness of cognitive rehabilitation in global cognitive status.

3.3.3. Attention

Five studies analyzed changes in attention after cognitive rehabilitation. The random-effects model showed a small and not significant effect size ($g = 0.36$, $p = 0.09$) with a 95% CI (-0.10 to 0.82). The heterogeneity test showed low levels of heterogeneity ($Q = 5.57$, $p = 0.23$; $I^2 = 28\%$) (Figure 4).

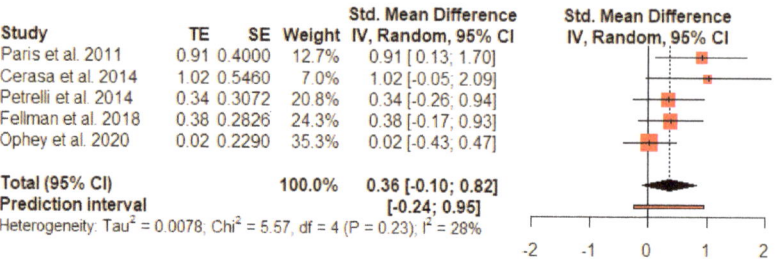

Figure 4. Effectiveness of cognitive rehabilitation in attention.

3.3.4. Working Memory

Six studies analyzed changes in working memory after cognitive rehabilitation. The random-effects model showed a moderate and statistically significant effect size ($g = 0.50$, $p = 0.02$) with a 95% CI (0.12 to 0.89). The heterogeneity test showed low levels of heterogeneity ($Q = 6.64$, $p = 0.25$; $I^2 = 25\%$) (Figure 5).

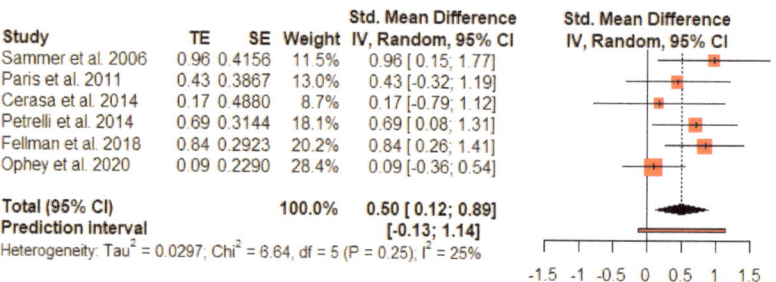

Figure 5. Effectiveness of cognitive rehabilitation in working memory.

3.3.5. Verbal Memory

Seven studies reported verbal memory measures after cognitive rehabilitation. The random-effects model showed a small and statistically significant effect size ($g = 0.41$, $p = 0.00$) with a 95% CI (0.17 to 0.65). The heterogeneity test showed low levels of heterogeneity ($Q = 4.20$, $p = 0.65$; $I^2 = 0\%$) (Figure 6).

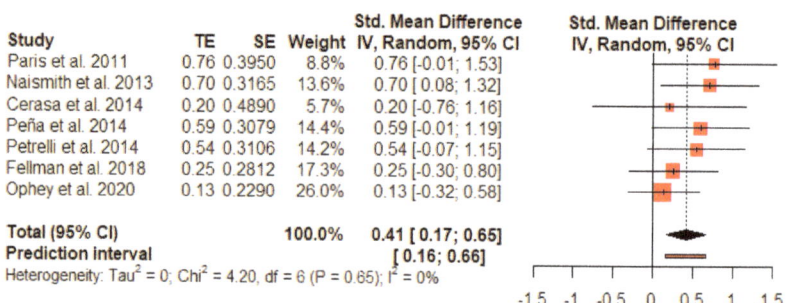

Figure 6. Effectiveness of cognitive rehabilitation in verbal memory.

3.3.6. Visual Memory

Five studies reported visual memory measures after cognitive rehabilitation. The random-effects model showed a small and not significant effect size ($g = 0.29$, $p = 0.08$) with a 95% CI (-0.07 to 0.66). The heterogeneity test showed low levels of heterogeneity ($Q = 3.47$, $p = 0.48$; $I^2 = 0\%$) (Figure 7).

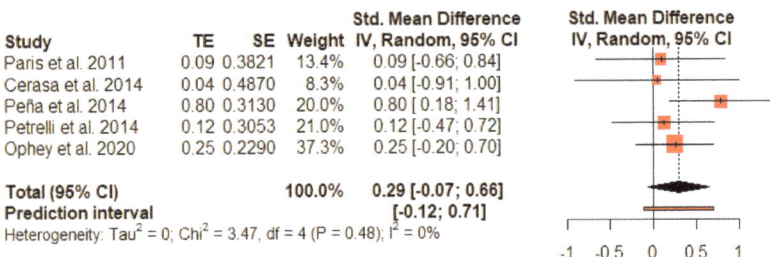

Figure 7. Efficacy of cognitive rehabilitation in visual memory.

3.3.7. Verbal Fluency

Six studies measured verbal fluency after cognitive rehabilitation. The random-effects model showed a small and not significant effect size ($g = 0.27$, $p = 0.11$) with a 95% CI (-0.09 to 0.63). The heterogeneity test showed low levels of heterogeneity ($Q = 5.20$, $p = 0.39$; $I^2 = 4$%) (Figure 8).

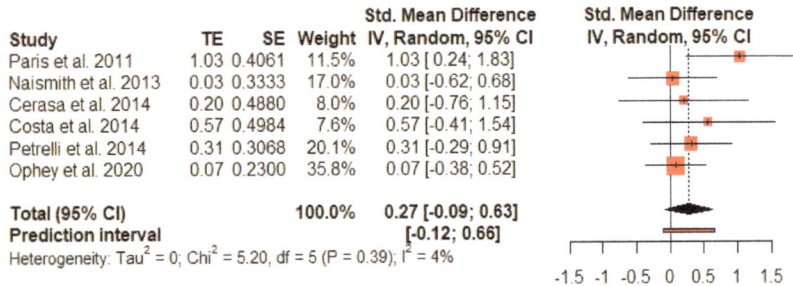

Figure 8. Effectiveness of cognitive rehabilitation in verbal fluency.

3.3.8. Executive Functions

Seven studies reported executive function measures. The random-effects model showed a small and statistically significant effect size ($g = 0.30$, $p = 0.04$) with a 95% CI (0.02 to 0.59). The heterogeneity test showed low levels of heterogeneity ($Q = 4.43$, $p = 0.62$; $I^2 = 0$%) (Figure 9).

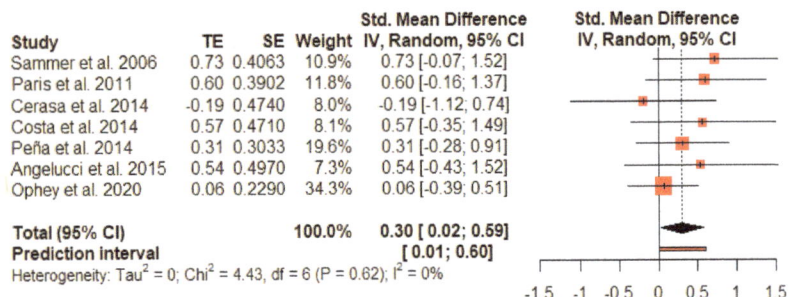

Figure 9. Effectiveness of cognitive rehabilitation in executive functions.

3.3.9. Visuospatial and Visuoconstructive Abilities

Four studies analyzed changes in visuospatial and visuoconstructive abilities after cognitive rehabilitation. The random-effects model showed no effect size ($g = 0.17$, $p = 0.11$) with a 95% CI (-0.04 to 0.38). The heterogeneity test showed low levels of heterogeneity ($Q = 0.51$, $p = 0.92$; $I^2 = 0$%) (Figure 10).

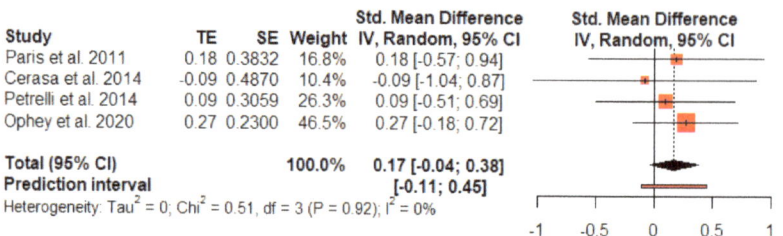

Figure 10. Effectiveness of cognitive rehabilitation in visuospatial and visuoconstructive abilities.

3.3.10. Processing Speed

Seven studies reported processing speed outcomes. The random-effects model showed a small and not significant effect size ($g = 0.24$, $p = 0.09$) with a 95% CI (-0.06 to 0.54). The heterogeneity test showed low levels of heterogeneity across the studies ($Q = 5.87$, $p = 0.44$; $I^2 = 0\%$) (Figure 11).

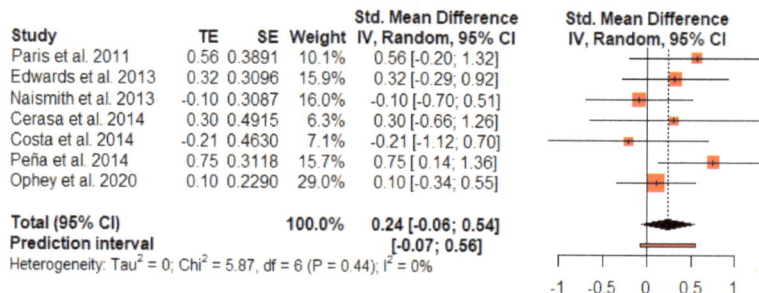

Figure 11. Effectiveness of cognitive rehabilitation in processing speed.

3.3.11. Others: Functionality, Depressive Symptoms and Quality of Life

Functionality was only reported in two studies, and so a meta-analysis could not be performed. Seven studies evaluated depressive symptoms after cognitive rehabilitation. Depressive symptoms showed a small and not significant effect size ($g = 0.24$, $p = 0.08$) with a 95% CI (-0.04 to 0.52). The heterogeneity test showed low levels of heterogeneity ($Q = 5.87$, $p = 0.44$; $I^2 = 0\%$) (Figure 12).

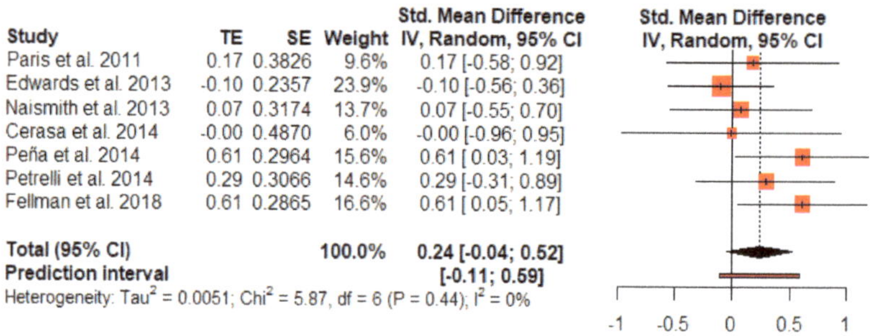

Figure 12. Effectiveness of cognitive rehabilitation in depressive symptoms.

Only three studies reported quality of life outcomes. The random-effects model showed no effect size ($g = -0.07$, $p = 0.64$) with a broad 95% CI (-0.68 to 0.53). The heterogeneity test showed low levels of heterogeneity across the studies ($Q = 0.88$, $p = 0.64$; $I^2 = 0\%$) (Figure 13).

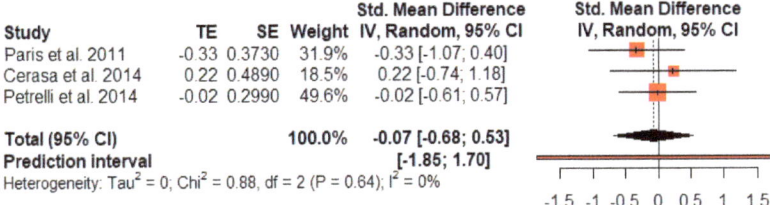

Figure 13. Effectiveness of cognitive rehabilitation in quality of life.

3.4. Moderator Analyses

Moderator analyses were performed to explore possible parameters that may explain the differences between the effect sizes obtained. The mixed-effects model meta-regression analyses were conducted with the overall cognitive function effect sizes estimated as previously shown in Figure 2, and with the following predictor variables: participants' age and years of education, variables related to intervention time (number, frequency, and duration of sessions), the modality of delivering the cognitive training (pencil and paper or computer), baseline global cognitive scores and PD patient-related features (disease duration, UPDRS III [26] and H&Y scale [27]) (See Table 2).

Table 2. Results of overall cognitive function meta-regression analyses.

Model Number	Predictor Variables	k	df	$F_{moderator}$	$Q_{residual}$	R^2	β	p
1	Age of participants	10	8	3.96	2.70	0%	0.04	0.08
2	Years of education	9	7	4.45	4.45	0%	−0.03	0.07
3	H&Y	8	6	2.03	2.79	0%	0.66	0.20
4	Duration of PD (years)	9	7	1.10	2.36	0%	0.01	0.32
5	Baseline global cognitive scores	10	8	0.30	3.90	0%	0.00	0.60
6	Total number of conducted sessions	10	8	0.02	4.03	0%	−0.00	0.89
7	Training session duration (min)	10	8	0.02	4.03	0%	0.01	0.87
8	Frequency of weekly sessions	9	7	1.72	2.19	0%	−0.08	0.23
9	UPDRS-III	8	6	0.03	2.4	0%	0.01	0.87
10	Tools for cognitive training (pencil & paper or computer)	10	7	1.71	2.71	0%	−0.12	0.24
11	Age × Years of education	9	5	2.71	1.04	0%	0.01	0.15
12	Duration of PD × H&Y	8	4	1.70	1.64	0%	−0.06	0.30
13	H&Y × UPDRS-III	6	2	0.43	1.05	0%	−1.54	0.75
14	Total number of sessions conducted × Training session duration (min)	10	6	4.04	1.33	0%	0.00	0.07
15	Total number of sessions conducted × Frequency of weekly sessions	9	5	4.41	0.75	0%	−0.02	0.04 *
16	Training session duration (min) × Frequency of weekly sessions	9	5	2.21	1.17	0%	0.01	0.20

Note: k = number of studies; $F_{moderator}$ = test of moderators; $Q_{residual}$ = test for residual heterogeneity; R^2 = amount of heterogeneity accounted for; β = estimate; * = $p < 0.05$; PD = Parkinson's disease; H&Y = Hoehn and Yahr scale; UPDRS-III = Unified Parkinson's Disease Rating Scale-part III.

No significant effects were found among the main effects of the predictor variables (models 1 to 10). We also tested the interaction between predictor variables (models 11 to 16) through a meta-regression analysis. Models 11, 12, 13, 14 and 16 showed no significant interactions. In contrast, the interaction between the number of sessions conducted and frequency of weekly sessions (model 15) was statistically significant and negatively associated with the overall cognitive function effect sizes ($F(3, 5) = 4.4$; $\beta = -0.02$; $p = 0.04$). These results indicated that the number of sessions in a cognitive rehabilitation programme could influence the effect sizes obtained when the weekly frequency of these sessions is also taken into account. Nonetheless, this interaction did not explain the possible heterogeneity between the different effect sizes ($R^2 = 0\%$).

3.5. Publication Bias

Funnel plots and Eggers regression test were performed to analyze the presence of publication bias.

The funnel plot of overall cognitive functions, global cognitive status, cognitive subdomains, depressive symptoms and quality of life showed no evidence of asymmetry (see Figure S1). In addition, the results obtained from Egger's regression test were not significant for most of the variables ($p > 0.15$), although a significant result was found in the attention domain ($p = 0.01$). However, Egger's test does not provide sufficient information for global cognitive status, cognitive subdomains, depressive symptoms and quality of life, as there are fewer than 10 studies in each of the domains [48]. Additionally, although most of the results indicate low levels of publication bias, it is necessary to consider the levels in isolation and to consider the presence of certain levels of publication bias.

3.6. Sensitivity Analyses

Sensitivity analyses were conducted to examine whether the previously obtained results would change if Naismith and colleagues' non-randomized study [39] was excluded from the analyses. Therefore, the analyses were carried out on the verbal memory, verbal fluency, executive function and processing speed cognitive subdomains. The sensitivity analyses showed small changes in the effect sizes of verbal memory (from $g = 0.41$, $p = 0.00$; to $g = 0.37$, $p = 0.01$), verbal fluency (from $g = 0.27$, $p = 0.11$; to $g = 0.32$, $p = 0.11$) and executive function (from $g = 0.30$, $p = 0.04$; to $g = 0.30$, $p = 0.03$) domains. Despite this, the exclusion of the non-randomized study did not significantly change the size nor the significance of the previous domains. The exception was observed in the processing speed cognitive domain, which, regardless of continuing to have a small effect size (from $g = 0.24$ to $g = 0.31$), becomes marginally significant (from $p = 0.09$ to $p = 0.06$) (see Figure S2).

4. Discussion

The aim of this study was to conduct a systematic review and meta-analysis of the literature regarding the effectiveness of cognitive rehabilitation in PD, not only at a cognitive level but also in functionality, depressive symptomatology and quality of life.

The systematic review indicated that the cognitive domains that most frequently improved after cognitive rehabilitation in PD were attention, working memory, verbal memory, executive functions and processing speed. Despite the considerable diversity and variability in intervention strategies, studies revealed cognitive improvements in at least one cognitive domain. Thus, cognitive rehabilitation has a positive impact on the cognition of PD patients, regardless of intervention method, duration and frequency [11].

The main results obtained from the meta-analysis showed moderate improvements in global cognitive status ($g = 0.55$) and working memory ($g = 0.50$). Small but significant improvements were found in verbal memory ($g = 0.41$), overall cognitive functions ($g = 0.39$) and executive functions ($g = 0.30$). Attention ($g = 0.36$), visual memory ($g = 0.29$), verbal fluency ($g = 0.27$) and processing speed ($g = 0.24$) showed a small non-significant effect and visuospatial and visuoconstructive abilities ($g = 0.17$) showed no effect. However, it should be noted that small effect sizes also report improvements after cognitive rehabilitation.

It is important to highlight that there was a moderate effect on global cognitive status after cognitive rehabilitation, and so it could be interesting to include global screening tests as outcome measures in the rehabilitation studies and not only to report them at baseline, in order to evaluate the differences between groups. On the other hand, the small effect size of overall cognitive functions showed in this meta-analysis may be due to the data analysis criteria applied in the article, which was based on the average of the global cognitive status and the cognitive subdomains of studies that had reported at least two cognitive variables.

Memory was one of the most frequently trained domains during the cognitive rehabilitation (5 of 12 studies), and was usually trained with a general approach, rather than being divided into verbal and visual memory domains. However, working memory was trained independently in some of the studies (four studies) and the results obtained from our meta-analysis showed a moderate and significant effect in this cognitive subdomain. In the case of the verbal memory and visual memory domains, 7 of the 12 studies included reported verbal memory measures and five reported visual memory. However, only four studies (two for verbal memory and two for visual memory) found significant improvements after rehabilitation. In this meta-analysis, we analyzed the effect sizes of verbal and visual memory independently, obtaining a small and significant effect size for verbal memory, although a small but non-significant effect size was found for visual memory. A meta-analysis performed in PD patients with MCI or dementia also obtained small effect sizes in verbal and visual memory [19]. Other meta-analyses analyzed improvements in memory using a general memory domain in which they also found a small effect after cognitive rehabilitation [17,18]. Regarding executive functions and processing speed, both domains were also two of the most frequently trained functions in cognitive rehabilitation (6–7/12 studies). The results obtained from our meta-analysis showed a small and significant effect size on executive functions, while processing speed showed a small and non-significant effect size. However, the small and significant effect size obtained in executive functions, and the small and not significant effect size in processing speed, may be due to the fact that executive functions and processing speed were two of the domains with the greatest variability among the assessment measures used. The effect sizes obtained in executive functions were similar to the meta-analysis performed in PD patients with MCI or dementia [19]. However, the meta-analyses conducted, respectively, by Leung and Lawrence [17,18] obtained moderate effect sizes in executive functions and small sizes in processing speed. This is the first meta-analysis of cognitive rehabilitation in PD that has analyzed the effects of verbal fluency after intervention and our results showed a small effect size in this domain. These results may have been obtained because although six studies reported verbal fluency measures, only one study showed improvements, specifically in semantic fluency.

Furthermore, changes in functionality, depressive symptoms and quality of life are also reported via transference effects [14], even though these functions have not been directly trained. A systematic review showed that one study has reflected the benefits of cognitive rehabilitation on the depressive symptomatology of people with PD. The small effect size ($g = 0.24$) obtained in the meta-analysis supports the results obtained from the systematic review, in which most of the studies that assessed depressive symptoms reported that the patients with PD obtained similar scores to those obtained at the beginning of the cognitive intervention. Regarding quality of life, no evidence was found after cognitive training. Therefore, further studies that include quality of life, functionality and mood as outcome variables need to be conducted.

There were low levels of heterogeneity and publication bias in most of the outcomes analyzed. Besides, we carried out moderator analyses only for the overall cognitive functions, and the results suggest that the interaction between the number of sessions conducted and the frequency of sessions in a cognitive training program could be relevant variables to take into account when applying and designing a cognitive rehabilitation program. However, none of them could explain the differences between the effect sizes obtained.

There are several limitations in this systematic review and meta-analysis study. First, the small number of studies that met the inclusion criteria for this meta-analysis limited the precision of the publication bias. In addition, the lack of data or the use of different methods in the analyses limits the possibility of making a comparison between all the studies included in the systematic review. On the one hand, the variability of trained cognitive functions allows studies divided by different cognitive domains to be compared, although not all the cognitive domains were trained in all the studies and so, in some cases, the comparison would be limited. On the other hand, some of the studies measured the cognitive domains differently. Therefore, when the specific cognitive domains were grouped according to the tests used, only studies that reported those tests independently could be included.

5. Importance of Cognitive Rehabilitation in Personalized Medicine

Personalized medicine refers to the idea that treatment strategies could be influenced by age, personality, lifestyle, genetic factors, pharmacoeconomics, pharmacogenetics and comorbidity [10,49]. Personalized medicine seeks to consider these aspects in order to develop individualized treatment strategies for each person with PD [10,49]. In this line, cognitive rehabilitation is proposed as an option in personalized medicine strategy to manage cognitive impairment [10,49], and it can be administered, along with other pharmacological therapies, to improve cognitive impairment [50].

This systematic review and meta-analysis showed the effectiveness of cognitive rehabilitation in PD. It is important to analyze the variables that influence the cognitive rehabilitation process itself in order to elucidate which are the best components of a successful cognitive rehabilitation program. Some of these variables are: age, years of education, the variables related to the time of intervention (number, frequency and duration of sessions), the modality of the cognitive training (pencil and paper or computer), the baseline global cognitive scores and PD patient-related features (disease duration, UPDRS and H&Y stages). However, in the regression analysis of our meta-analysis, none of these variables showed a percentage of variance accounted for in the effect sizes. Studies should continue reporting the specific methodology used and provide as much detailed information as possible to further investigate these aspects. Regarding age, studies in neuropsychiatric diseases such as schizophrenia showed that younger participants obtained a greater benefit from cognitive rehabilitation [51,52]. In PD studies, the groups that perform cognitive rehabilitation activities usually have a similar average age, which allows for more accurate comparison between groups. However, further studies are needed that analyze the age factor, because the age at the time of the diagnosis, the cognitive impairment associated with age and the age at the time of the intervention are all variables that could influence the cognitive rehabilitation process. In addition, it is important to start cognitive rehabilitation as early as possible in order to manage the cognitive deficits in PD patients. Most studies focus on participants at the early stages of the disease (H&Y stages ≤3), since the application of treatment before the onset of dementia could increase or maintain cognitive outcomes over time [12]. However, few studies focus on analyzing the impact of cognitive rehabilitation in more advanced stages of the disease, including patients with PD dementia. Previous meta-analyses [17,18], as well as our meta-analysis, focused on analyzing the impact of cognitive rehabilitation in PD without dementia and found evidence of cognitive improvement. In PD patients with dementia, no evidence of improvement has been found after cognitive rehabilitation [19]. Therefore, it is very important to start the cognitive intervention before the appearance of cognitive deterioration. However, it would be interesting to continue investigating the effects of cognitive rehabilitation in PD-MCI and dementia, and to observe whether, despite the presence of dementia, it is possible to maintain or reduce the progression of cognitive deficits.

Active lifestyle and personality are two determining factors in the cognitive rehabilitation process. Participating in a specific cognitive rehabilitation program requires the availability of sufficient time for attending sessions and performing cognitive activities at set times. A proactive, active lifestyle and a positive attitude can help in increasing attendance and participation in cognitive rehabilitation sessions and achieving positive results. A study conducted in older adults at risk of dementia analyzed the relationship between self-reported lifestyle and cognitive changes associated with cognitive and physical rehabilitation [53]. The authors showed that individuals with a more active lifestyle demonstrated a favorable change in cognitive performance during the study period compared to individuals with a less active lifestyle, regardless of the group to which they belonged (experimental or control groups) [53]. In addition, the personality of each individual may also influence participation in their rehabilitation program, as well as how comfortable they feel with therapy (group or individual). A common component regarding PD patients' personal factors is whether intervention groups should be homogeneous or heterogeneous. Homogeneous groups can facilitate the integration of each participant more easily because all members experience similar conditions. However, it is sometimes necessary to consider that heterogeneous groups can encourage companionship and prompt people to help each other.

Finally, another important variable to consider in personalized medicine is genetics. In our meta-analysis, the included studies were focused on idiopathic PD, without mentioning genetic variants of PD. However, PD is a heterogeneous disease in which 3–5% of cases are affected by a genetic variant [54], which contributes to clinical variability, in some cases also including a predisposition to cognitive impairment and dementia [55]. Therefore, further studies should be conducted to analyze the effect of cognitive rehabilitation in genetic PD, especially in patients with a mutation known to cause a higher predisposition to cognitive impairment.

6. Conclusions

The review of available studies along with the effect sizes obtained in the meta-analysis would seem to support the fact that cognitive rehabilitation may be beneficial in improving cognitive functions in PD patients. However, there are not many studies that assess functionality and quality of life after cognitive rehabilitation. Therefore, more studies are needed to analyze the effectiveness of cognitive rehabilitation in patients with PD at the cognitive level and on the instrumental activities of daily living, functionality and quality of life. In addition, it would be interesting to analyze individual factors such as age, lifestyle, personality and genetic factors, which may be applicable to personalized medicine, in order to design more specific and individualized interventions. On the other hand, cognitive impairment, dysfunctionality and disease progression in people with PD are determining factors in the quality of life of patients and their family caregivers, resulting in major changes in their lives and creating a future need for long-term care. This care is usually provided by a family member [56], leading to possible physical, emotional and psychosocial problems for the caregivers themselves [57]. It is necessary to include treatment that takes a holistic approach to the disease, and thus, incorporating systems of psychoeducation and measurement of clinical symptoms may be beneficial for people with PD and their family caregivers.

Supplementary Materials: The following are available online at https://www.mdpi.com/article/10.3390/jpm11050429/s1, Figure S1: Funnel plot asymmetry of publication bias, Figure S2: Forest plot of sensitive analysis: Effect sizes of randomized controlled trials, Table S1: Search strategy, Table S2: Methodological quality and risk of bias, Table S3: Outcomes and assessment included in the meta-analysis.

Author Contributions: Conceptualization, I.S.-L., Y.B.-B., O.L.-J., N.O., J.P. and N.I.-B.; Formal analysis, Y.B.-B.; Funding acquisition, I.S.-L., N.O. and N.I.-B.; Investigation, I.S.-L. and Y.B.-B.; Methodology, I.S.-L. and Y.B.-B.; Project administration, N.I.-B.; Supervision, O.L.-J., N.O., J.P. and N.I.-B.; Writing—original draft, I.S.-L.; Writing—review and editing, I.S.-L., Y.B.-B., O.L.-J., N.O., J.P. and N.I.-B. All authors have read and agreed to the published version of the manuscript.

Funding: This study was funded by the BBK foundation (P201902032-12/1284), the Department of Education of the Basque Government (IT946-16) and a Research Staff Training Programme Grant from the Basque Government (PRE_2018_1_0379).

Institutional Review Board Statement: Ethical review and approval was not required for this study because it is a meta-analysis based on previously published studies.

Informed Consent Statement: Not applicable.

Data Availability Statement: All relevant data are included in the study and supplementary information.

Conflicts of Interest: The authors declare no conflict of interest.

References

1. Poewe, W.; Seppi, K.; Tanner, C.M.; Halliday, G.M.; Brundin, P.; Volkmann, J.; Schrag, A.-E.; Lang, A.E. Parkinson disease. *Nat. Rev. Dis. Prim.* **2017**, *3*, 17013. [CrossRef] [PubMed]
2. Schapira, A.H.; Chaudhuri, K.R.; Jenner, P. Non-motor features of Parkinson disease. *Nat. Rev. Neurosci.* **2017**, *18*, 435–450. [CrossRef] [PubMed]
3. Emre, M.; Aarsland, D.; Brown, R.; Burn, D.J.; Duyckaerts, C.; Mizuno, Y.; Broe, G.A.; Cummings, J.; Dickson, D.W.; Gauthier, S.; et al. Clinical diagnostic criteria for dementia associated with Parkinson's disease. *Mov. Disord.* **2007**, *22*, 1689–1707. [CrossRef] [PubMed]
4. Baiano, C.; Barone, P.; Trojano, L.; Santangelo, G. Prevalence and clinical aspects of mild cognitive impairment in Parkinson's disease: A meta-analysis. *Mov. Disord.* **2020**, *35*, 45–54. [CrossRef] [PubMed]
5. Svenningsson, P.; Westman, E.; Ballard, C.; Aarsland, D. Cognitive impairment in patients with Parkinson's disease: Diagnosis, biomarkers, and treatment. *Lancet Neurol.* **2012**, *11*, 697–707. [CrossRef]
6. Aarsland, D.; Creese, B.; Politis, M.; Chaudhuri, K.R.; Ffytche, D.H.; Weintraub, D.; Ballard, C. Cognitive decline in Parkinson disease. *Nat. Rev. Neurol.* **2017**, *13*, 217–231. [CrossRef] [PubMed]
7. Sasikumar, S.; Strafella, A.P. Imaging mild cognitive impairment and dementia in Parkinson's disease. *Front. Neurol.* **2020**, *11*, 1–8. [CrossRef] [PubMed]
8. Hely, M.A.; Reid, W.G.; Adena, M.A.; Halliday, G.M.; Morris, J.G. The Sydney multicenter study of Parkinson's disease: The inevitability of dementia at 20 years. *Mov. Disord.* **2008**, *23*, 837–844. [CrossRef] [PubMed]
9. Van de Weijer, S.; Hommel, A.; Bloem, B.; Nonnekes, J.; De Vries, N. Promising non-pharmacological therapies in PD: Targeting late stage disease and the role of computer based cognitive training. *Park. Relat. Disord.* **2018**, *46*, S42–S46. [CrossRef] [PubMed]
10. Titova, N.; Chaudhuri, K.R. Personalized medicine in Parkinson's disease: Time to be precise. *Mov. Disord.* **2017**, *32*, 1147–1154. [CrossRef] [PubMed]
11. Alzahrani, H.; Venneri, A. Cognitive rehabilitation in Parkinson's disease: A systematic review. *J. Park. Dis.* **2018**, *8*, 233–245. [CrossRef] [PubMed]
12. Biundo, R.; Weis, L.; Fiorenzato, E.; Antonini, A. Cognitive rehabilitation in Parkinson's disease: Is it feasible? *Arch. Clin. Neuropsychol.* **2017**, *32*, 840–860. [CrossRef] [PubMed]
13. Couture, M.; Giguère-Rancourt, A.; Simard, M. The impact of cognitive interventions on cognitive symptoms in idiopathic Parkinson's disease: A systematic review. *Aging Neuropsychol. Cogn.* **2018**, *26*, 637–659. [CrossRef] [PubMed]
14. Díez-Cirarda, M.; Ibarretxe-Bilbao, N.; Peña, J.; Ojeda, N. Neurorehabilitation in Parkinson's disease: A critical review of cognitive rehabilitation effects on cognition and brain. *Neural Plast.* **2018**, *2018*, 1–12. [CrossRef] [PubMed]
15. Hindle, J.V.; Petrelli, A.; Clare, L.; Kalbe, E. Nonpharmacological enhancement of cognitive function in Parkinson's disease: A systematic review. *Mov. Disord.* **2013**, *28*, 1034–1049. [CrossRef] [PubMed]
16. Glizer, D.; MacDonald, P.A. Cognitive training in Parkinson's disease: A review of studies from 2000 to 2014. *Park. Dis.* **2016**, *2016*, 1–19. [CrossRef] [PubMed]
17. Lawrence, B.J.; Gasson, N.; Bucks, R.S.; Troeung, L.; Loftus, A.M. Cognitive training and noninvasive brain stimulation for cognition in Parkinson's disease: A meta-analysis. *Neurorehabil. Neural Repair* **2017**, *31*, 597–608. [CrossRef] [PubMed]
18. Leung, I.H.; Walton, C.C.; Hallock, H.; Lewis, S.J.; Valenzuela, M.; Lampit, A. Cognitive training in Parkinson disease. *Neurology* **2015**, *85*, 1843–1851. [CrossRef] [PubMed]
19. Orgeta, V.; McDonald, K.R.; Poliakoff, E.; Hindle, J.V.; Clare, L.; Leroi, I. Cognitive training interventions for dementia and mild cognitive impairment in Parkinson's disease. *Cochrane Database Syst. Rev.* **2020**, *2*, CD011961. [CrossRef] [PubMed]
20. Vlagsma, T.T.; Koerts, J.; Fasotti, L.; Tucha, O.; Van Laar, T.; Dijkstra, H.; Spikman, J.M. Parkinson's patients' executive profile and goals they set for improvement: Why is cognitive rehabilitation not common practice? *Neuropsychol. Rehabil.* **2015**, *26*, 216–235. [CrossRef]
21. Page, M.J.; Moher, D.; Bossuyt, P.M.; Boutron, I.; Hoffmann, T.C.; Mulrow, C.D.; Shamseer, L.; Tetzlaff, J.M.; Akl, E.; Brennan, S.; et al. PRISMA 2020 explanation and elaboration: Updated guidance and exemplars for reporting systematic reviews. *BMJ* **2021**, *372*, n160. [CrossRef] [PubMed]
22. Sterne, J.A.C.; Savović, J.; Page, M.J.; Elbers, R.G.; Blencowe, N.S.; Boutron, I.; Cates, C.J.; Cheng, H.-Y.; Corbett, M.S.; Eldridge, S.M.; et al. RoB 2: A revised tool for assessing risk of bias in randomised trials. *BMJ* **2019**, *366*, l4898. [CrossRef] [PubMed]
23. Sterne, J.A.; Hernán, M.A.; Reeves, B.C.; Savović, J.; Berkman, N.D.; Viswanathan, M.; Henry, D.; Altman, D.G.; Ansari, M.T.; Boutron, I.; et al. ROBINS-I: A tool for assessing risk of bias in non-randomised studies of interventions. *BMJ* **2016**, *355*, i4919. [CrossRef] [PubMed]
24. Higgins, J.P.T.; Savović, J.; Page, M.J.; Elbers, R.G.; Sterne, J.A.C. Chapter 8: Assessing risk of bias in a randomized trial. In *Cochrane Handbook for Systematic Reviews of Interventions*; Higgins, J.P.T., Thomas, J., Chandler, J., Cumpston, M., Li, T., Page, M.J., Welch, V.A., Eds.; Version 6.2 (Updated February 2021); 2021; Available online: www.training.cochrane.org/handbook (accessed on 30 April 2021).

25. Maher, C.G.; Sherrington, C.; Herbert, R.D.; Moseley, A.M.; Elkins, M. Reliability of the PEDro scale for rating quality of randomized controlled trials. *Phys. Ther.* **2003**, *83*, 713–721. [CrossRef] [PubMed]
26. Martínez-Martín, P.; Gil-Nagel, A.; Gracia, L.M.; Gómez, J.B.; Martínez-Sarriés, J.; Bermejo, F. The Cooperative Multicentric Group Unified Parkinson's disease rating scale characteristics and structure. *Mov. Disord.* **1994**, *9*, 76–83. [CrossRef] [PubMed]
27. Hoehn, M.M.; Yahr, M.D. Parkinsonism: Onset, progression, and mortality. *Neurology* **1967**, *17*, 427–442. [CrossRef] [PubMed]
28. Cohen, J. *Statistical Power Analysis for the Behavioral Sciences*; Routledge Academic: New York, NY, USA, 1988.
29. Cumming, G. *Understanding the New Statistics: Effect Sizes, Confidence Intervals, and Meta-Analysis*; Routledge: New York, NY, USA, 2012.
30. Huedo-Medina, T.B.; Sánchez-Meca, J.; Marín-Martínez, F.; Botella, J. Assessing heterogeneity in meta-analysis: Q statistic or I^2 index? *Psychol. Methods* **2006**, *11*, 193–206. [CrossRef] [PubMed]
31. Harrer, M.; Cuijpers, P.; Furukawa, T.; Ebert, D.D. *Doing Meta-Analysis in R: A Hands-on Guide*; Chapman and Hall/CRC: Boca Raton, FL, USA, 2019. [CrossRef]
32. Cheung, M.W.-L.; Vijayakumar, R. A Guide to Conducting a Meta-Analysis. *Neuropsychol. Rev.* **2016**, *26*, 121–128. [CrossRef] [PubMed]
33. Dickersin, K. The existence of publication bias and risk factors for its occurrence. *JAMA* **1990**, *263*, 1385–1389. [CrossRef] [PubMed]
34. Rothstein, H.R.; Sutton, A.J.; Borenstein, M. *Publication Bias in Meta-Analysis*; John Wiley and Sons: Hoboken, NJ, USA, 2006; pp. 1–7.
35. Egger, M.C.M.; Smith, G.D.; Schneider, M.; Minder, C. Bias in meta-analysis detected by a simple, graphical test. *Br. Med. J.* **1997**, *315*, 629–634. [CrossRef] [PubMed]
36. Sammer, G.; Reuter, I.; Hullmann, K.; Kaps, M.; Vaitl, D. Training of executive functions in Parkinson's disease. *J. Neurol. Sci.* **2006**, *248*, 115–119. [CrossRef] [PubMed]
37. París, A.P.; Saleta, H.G.; Maraver, M.D.L.C.C.; Silvestre, E.; Freixa, M.G.; Torrellas, C.P.; Pont, S.A.; Nadal, M.F.; Garcia, S.A.; Bartolomé, M.V.P.; et al. Blind randomized controlled study of the efficacy of cognitive training in Parkinson's disease. *Mov. Disord.* **2011**, *26*, 1251–1258. [CrossRef] [PubMed]
38. Edwards, J.D.; Hauser, R.A.; O'Connor, M.L.; Valdés, E.G.; Zesiewicz, T.A.; Uc, E.Y. Randomized trial of cognitive speed of processing training in Parkinson disease. *Neurology* **2013**, *81*, 1284–1290. [CrossRef]
39. Naismith, S.L.; Mowszowski, L.; Diamond, K.; Lewis, S.J. Improving memory in Parkinson's disease: A healthy brain ageing cognitive training program. *Mov. Disord.* **2013**, *28*, 1097–1103. [CrossRef] [PubMed]
40. Cerasa, A.; Gioia, M.C.; Salsone, M.; Donzuso, G.; Chiriaco, C.; Realmuto, S.; Nicoletti, A.; Bellavia, G.; Banco, A.; D'Amelio, M.; et al. Neurofunctional correlates of attention rehabilitation in Parkinson's disease: An explorative study. *Neurol. Sci.* **2014**, *35*, 1173–1180. [CrossRef] [PubMed]
41. Costa, A.; Peppe, A.; Serafini, F.; Zabberoni, S.; Barban, F.; Caltagirone, C.; Carlesimo, G.A. Prospective memory performance of patients with Parkinson's disease depends on shifting aptitude: Evidence from cognitive rehabilitation. *J. Int. Neuropsychol. Soc.* **2014**, *20*, 717–726. [CrossRef] [PubMed]
42. Peña, J.; Ibarretxe-Bilbao, N.; García-Gorostiaga, I.; Gomez-Beldarrain, M.A.; Díez-Cirarda, M.; Ojeda, N. Improving functional disability and cognition in Parkinson disease: Randomized controlled trial. *Neurology* **2014**, *83*, 2167–2174. [CrossRef] [PubMed]
43. Petrelli, A.; Kaesberg, S.; Barbe, M.T.; Timmermann, L.; Fink, G.R.; Kessler, J.; Kalbe, E. Effects of cognitive training in Parkinson's disease: A randomized controlled trial. *Park. Relat. Disord.* **2014**, *20*, 1196–1202. [CrossRef] [PubMed]
44. Eangelucci, F.; Epeppe, A.; Carlesimo, G.A.; Eserafini, F.; Ezabberoni, S.; Ebarban, F.; Eshofany, J.; Ecaltagirone, C.; Ecosta, A. A pilot study on the effect of cognitive training on BDNF serum levels in individuals with Parkinson's disease. *Front. Hum. Neurosci.* **2015**, *9*, 130. [CrossRef] [PubMed]
45. Fellman, D.; Salmi, J.; Ritakallio, L.; Ellfolk, U.; Rinne, J.O.; Laine, M. Training working memory updating in Parkinson's disease: A randomised controlled trial. *Neuropsychol. Rehabil.* **2018**, *30*, 673–708. [CrossRef] [PubMed]
46. Bernini, S.; Panzarasa, S.; Barbieri, M.; Sinforiani, E.; Quaglini, S.; Tassorelli, C.; Bottiroli, S. A double-blind randomized controlled trial of the efficacy of cognitive training delivered using two different methods in mild cognitive impairment in Parkinson's disease: Preliminary report of benefits associated with the use of a computerized tool. *Aging Clin. Exp. Res.* **2020**, 1–9. [CrossRef] [PubMed]
47. Ophey, A.; Giehl, K.; Rehberg, S.; Eggers, C.; Reker, P.; van Eimeren, T.; Kalbe, E. Effects of working memory training in patients with Parkinson's disease without cognitive impairment: A randomized controlled trial. *Park. Relat. Disord.* **2020**, *72*, 13–22. [CrossRef] [PubMed]
48. Sterne, J.A.C.; Sutton, A.J.; Ioannidis, J.P.A.; Terrin, N.; Jones, D.R.; Lau, J.; Carpenter, J.; Rücker, G.; Harbord, R.M.; Schmid, C.H.; et al. Recommendations for examining and interpreting funnel plot asymmetry in meta-analyses of randomised controlled trials. *BMJ* **2011**, *343*, d4002. [CrossRef] [PubMed]
49. Titova, N.; Chaudhuri, K.R. Personalized medicine and nonmotor symptoms in Parkinson's diseas. *Int. Rev. Neurobiol.* **2017**, *134*, 1257–1281. [PubMed]
50. Calleo, J.; Burrows, C.; Levin, H.; Marsh, L.; Lai, E.; York, M.K. Cognitive rehabilitation for executive dysfunction in Parkinson's disease: Application and current directions. *Park. Dis.* **2011**, *2012*, 1–6. [CrossRef]

51. Wykes, T.; Reeder, C.; Landau, S.; Matthiasson, P.; Haworth, E.; Hutchinson, C. Does age matter? Effects of cognitive rehabilitation across the age span. *Schizophr. Res.* **2009**, *113*, 252–258. [CrossRef] [PubMed]
52. Kontis, D.; Huddy, V.; Reeder, C.; Landau, S.; Wykes, T. Effects of age and cognitive reserve on cognitive remediation therapy outcome in patients with schizophrenia. *Am. J. Geriatr. Psychiatry* **2013**, *21*, 218–230. [CrossRef] [PubMed]
53. Küster, O.C.; Fissler, P.; Laptinskaya, D.; Thurm, F.; Scharpf, A.; Woll, A.; Kolassa, S.; Kramer, A.F.; Elbert, T.; Von Arnim, C.A.F.; et al. Cognitive change is more positively associated with an active lifestyle than with training interventions in older adults at risk of dementia: A controlled interventional clinical trial. *BMC Psychiatry* **2016**, *16*, 315. [CrossRef]
54. Klein, C.; Westenberger, A. Genetics of Parkinson's disease. *Cold Spring Harb. Perspect. Med.* **2012**, *2*, a008888. [CrossRef] [PubMed]
55. Fagan, E.S.; Pihlstrøm, L. Genetic risk factors for cognitive decline in Parkinson's disease: A review of the literature. *Eur. J. Neurol.* **2017**, *24*, 561-e20. [CrossRef] [PubMed]
56. Peters, M.; Fitzpatrick, R.; Doll, H.; Playford, D.; Jenkinson, C. Does self-reported well-being of patients with Parkinson's disease influence caregiver strain and quality of life? *Park. Relat. Disord.* **2011**, *17*, 348–352. [CrossRef] [PubMed]
57. Martínez-Martín, P.; Rodríguez-Blázquez, C.; Forjaz, M.J. Quality of life and burden in caregivers for patients with Parkinson's disease: Concepts, assessment and related factors. *Expert Rev. Pharm. Outcomes Res.* **2012**, *12*, 221–230. [CrossRef] [PubMed]

Advancing Personalized Medicine in Common Forms of Parkinson's Disease through Genetics: Current Therapeutics and the Future of Individualized Management

Xylena Reed [1,†], Artur Schumacher-Schuh [2,3,†], Jing Hu [4,†] and Sara Bandres-Ciga [1,*,†]

1. Laboratory of Neurogenetics, National Institute on Aging, National Institutes of Health, 35 Convent Drive, Room 1A-211, Bethesda, MD 20892-3707, USA; xylena.reed@nih.gov
2. Serviço de Neurologia, Hospital de Clínicas de Porto Alegre, Rua Ramiro Barcelos 2350, Porto Alegre, RS 90035-003, Brazil; schuh.afs@gmail.com
3. Departamento de Farmacologia, Universidade Federal do Rio Grande do Sul, Rua Sarmento Leite, 500 sala 305, Porto Alegre, RS 90050-170, Brazil
4. Simpson Querrey Center for Neurogenetics, Ken and Ruth Davee Department of Neurology, Northwestern University Feinberg School of Medicine, Chicago, IL 60611, USA; jing.hu@northwestern.edu
* Correspondence: sara.bandresciga@nih.gov; Tel.: +1-301-841-5295
† All the authors contributed equally to this work.

Abstract: Parkinson's disease (PD) is a condition with heterogeneous clinical manifestations that vary in age at onset, rate of progression, disease course, severity, motor and non-motor symptoms, and a variable response to antiparkinsonian drugs. It is considered that there are multiple PD etiological subtypes, some of which could be predicted by genetics. The characterization and prediction of these distinct molecular entities provides a growing opportunity to use individualized management and personalized therapies. Dissecting the genetic architecture of PD is a critical step in identifying therapeutic targets, and genetics represents a step forward to sub-categorize and predict PD risk and progression. A better understanding and separation of genetic subtypes has immediate implications in clinical trial design by unraveling the different flavors of clinical presentation and development. Personalized medicine is a nascent area of research and represents a paramount challenge in the treatment and cure of PD. This manuscript summarizes the current state of precision medicine in the PD field and discusses how genetics has become the engine to gain insights into disease during our constant effort to develop potential etiological based interventions.

Keywords: precision medicine; Parkinson's disease; genetics; clinical trials

1. Introduction

Personalized medicine, also referred to as precision or stratified medicine, is a medical model that uses an individual's biological profile to guide decisions made in regard to the prevention, diagnosis, and treatment of a disease [1]. Based on each patient's unique molecular makeup, clinical information and personal preferences, it aims to overcome the limitations of traditional medicine by providing better diagnoses with earlier intervention. Combining all of this individual data allows for more efficient drug development and the advancement of more targeted therapies, by selecting the optimal treatment for a specific patient. The genomic, epigenomic, transcriptomic, and proteomic profile of an individual plays a crucial role in understanding how well a patient will respond to a certain treatment.

In the Parkinson's disease (PD) field, precision medicine is a nascent and exciting area of research that ultimately aims to achieve an appropriate disease-modifying treatment, with the right dose, at the right time in a specific patient. The link of PD to α-synuclein was the first decisive proof of a genetic defect leading to disease [2]. Later on, the first PD genome-wide association studies (GWAS) identified *SNCA* [3] as one of the major genes driving risk for sporadic PD, linking both familial and sporadic forms. Abnormal α-synuclein is a histopathological hallmark of PD patients, but also patients with other neurodegenerative conditions, collectively termed synucleinopathies, making this target promising. However, the fact that PD patients harbouring genetic defects in genes such as *PRKN* do not present with Lewy body pathology, strengthens the notion that distinct entities and multiple overlapping etiologies are at play.

So far, our limited understanding of how common forms of PD start and progress at the cellular and molecular level alongside the challenge of establishing methods for early preclinical diagnosis have hampered the development of PD modifying therapies able to prevent, stop or slow down the neurodegenerative process. However, the future holds promise. Using genetics to stratify patients can help predict success in the clinic, and drugs targeting proteins with a genetic connection to disease are more likely to be approved [4].

Clinical trials targeting genetic forms of PD, such as patients with variants in *LRRK2* and *GBA* have already been initialized, highlighting the rapid progress made in the field in the past two decades [5]. As we piece together the complex molecular puzzle of PD by unraveling the underlying pathophysiology, our hope is that novel etiological based therapies will emerge. More studies will need to be done to understand whether these therapies would be useful only for specific variant carriers or if they could also be beneficial in some forms of idiopathic PD.

On another front, drugs currently used that have significant side effects in some individuals could be used more wisely to obtain more benefits with fewer adverse events when guided by genomic information. However, identifying the right treatment for a specific patient remains a daunting challenge. PD is a widely heterogeneous disease, and numerous etiological subtypes might exist. Therefore, treating PD as one disease with a single solution will only lead to failure. Increasing evidence suggests that defining subclasses of PD and developing tools to predict the course of the disease has the potential to significantly improve cohort selection in clinical trials, reduce their cost, and increase the ability of such trials to detect treatment effects [6]. On the whole, pure monogenic forms of PD are rare and although variants in genes like *SNCA*, *PINK1*, *PRKN*, and *DJ1* are well established causes of disease it would be difficult to collect enough patients to create an appropriately powered clinical trial in these populations. For this reason, in this review we will focus on more common forms of disease including those with variants in known risk factors, like *LRRK2* and *GBA*, as well as idiopathic forms of PD where the exact cause is not known but it is thought to be a combination of genetic and environmental factors. Current estimates of PD heritability have revealed that the contribution of genetic factors to PD phenotype is about 22% indicating that stratifying patients by genomic factors is possible [7,8].

Just as important as knowing the right drug is knowing the right time in disease development to provide treatment before irreversible brain damage occurs. With current diagnostic tools, by the time there is a clinical manifestation of PD, a substantial number of dopaminergic neurons have already been permanently lost, so even if the right therapeutic is applied to the right patient, it is too late for a full recovery of motor symptoms. Using personalized medicine to examine the specific genetic context can also help identify individuals at higher risk of developing PD before symptoms appear.

This manuscript summarizes the current state of the role of genetics in precision medicine in common forms of PD. We will discuss how genetics has become the engine to gain insights into PD etiology during our constant effort to develop potential etiological based interventions.

2. Genetics as a Tool to Improve Current Symptomatic Treatment

The symptomatic treatment available for PD targets the motor symptoms induced by the dopaminergic deficit due to the degeneration of the substantia nigra. Nevertheless, the disease affects other systems and regions in the brain, which leads to a myriad of levodopa-resistant motor and non-motor symptoms for which we do not have well-established pharmacological interventions. Despite this limitation, PD is the only neurodegenerative disorder with a symptomatic treatment that provides a substantial benefit. Since the introduction of levodopa in the 1960s, it has changed the natural history of PD and remains the gold standard of treatment [9]. However, the pharmacological response is variable and, as the disease progresses, higher doses of levodopa are required. Moreover, complications induced by chronic treatment can develop over time, including motor fluctuations and dyskinesia, which affect almost half of the patients after five years of treatment and nearly all in the long term [10–12]. This situation impairs the patient's quality of life and demands more costly and complex therapeutic regimens.

Pharmacogenetics assumes that the variability in the pharmacological response observed in the clinic, can be partially explained by genetics, envisioning a scenario where a patient's genotype can assist in drug prescription. It is speculated that genetics accounts for 60–90% of the variability in the pharmacokinetics and pharmacodynamics of antiparkinsonian drugs [13]. Despite this, there is a lack of studies with robust designs that enable strong pharmacogenetic recommendations for these drugs. Most of the pharmacogenetics studies in PD were conducted in a "pre-genomic" era when variants in candidate genes were nominated with a hypothesis-driven approach [14,15].

Polymorphisms in genes related to dopamine metabolism, like *COMT*, *MAOB*, *SLC6A3*, and *DRD2*, were the natural candidates. Several phenotypes related to drug effect were studied, including levodopa response, dyskinesia, sleep disturbances, and hallucination. For example, COMT V158M, a polymorphism that alters enzyme activity, was associated with levodopa and COMT inhibitor response, while variants in the *DRD2* gene were associated with levodopa-induced dyskinesia [16]. However, these studies had small sample sizes, lacked independent replication and did not correct for multiple comparisons. The variant selection was not consistent, and the outcome assessment varied among them preventing any clear pharmacogenetic recommendations for clinicians [14].

The next frontier is pharmacogenomics, which is based largely on the data provided by genome-wide association studies (GWAS). GWAS uses genotyping arrays to identify variants that are associated with a particular phenotype by comparing the frequency of thousands of variants between cases and controls. This approach can assess the effect of genetics on pharmacological variability for a particular trait (in this case, a specific pharmacological response) using a hypothesis-free strategy. Pioneers of this approach in the pharmacogenomics of PD were two studies conducted in the same cohort that evaluated the effects of caffeine and smoking in 1458 patients with PD and 931 healthy controls [17,18]. The authors reported a gene-caffeine and gene-smoking interaction on PD risk at the risk loci *GRIN2A* and *SV2C*, respectively. In another study, Ryu et al. performed a GWAS to evaluate motor fluctuation and levodopa-induced dyskinesia in 741 Korean PD patients [19]. They identified a variant in the *GALNT14* gene associated with dyskinesia (odds ratio of 5.5, 95% CI = 2.9–10.3, $p = 7.88 \times 10^{-9}$), which can potentially predict patients more prone to this complication and may provide glimpses on how to disentangle its pathophysiology. In another study, Prud'hon et al. investigated impulse control disorder (ICD), a significant adverse effect caused by dopamine agonists in PD [20]. Here they compared exome sequencing of two groups of individuals with extreme phenotypes for ICD and found an enrichment of variants in brain-expressed genes of the adenylate cyclase-activating pathway. Using these genes as targets in future studies and clinical trials could lead to better symptomatic treatment options.

There is a growing interest regarding the effect of microbiome on diseases, particularly for PD [21]. Beyond its pathophysiological implications, drug-microbiome interactions can also influence therapeutics. COMT inhibitors, anticholinergics, and levodopa were associated with changes in the microbiome [22]. Gut bacteria, precisely some *Enterococcus* strains carrying the *tdc* gene, can exhibit tyrosine decarboxylase activity, which can convert levodopa to dopamine and decrease the levels of drug in plasma [23]. The amount of the *tdc* gene was correlated with disease duration and higher levodopa doses. Another study found that *Eggerthella* strains can contribute to levodopa degradation, and a single nucleotide variant in this bacteria can predict their enzymatic activity [24]. Interestingly, human decarboxylase inhibitors used in conjunction with levodopa, like carbidopa, do not affect the bacteria enzymatic activity. AFMT, a small-molecule that inhibits bacteria decarboxylase, was suggested as an innovative therapeutic approach. These bacteria or the *tdc* gene may potentially be used as biomarkers to predict or stratify patients who are more responsive to levodopa or more prone to develop levodopa-induced motor complications. This also suggests that the inactivation of the *tdc* gene is a potential future therapeutic target to improve the levodopa response.

Although deep brain stimulation therapy (DBS) is not generally considered a personalized genomics approach, there is evidence that PD patients have varied responses to DBS depending on their genetic background. So far, studies assessing DBS outcomes in patients carrying variants in specific genes are limited in size, but it has been reported that in patients with *LRRK2* variants, outcomes of DBS are similar to cases without known variants [25,26], whereas less favorable outcomes are seen in patients carrying variants in *GBA* [27,28].

As we work towards discovering disease-modifying strategies, it is unlikely that current antiparkinsonian symptomatic treatments, like levodopa and DBS, will lose their importance in the medium term for most patients. However, the goal to achieve a personalized approach for PD is still elusive, in part because evidence from "pre-genomic" era studies is inconclusive. There should be an effort to collect replication cohorts with larger samples and deep phenotyping to derive consistent pharmacogenetics recommendations. The current efforts to increase the power of GWAS for PD risk could also benefit by taking into account the importance of collecting information regarding pharmacological response. Finally, understanding the influence of the microbiome on levodopa metabolism may provide another front to personalize treatments in common forms of PD.

3. Genetics Nominates Promising Targets: *LRRK2* and *GBA* Clinical Trials

Despite the remarkable effects of the current treatments and drugs on the symptoms of PD, genetics has played a key role in nominating causative genes or genetic risk factors as targets for different genetic subtypes of PD. Leucine-rich repeat kinase 2 (*LRRK2*) variants are the most common cause of monogenic PD and one of the most common risk factors for idiopathic PD with a variable penetrance between 50–70% [29,30]. The LRRK2 protein exhibits both kinase and GTPase functions, and mounting evidence has shown that known pathogenic *LRRK2* variants increase the kinase activity. The most common PD-linked variant, LRRK2 G2019S, leads to a two-to-threefold increase in kinase activity which is hypothesized to be an underlying molecular mechanism responsible for the development of PD [31]. This gain-of-function implies that utilizing LRRK2 kinase inhibitors may have neuroprotective effects in PD [32,33].

Following positive preclinical experiments, two small molecule inhibitors of LRRK2 developed by Denali Therapeutics, DNL201 and DNL151, are currently in clinical trials [34,35]. A phase 1b, randomized, multicenter, double-blind placebo-controlled clinical trial of DNL201 (NCT04056689) included 29 patients with mild to moderate PD, with or without *LRRK2* variants. The results indicated that levels of LRRK2 phospho Serine-935 and phospho-RAB10 in the blood of PD patients were each decreased by more than 50% at both doses. Meanwhile, a biomarker of lysosomal function, BMP (22:6-bis-monoacylglycerophosphate), was increased by 20% and 60% in urine at the low and high dose, respectively [36]. Similar trials (NCT04056689) of DNL151 followed and have also met safety and biomarker goals. Given a more flexible dosing regimen, Denali intends to choose DNL151 to advance into phase 2/3 clinical trials in PD patients.

Since genetic studies have indicated no association of LRRK2 loss of function alleles with PD, [37] another approach now entering clinical trials is the use of antisense oligonucleotides (ASOs) to reduce the levels of active LRRK2 protein [38,39]. ASOs are promising therapeutic approaches that aim at directly and chronically decrease LRRK2 kinase activity by editing out the parts of the mRNA known to contain disease associated variants. A phase 1 clinical trial using BIIB094, an ASO to LRRK2, is currently underway to assess its safety, tolerability, and pharmacokinetics in PD patients (NCT03976349). This unique and novel approach is thought to be key to develop a long-term, effective and stable therapeutic treatment decreasing LRRK2 kinase activity and alleviating LRRK2-associated neuronal dysfunction in PD.

As the most common genetic risk factor for PD, *GBA* variants are found in 7–10% of patients with PD [40,41]. Inheriting two copies of defective *GBA* causes Gaucher Disease (GD) with varying severity depending on where the variant is located. Carriers of severe *GBA* variants have an age at onset (AAO) for PD roughly five years earlier and around a three to fourfold increase in PD risk, compared with mild *GBA* variants carriers [42]. Furthermore, severe *GBA* variants appear to be associated with higher risk of cognitive impairment and aggressive cognitive decline [43,44]. There are two common *GBA* variants associated with PD risk which do not cause GD, p.E326K and p.T369M, that may modify GCase activity to a lower level than GD associated variants. It is well established that GD phenotype can also increase the risk for PD [45]. Growing evidence supports the notion that heterozygous PD-related *GBA* variants affect multiple PD pathways [46] (shown in Figure 1) by reducing glucocerebrosidase (GCase) activity in the lysosome, leading to altered lipid metabolism, aggregation of a-synuclein (α-syn) and impaired neuronal transmission. Furthermore, aggregates of α-synuclein inhibit normal GCase activity by restricting GCase transport, thereby causing a pathogenic feedback loop [47]. Current approaches targeting GBA include GCase substrate reduction, gene therapy, small molecule chaperones and enzyme activators.

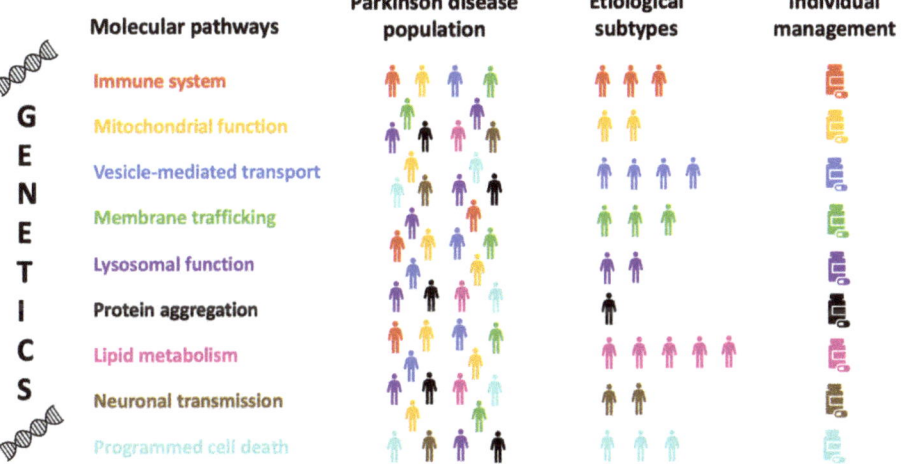

Figure 1. The role of genetics to define subtypes of Parkinson's disease and to develop potential etiological based interventions. This figure serves as an example showing that certain molecular pathways within the same disease can be significantly enriched in different individuals. These pathways may eventually become targets for personalized based interventions.

The MOVES-PD study, a randomized, multicenter, double-blind, placebo-controlled trial, was conducted to evaluate the ability of the glucosylceramide synthase inhibitor Venglustat (GZ/SAR402671) to target substrate reduction in PD patients carrying *GBA* variants (NCT02906020). Part 1 of the phase II trial results revealed that Venglustat safely achieves a dose-dependent reduction of glucosylceramide levels in plasma and cerebrospinal fluid (CSF), however, the most recent earnings report by Sanofi suggests that the trial did not meet the primary goals and has been discontinued. An ongoing Phase 1/2a trial launched by Prevail Therapeutics in early 2020, employs an AAV9-based dosage of PR001A in PD patients with at least one pathogenic *GBA* variant (NCT04127578) to assess its long term (five years) safety and efficacy. A recently reported phase II open label clinical trial of Ambroxol, a GCase chaperone that has previously been used to treat respiratory symptoms, in PD patients with or without GBA variants, demonstrated a decrease in CSF GCase enzyme activity [48]. Although the drug appears safe and well-tolerated, placebo-controlled clinical trials are needed to further confirm their findings. Another single-centre, randomized, double-blind, placebo-controlled trial of Ambroxol is currently in phase II (NCT02914366) [49].

A small molecule activator of GCase (LTI-291) has been under investigation in a phase Ib clinical trial in patients with *GBA* variants conducted by Lysosomal Therapeutics (Trialregister.nl ID: NTR7299). Furthermore, RTB101, an inhibitor of the mammalian target of rapamycin complex 1 (mTORC1), has been tested in a randomized, double-blind, placebo-controlled phase 1b/2a trial of RTB101 alone and in combination with Sirolimus (another inhibitor of mTOR often used an immunosuppressive agent) to be used in PD patients with or without *GBA* variants (ANZCTR ID: ACTR N12619000372189). Interim data from this study revealed that RTB101 was well tolerated and crossed the blood-brain barrier (BBB).

4. Genetics as a Tool to Nominate Networks to Be Targeted in Therapeutic Development

Genetics can be used in multiple ways to identify potential genes, proteins, pathways, and networks that may be involved in the pathogenesis of PD and could potentially be therapeutically targeted [50]. The simplest way of identifying targets using genetics is by examining genes known to cause disease or increase risk, like *LRRK2* and *GBA*, using linkage and sequencing studies in families and sporadic cases. Robak et al. expanded this strategy to a larger gene-set using burden analysis in a combination of data from whole exome sequencing (WES) and genotyping of 54 known lysosomal storage disease (LSD) genes to show there is a significant increase in the burden of LSD variants in PD [51]. This association remained significant in multiple cohorts even when GBA was excluded.

Another genetics tool that can be used to select potential therapeutic targets is by identifying variants that are associated with PD risk through GWAS. The latest and largest GWAS meta-analyses have identified over 90 genetic loci harboring common variants that are associated with both PD risk and progression [7,52,53]. Burden analyses examining coding variants are now regularly combined with GWAS results to prioritize genes at a locus that is associated with PD [54]. However, the non-coding portion of the genome is significantly larger than protein coding regions so it is unusual that a specific gene is identified by GWAS. This makes nomination of specific therapeutic targets at a GWAS locus very difficult [55]. In general, the effects exerted by individual GWAS variants are quite small, but when they are combined to determine a polygenic risk score (PRS) they can be used to further stratify cases from low to high risk [56–58]. PRS is defined as a model that sums the contribution of multiple risk variants of variable magnitude of effect, as determined by GWAS summary statistics. The 90 risk loci identified in the most recent PD meta-analysis are associated with higher relative risk of developing PD, with those individuals in the top 10% of PRS being nearly six-fold more likely to develop PD than those in the bottom 10% [7]. In the first major study on PRS in PD, Ibanez et al. showed that PRS in cases, excluding variants in known familial or risk genes, associated with PD status and age at onset but not with the levels of three predicted CSF biomarkers [56].

Instead of focusing on a single variant or PRS, genetic data can be integrated with transcriptomic, proteomic and protein-protein interaction (PPI) networks to nominate affected biological pathways that a single data type might miss [59,60]. A recent study examined the association of 2199 pre-defined gene sets grouped by biological process with PD by assigning a Polygenic Effect Score (PES) to each gene-set and then performing an association study [59]. The authors identified a wide range of gene-sets that were associated with PD. Further analysis using Mendelian randomization in genome-wide expression and methylation datasets identified genes with quantitative trait loci (QTL) for expression in blood and brain, as well as changes in methylation at multiple CpG sites that are associated with PD risk. This unbiased and data-driven study provided a foundational resource for the PD community through a publicly available pathways browser. Pathways previously implicated by genetics and functional studies also found to be significant in this study include endocytic trafficking [61,62], autophagic-lysosomal function [51,63], mitochondrial function [64,65], protein aggregation [66], neuronal transmission [67], lipid metabolism [68,69], and certain inflammatory pathways [70,71] (Figure 1). It has also been shown that similar pathways can be deficient in both familial and common forms of PD [51,62] and multiple networks can overlap or a single pathway can act alone. Interestingly, some of the nominated gene-sets span the etiological risk spectrum in which both common and rare variation contribute to PD susceptibility.

Combining all genomic, transcriptomic and proteomic data to identify affected pathways in PD allows individuals without variants in known risk factors to be stratified by the pathways thought to be involved in their subtype of disease. Examining pathways instead of genes also suggests that other members of the pathway could be used as therapeutic targets even if the associated gene is not druggable (Figure 1). For example, the RTB101/rapamycin clinical trial described previously (ANZCTR ID: ACTR N12619000372189) targets the mTOR complex, which is not itself associated with PD, but is involved in a signaling pathway that regulates autophagy and has been shown to rescue dopaminergic neuron degeneration in some PD models [72]. Examining the genetic networks associated with PD and employing drug repositioning to target them may be a way to quickly increase the number of PD therapeutics available in the future.

The integration of genetic (like GWAS) and transcriptomic (e.g., RNA-sequencing) data can further inform the development of personalized medicine for the diagnosis and treatment of PD. These two data types can yield biological insight into candidate genes and pathways for the development of targeted therapeutics. When multi-omics data types such as these are combined, we can begin to gain mechanistic insights. Recent studies have aimed at linking the genes underlying GWAS loci to functional consequences by leveraging large-scale transcriptomic datasets to prioritize genes by using a transcriptome-wide association study (TWAS) [73]. Another way to integrate these data types uses colocalization and weighted gene coexpression network analysis to identify candidate genes [74]. These comprehensive and unbiased explorations provide a strong foundation for further mechanistic studies that can help functionally characterize therapeutic targets and plan clinical trials.

5. Genetics Informs Parkinson's Disease Subtyping

Understanding the etiological heterogeneity of PD is widely recognized as a critical step in achieving personalized and disease-modifying approaches. The first attempts to subtype PD used clinical information, like age at onset. In fact, early-onset patients, as compared to late-onset, tend to exhibit a slower disease progression, less severe clinical course and a higher risk of developing levodopa-induced dyskinesia [75]. Subtyping PD according to motor and non-motor symptoms is also a common approach, either using pre-defined clinical criteria or a data-driven approach. Its utility has been questioned since the first strategy does not seem to be stable along the disease course, and the latter lacks reproducibility [76,77]. Despite these limitations, a subgroup of PD with tremor-dominant symptoms is widely recognized, in opposition to a group with less tremor and more akinetic and gait dysfunction [78]. The next frontier to delineate PD heterogeneity must incorporate more objective measures such as biomarkers and deep-phenotyping information to define biological subtypes suitable for personalized interventions [79].

Developing strategies for diagnosis of the prodromal phase of PD and identifying biomarkers that are able to measure its progression are essential in the search for new therapies. Studies suggest that by the time of diagnosis, patients already show a neuronal loss of 40–50% in the substantia nigra [80,81], explaining, at least in part, why previous trials have failed to find a disease-modifying effect [82,83]. Since 2015, the Movement Disorder Society has been proposing diagnostic research criteria to define prodromal PD [84]. Multiple clinical symptoms were included, like REM sleep behavior disorder, olfactory loss, constipation, and depression. In 2019, the criteria were updated [85], and genetics is now combined with clinical and other types of biomarkers to improve PD prediction. Carriers of rare highly-penetrant and pathogenic variants (like those in *SNCA*, *PRKN*, and *PINK1*) formed distinct prodromal monogenic PD subgroups. Variants of intermediate magnitude of effect in genes such as *GBA* and *LRRK2* were included considering their age-dependent penetrance. Finally, for common variants with low individual effect identified in previous GWAS studies, the criteria recommend calculating the PRS for a large sample series with genetic data and classifying patients according to the risk score distribution in the sample. A recent study has identified common non-coding SNPs within *GBA* regulating *GBA* expression in peripheral tissues [86]. Interestingly, the authors report that non-coding SNPs within *GBA* also coregulate potential modifier genes in the central nervous system and/or peripheral tissues, delaying disease onset by 5 years. Although the nominated variants need to be functionally validated, this promising approach opens the door for future disease stratification, personalized drug selection and the possible development or repurposing of novel drugs.

6. Conclusions and Future Directions

Symptomatic treatment with levodopa has been the norm in PD for more than fifty years despite its sometimes serious side effects. Until recently, efforts to improve treatment options have been slow. Although there is still much to learn about the molecular mechanisms underlying PD, significant progress is now being made towards the identification of potential therapeutic targets in this complex disease. Genetics has played a key role in increasing the number of recent and ongoing clinical trials. The random genetic assortment of patients in clinical trials represents an avoidable source of variance that is likely contributing to the high failure rate seen in PD trials. In fact, even within specific subgroups carrying known PD variants, large variation between patients still exists. Different variants within a specific gene can lead to differential effects on PD phenotypes, and as previously shown [87], this genetic imbalance affects clinical trial design. Acknowledging the limitation that understanding the exact effect of all human genetic variation on disease aetiology and drug response is not yet possible, at the minimum, balancing known disease risk variants should be performed. Using PRS to stratify patients by low and high risk could help identify drugs that will work in some forms of PD.

Stratified trial designs can be used to potentially increase the efficiency of a trial. This was evident in exemplary form in the relevant success attributable to the enrollment strategy of the Aducanumab trial in 2015 and deviations from this strategy being potentially related to less positive results in more recent development phases of the drug [88]. Using genetic, clinical, imaging or other molecular biomarkers to enroll patients that may have a higher probability to efficiently respond to an intervention is key to trial success and a central concept in stratified trials. Another aspect of using potential patient stratification to design more efficient trials, particularly in degenerative type diseases, is to identify patients early in the disease course where targetable cell types of interest are still functional or available and may be protected or rescued; too late in disease course irreparable or immutable damage may have already occurred.

Additionally, advancing target development by combining genomic, transcriptomic and proteomic data has broadened the search space for potential drugs. Focusing not just on monogenic or known risk factors but also the various pathways and networks implicated across the subtypes of idiopathic PD may soon increase the available therapeutic options. The numerous studies directed by genetics described here show that the age of personalized medicine in PD is fast approaching.

Author Contributions: Initial manuscript preparation: X.R., A.S.-S., J.H., S.B.-C. Manuscript editing and commentary: X.R., A.S.-S., J.H., S.B.-C. All authors have read and agreed to the published version of the manuscript.

Funding: This research was supported, in part, by the Intramural Research Program of the National Institutes of Health (National Institute on Aging, National Institute of Neurological Disorders and Stroke: project numbers 1ZIA-NS003154, Z01-AG000949-02, and Z01-ES10198.

Institutional Review Board Statement: Not applicable.

Informed Consent Statement: Not applicable.

Data Availability Statement: Not applicable.

Conflicts of Interest: The authors declare no conflict of interest.

References

1. Ashley, E.A. Towards precision medicine. *Nat. Rev. Genet.* **2016**, *17*, 507–522. [CrossRef]
2. Polymeropoulos, M.H.; Lavedan, C.; Leroy, E.; Ide, S.E.; Dehejia, A.; Dutra, A.; Pike, B.; Root, H.; Rubenstein, J.; Boyer, R.; et al. Mutation in the alpha-synuclein gene identified in families with Parkinson's disease. *Science* **1997**, *276*, 2045–2047. [CrossRef]
3. Simón-Sánchez, J.; Schulte, C.; Bras, J.M.; Sharma, M.; Gibbs, J.R.; Berg, D.; Paisan-Ruiz, C.; Lichtner, P.; Scholz, S.W.; Hernandez, D.G.; et al. Genome-wide association study reveals genetic risk underlying Parkinson's disease. *Nat. Genet.* **2009**, *41*, 1308–1312. [CrossRef]
4. Ho, D.; Quake, S.R.; McCabe, E.R.B.; Chng, W.J.; Chow, E.K.; Ding, X.; Gelb, B.D.; Ginsburg, G.S.; Hassenstab, J.; Ho, C.-M.; et al. Enabling Technologies for Personalized and Precision Medicine. *Trends Biotechnol.* **2020**, *38*, 497–518. [CrossRef] [PubMed]
5. Schneider, S.A.; Alcalay, R.N. Precision medicine in Parkinson's disease: Emerging treatments for genetic Parkinson's disease. *J. Neurol.* **2020**, *267*, 860–869. [CrossRef] [PubMed]
6. Faghri, F.; Hashemi, S.H.; Leonard, H.; Scholz, S.W.; Campbell, R.H.; Nalls, M.A.; Singleton, A.B. Predicting onset, progression, and clinical subtypes of Parkinson disease using machine learning. *bioRxiv* **2018**, 338913. [CrossRef]
7. Nalls, M.A.; Blauwendraat, C.; Vallerga, C.L.; Heilbron, K.; Bandres-Ciga, S.; Chang, D.; Tan, M.; Kia, D.A.; Noyce, A.J.; Xue, A.; et al. Identification of novel risk loci, causal insights, and heritable risk for Parkinson's disease: A meta-analysis of genome-wide association studies. *Lancet Neurol.* **2019**, *18*, 1091–1102. [CrossRef]
8. Goldman, S.M.; Marek, K.; Ottman, R.; Meng, C.; Comyns, K.; Chan, P.; Ma, J.; Marras, C.; Langston, J.W.; Ross, G.W.; et al. Concordance for Parkinson's disease in twins: A 20-year update. *Ann. Neurol.* **2019**, *85*, 600–605. [CrossRef]
9. Olanow, C.W.; Stocchi, F. Levodopa: A new look at an old friend. *Mov. Disord.* **2018**, *33*, 859–866. [CrossRef] [PubMed]
10. Manson, A.; Stirpe, P.; Schrag, A. Levodopa-induced-dyskinesias clinical features, incidence, risk factors, management and impact on quality of life. *J. Parkinsons. Dis.* **2012**, *2*, 189–198. [CrossRef] [PubMed]
11. Kelly, M.J.; Lawton, M.A.; Baig, F.; Ruffmann, C.; Barber, T.R.; Lo, C.; Klein, J.C.; Ben-Shlomo, Y.; Hu, M.T. Predictors of motor complications in early Parkinson's disease: A prospective cohort study. *Mov. Disord.* **2019**, *34*, 1174–1183. [CrossRef]
12. Stocchi, F.; Antonini, A.; Barone, P.; Tinazzi, M.; Zappia, M.; Onofrj, M.; Ruggieri, S.; Morgante, L.; Bonuccelli, U.; Lopiano, L.; et al. Early DEtection of wEaring off in Parkinson disease: The DEEP study. *Parkinsonism Relat. Disord.* **2014**, *20*, 204–211. [CrossRef]
13. Cacabelos, R. Parkinson's Disease: From Pathogenesis to Pharmacogenomics. *Int. J. Mol. Sci.* **2017**, *18*, 551. [CrossRef]
14. Schumacher-Schuh, A.F.; Rieder, C.R.M.; Hutz, M.H. Parkinson's disease pharmacogenomics: New findings and perspectives. *Pharmacogenomics* **2014**, *15*, 1253–1271. [CrossRef]
15. Payami, H. The emerging science of precision medicine and pharmacogenomics for Parkinson's disease. *Mov. Disord.* **2017**, *32*, 1139–1146. [CrossRef] [PubMed]
16. Titova, N.; Chaudhuri, K.R. Personalized medicine in Parkinson's disease: Time to be precise. *Mov. Disord.* **2017**, *32*, 1147–1154. [CrossRef] [PubMed]
17. Hamza, T.H.; Chen, H.; Hill-Burns, E.M.; Rhodes, S.L.; Montimurro, J.; Kay, D.M.; Tenesa, A.; Kusel, V.I.; Sheehan, P.; Eaaswarkhanth, M.; et al. Genome-wide gene-environment study identifies glutamate receptor gene GRIN2A as a Parkinson's disease modifier gene via interaction with coffee. *PLoS Genet.* **2011**, *7*, e1002237. [CrossRef] [PubMed]
18. Hill-Burns, E.M.; Singh, N.; Ganguly, P.; Hamza, T.H.; Montimurro, J.; Kay, D.M.; Yearout, D.; Sheehan, P.; Frodey, K.; McLear, J.A.; et al. A genetic basis for the variable effect of smoking/nicotine on Parkinson's disease. *Pharm. J.* **2013**, *13*, 530–537. [CrossRef] [PubMed]
19. Ryu, H.-S.; Park, K.W.; Choi, N.; Kim, J.; Park, Y.-M.; Jo, S.; Kim, M.-J.; Kim, Y.J.; Kim, J.; Kim, K.; et al. Genomic Analysis Identifies New Loci Associated with Motor Complications in Parkinson's Disease. *Front. Neurol.* **2020**, *11*, 570. [CrossRef] [PubMed]
20. Prud'hon, S.; Bekadar, S.; Rastetter, A.; Guégan, J.; Cormier-Dequaire, F.; Lacomblez, L.; Mangone, G.; You, H.; Daniau, M.; Marie, Y.; et al. Exome Sequencing Reveals Signal Transduction Genes Involved in Impulse Control Disorders in Parkinson's Disease. *Front. Neurol.* **2020**, *11*, 641. [CrossRef]
21. Elfil, M.; Kamel, S.; Kandil, M.; Koo, B.B.; Schaefer, S.M. Implications of the Gut Microbiome in Parkinson's Disease. *Mov. Disord.* **2020**, *35*, 921–933. [CrossRef]
22. Hill-Burns, E.M.; Debelius, J.W.; Morton, J.T.; Wissemann, W.T.; Lewis, M.R.; Wallen, Z.D.; Peddada, S.D.; Factor, S.A.; Molho, E.; Zabetian, C.P.; et al. Parkinson's disease and Parkinson's disease medications have distinct signatures of the gut microbiome. *Mov. Disord.* **2017**, *32*, 739–749. [CrossRef]

23. van Kessel, S.P.; Frye, A.K.; El-Gendy, A.O.; Castejon, M.; Keshavarzian, A.; van Dijk, G.; El Aidy, S. Gut bacterial tyrosine decarboxylases restrict levels of levodopa in the treatment of Parkinson's disease. *Nat. Commun.* **2019**, *10*, 310. [CrossRef] [PubMed]
24. Maini Rekdal, V.; Bess, E.N.; Bisanz, J.E.; Turnbaugh, P.J.; Balskus, E.P. Discovery and inhibition of an interspecies gut bacterial pathway for Levodopa metabolism. *Science* **2019**, *364*. [CrossRef]
25. Greenbaum, L.; Israeli-Korn, S.D.; Cohen, O.S.; Elincx-Benizri, S.; Yahalom, G.; Kozlova, E.; Strauss, H.; Molshatzki, N.; Inzelberg, R.; Spiegelmann, R.; et al. The LRRK2 G2019S mutation status does not affect the outcome of subthalamic stimulation in patients with Parkinson's disease. *Parkinsonism Relat. Disord.* **2013**, *19*, 1053–1056. [CrossRef] [PubMed]
26. Schüpbach, M.; Lohmann, E.; Anheim, M.; Lesage, S.; Czernecki, V.; Yaici, S.; Worbe, Y.; Charles, P.; Welter, M.-L.; Pollak, P.; et al. Subthalamic nucleus stimulation is efficacious in patients with Parkinsonism and LRRK2 mutations. *Mov. Disord.* **2007**, *22*, 119–122. [CrossRef]
27. Angeli, A.; Mencacci, N.E.; Duran, R.; Aviles-Olmos, I.; Kefalopoulou, Z.; Candelario, J.; Rusbridge, S.; Foley, J.; Pradhan, P.; Jahanshahi, M.; et al. Genotype and phenotype in Parkinson's disease: Lessons in heterogeneity from deep brain stimulation. *Mov. Disord.* **2013**, *28*, 1370–1375. [CrossRef] [PubMed]
28. Lythe, V.; Athauda, D.; Foley, J.; Mencacci, N.E.; Jahanshahi, M.; Cipolotti, L.; Hyam, J.; Zrinzo, L.; Hariz, M.; Hardy, J.; et al. GBA-Associated Parkinson's Disease: Progression in a Deep Brain Stimulation Cohort. *J. Parkinsons. Dis.* **2017**, *7*, 635–644. [CrossRef] [PubMed]
29. Healy, D.G.; Falchi, M.; O'Sullivan, S.S.; Bonifati, V.; Durr, A.; Bressman, S.; Brice, A.; Aasly, J.; Zabetian, C.P.; Goldwurm, S.; et al. Phenotype, genotype, and worldwide genetic penetrance of LRRK2-associated Parkinson's disease: A case-control study. *Lancet Neurol.* **2008**, *7*, 583–590. [CrossRef]
30. Tolosa, E.; Vila, M.; Klein, C.; Rascol, O. LRRK2 in Parkinson disease: Challenges of clinical trials. *Nat. Rev. Neurol.* **2020**, *16*, 97–107. [CrossRef] [PubMed]
31. Jaleel, M.; Nichols, R.J.; Deak, M.; Campbell, D.G.; Gillardon, F.; Knebel, A.; Alessi, D.R. LRRK2 phosphorylates moesin at threonine-558: Characterization of how Parkinson's disease mutants affect kinase activity. *Biochem. J.* **2007**, *405*, 307–317. [CrossRef]
32. Estrada, A.A.; Liu, X.; Baker-Glenn, C.; Beresford, A.; Burdick, D.J.; Chambers, M.; Chan, B.K.; Chen, H.; Ding, X.; DiPasquale, A.G.; et al. Discovery of highly potent, selective, and brain-penetrable leucine-rich repeat kinase 2 (LRRK2) small molecule inhibitors. *J. Med. Chem.* **2012**, *55*, 9416–9433. [CrossRef]
33. Fell, M.J.; Mirescu, C.; Basu, K.; Cheewatrakoolpong, B.; DeMong, D.E.; Ellis, J.M.; Hyde, L.A.; Lin, Y.; Markgraf, C.G.; Mei, H.; et al. MLi-2, a Potent, Selective, and Centrally Active Compound for Exploring the Therapeutic Potential and Safety of LRRK2 Kinase Inhibition. *J. Pharmacol. Exp. Ther.* **2015**, *355*, 397–409. [CrossRef] [PubMed]
34. Fuji, R.N.; Flagella, M.; Baca, M.; Baptista, M.A.S.; Brodbeck, J.; Chan, B.K.; Fiske, B.K.; Honigberg, L.; Jubb, A.M.; Katavolos, P.; et al. Effect of selective LRRK2 kinase inhibition on nonhuman primate lung. *Sci. Transl. Med.* **2015**, *7*, 273ra15. [CrossRef]
35. Baptista, M.A.S.; Merchant, K.; Barrett, T.; Bhargava, S.; Bryce, D.K.; Ellis, J.M.; Estrada, A.A.; Fell, M.J.; Fiske, B.K.; Fuji, R.N.; et al. LRRK2 inhibitors induce reversible changes in nonhuman primate lungs without measurable pulmonary deficits. *Sci. Transl. Med.* **2020**, *12*. [CrossRef]
36. DENALI. Available online: https://denalitherapeutics.gcs-web.com/ (accessed on 11 February 2021).
37. Blauwendraat, C.; Reed, X.; Kia, D.A.; Gan-Or, Z.; Lesage, S.; Pihlstrøm, L.; Guerreiro, R.; Gibbs, J.R.; Sabir, M.; Ahmed, S.; et al. Frequency of Loss of Function Variants in LRRK2 in Parkinson Disease. *JAMA Neurol.* **2018**, *75*, 1416–1422. [CrossRef]
38. Zhao, H.T.; John, N.; Delic, V.; Ikeda-Lee, K.; Kim, A.; Weihofen, A.; Swayze, E.E.; Kordasiewicz, H.B.; West, A.B.; Volpicelli-Daley, L.A. LRRK2 Antisense Oligonucleotides Ameliorate α-Synuclein Inclusion Formation in a Parkinson's Disease Mouse Model. *Mol. Ther. Nucleic Acids* **2017**, *8*, 508–519. [CrossRef]
39. Korecka, J.A.; Thomas, R.; Hinrich, A.J.; Moskites, A.M.; Macbain, Z.K.; Hallett, P.J.; Isacson, O.; Hastings, M.L. Splice-Switching Antisense Oligonucleotides Reduce LRRK2 Kinase Activity in Human LRRK2 Transgenic Mice. *Mol. Ther. Nucleic Acids* **2020**, *21*, 623–635. [CrossRef]
40. Clark, L.N.; Ross, B.M.; Wang, Y.; Mejia-Santana, H.; Harris, J.; Louis, E.D.; Cote, L.J.; Andrews, H.; Fahn, S.; Waters, C.; et al. Mutations in the glucocerebrosidase gene are associated with early-onset Parkinson disease. *Neurology* **2007**, *69*, 1270–1277. [CrossRef] [PubMed]
41. Sidransky, E.; Nalls, M.A.; Aasly, J.O.; Aharon-Peretz, J.; Annesi, G.; Barbosa, E.R.; Bar-Shira, A.; Berg, D.; Bras, J.; Brice, A.; et al. Multicenter analysis of glucocerebrosidase mutations in Parkinson's disease. *N. Engl. J. Med.* **2009**, *361*, 1651–1661. [CrossRef] [PubMed]
42. Gan-Or, Z.; Amshalom, I.; Kilarski, L.L.; Bar-Shira, A.; Gana-Weisz, M.; Mirelman, A.; Marder, K.; Bressman, S.; Giladi, N.; Orr-Urtreger, A. Differential effects of severe vs mild GBA mutations on Parkinson disease. *Neurology* **2015**, *84*, 880–887. [CrossRef]
43. Liu, G.; Boot, B.; Locascio, J.J.; Jansen, I.E.; Winder-Rhodes, S.; Eberly, S.; Elbaz, A.; Brice, A.; Ravina, B.; van Hilten, J.J.; et al. Specifically neuropathic Gaucher's mutations accelerate cognitive decline in Parkinson's. *Ann. Neurol.* **2016**, *80*, 674–685. [CrossRef]
44. Cilia, R.; Tunesi, S.; Marotta, G.; Cereda, E.; Siri, C.; Tesei, S.; Zecchinelli, A.L.; Canesi, M.; Mariani, C.B.; Meucci, N.; et al. Survival and dementia in GBA-associated Parkinson's disease: The mutation matters. *Ann. Neurol.* **2016**, *80*, 662–673. [CrossRef]

45. Lwin, A.; Orvisky, E.; Goker-Alpan, O.; LaMarca, M.E.; Sidransky, E. Glucocerebrosidase mutations in subjects with parkinsonism. *Mol. Genet. Metab.* **2004**, *81*, 70–73. [CrossRef] [PubMed]
46. Westbroek, W.; Gustafson, A.M.; Sidransky, E. Exploring the link between glucocerebrosidase mutations and parkinsonism. *Trends Mol. Med.* **2011**, *17*, 485–493. [CrossRef] [PubMed]
47. Barkhuizen, M.; Anderson, D.G.; Grobler, A.F. Advances in GBA-associated Parkinson's disease–Pathology, presentation and therapies. *Neurochem. Int.* **2016**, *93*, 6–25. [CrossRef]
48. Mullin, S.; Smith, L.; Lee, K.; D'Souza, G.; Woodgate, P.; Elflein, J.; Hällqvist, J.; Toffoli, M.; Streeter, A.; Hosking, J.; et al. Ambroxol for the Treatment of Patients With Parkinson Disease With and Without Glucocerebrosidase Gene Mutations: A Nonrandomized, Noncontrolled Trial. *JAMA Neurol.* **2020**, *77*, 427–434. [CrossRef] [PubMed]
49. Silveira, C.R.A.; MacKinley, J.; Coleman, K.; Li, Z.; Finger, E.; Bartha, R.; Morrow, S.A.; Wells, J.; Borrie, M.; Tirona, R.G.; et al. Ambroxol as a novel disease-modifying treatment for Parkinson's disease dementia: Protocol for a single-centre, randomized, double-blind, placebo-controlled trial. *BMC Neurol.* **2019**, *19*, 20. [CrossRef]
50. Hall, A.; Bandres-Ciga, S.; Diez-Fairen, M.; Quinn, J.P.; Billingsley, K.J. Genetic Risk Profiling in Parkinson's Disease and Utilizing Genetics to Gain Insight into Disease-Related Biological Pathways. *Int. J. Mol. Sci.* **2020**, *21*, 7332. [CrossRef]
51. Robak, L.A.; Jansen, I.E.; van Rooij, J.; Uitterlinden, A.G.; Kraaij, R.; Jankovic, J.; International Parkinson's Disease Genomics Consortium (IPDGC); Heutink, P.; Shulman, J.M. Excessive burden of lysosomal storage disorder gene variants in Parkinson's disease. *Brain* **2017**, *140*, 3191–3203. [CrossRef] [PubMed]
52. Blauwendraat, C.; Reed, X.; Krohn, L.; Heilbron, K.; Bandres-Ciga, S.; Tan, M.; Gibbs, J.R.; Hernandez, D.G.; Kumaran, R.; Langston, R.; et al. Genetic modifiers of risk and age at onset in GBA associated Parkinson's disease and Lewy body dementia. *Brain* **2020**, *143*, 234–248. [CrossRef] [PubMed]
53. Tan, M.M.X.; Lawton, M.A.; Jabbari, E.; Reynolds, R.H.; Iwaki, H.; Blauwendraat, C.; Kanavou, S.; Pollard, M.I.; Hubbard, L.; Malek, N.; et al. Genome-Wide Association Studies of Cognitive and Motor Progression in Parkinson's Disease. *Mov. Disord.* **2020**. [CrossRef] [PubMed]
54. Grenn, F.P.; Kim, J.J.; Makarious, M.B.; Iwaki, H.; Illarionova, A.; Brolin, K.; Kluss, J.H.; Schumacher-Schuh, A.F.; Leonard, H.; Faghri, F.; et al. The Parkinson's Disease Genome-Wide Association Study Locus Browser. *Mov. Disord.* **2020**, *35*, 2056–2067. [CrossRef] [PubMed]
55. Ohnmacht, J.; May, P.; Sinkkonen, L.; Krüger, R. Missing heritability in Parkinson's disease: The emerging role of non-coding genetic variation. *J. Neural Transm.* **2020**, *127*, 729–748. [CrossRef]
56. Ibanez, L.; Dube, U.; Saef, B.; Budde, J.; Black, K.; Medvedeva, A.; Del-Aguila, J.L.; Davis, A.A.; Perlmutter, J.S.; Harari, O.; et al. Parkinson disease polygenic risk score is associated with Parkinson disease status and age at onset but not with alpha-synuclein cerebrospinal fluid levels. *BMC Neurol.* **2017**, *17*, 198. [CrossRef]
57. Paul, K.C.; Schulz, J.; Bronstein, J.M.; Lill, C.M.; Ritz, B.R. Association of Polygenic Risk Score With Cognitive Decline and Motor Progression in Parkinson Disease. *JAMA Neurol.* **2018**, *75*, 360–366. [CrossRef]
58. Lee, M.J.; Pak, K.; Kim, J.H.; Kim, Y.J.; Yoon, J.; Lee, J.; Lyoo, C.H.; Park, H.J.; Lee, J.-H.; Jung, N.-Y. Effect of polygenic load on striatal dopaminergic deterioration in Parkinson disease. *Neurology* **2019**, *93*, e665–e674. [CrossRef]
59. Bandres-Ciga, S.; Saez-Atienzar, S.; Kim, J.J.; Makarious, M.B.; Faghri, F.; Diez-Fairen, M.; Iwaki, H.; Leonard, H.; Botia, J.; Ryten, M.; et al. Large-scale pathway specific polygenic risk and transcriptomic community network analysis identifies novel functional pathways in Parkinson disease. *Acta Neuropathol.* **2020**, *140*, 341–358. [CrossRef]
60. Siitonen, A.; Kytövuori, L.; Nalls, M.A.; Gibbs, R.; Hernandez, D.G.; Ylikotila, P.; Peltonen, M.; Singleton, A.B.; Majamaa, K. Finnish Parkinson's disease study integrating protein-protein interaction network data with exome sequencing analysis. *Sci. Rep.* **2019**, *9*, 18865. [CrossRef]
61. Bandres-Ciga, S.; Saez-Atienzar, S.; Bonet-Ponce, L.; Billingsley, K.; Vitale, D.; Blauwendraat, C.; Gibbs, J.R.; Pihlstrøm, L.; Gan-Or, Z.; International Parkinson's Disease Genomics Consortium (IPDGC); et al. The endocytic membrane trafficking pathway plays a major role in the risk of Parkinson's disease. *Mov. Disord.* **2019**, *34*, 460–468. [CrossRef]
62. Fasano, D.; Parisi, S.; Pierantoni, G.M.; De Rosa, A.; Picillo, M.; Amodio, G.; Pellecchia, M.T.; Barone, P.; Moltedo, O.; Bonifati, V.; et al. Alteration of endosomal trafficking is associated with early-onset parkinsonism caused by SYNJ1 mutations. *Cell Death Dis.* **2018**, *9*, 385. [CrossRef]
63. Hopfner, F.; Mueller, S.H.; Szymczak, S.; Junge, O.; Tittmann, L.; May, S.; Lohmann, K.; Grallert, H.; Lieb, W.; Strauch, K.; et al. Rare Variants in Specific Lysosomal Genes Are Associated With Parkinson's Disease. *Mov. Disord.* **2020**, *35*, 1245–1248. [CrossRef]
64. Billingsley, K.J.; Barbosa, I.A.; Bandrés-Ciga, S.; Quinn, J.P.; Bubb, V.J.; Deshpande, C.; Botia, J.A.; Reynolds, R.H.; Zhang, D.; Simpson, M.A.; et al. Mitochondria function associated genes contribute to Parkinson's Disease risk and later age at onset. *Npj Parkinsons Dis.* **2019**, *5*, 8. [CrossRef]
65. Zanin, M.; Santos, B.F.R.; Antony, P.M.A.; Berenguer-Escuder, C.; Larsen, S.B.; Hanss, Z.; Barbuti, P.A.; Baumuratov, A.S.; Grossmann, D.; Capelle, C.M.; et al. Mitochondria interaction networks show altered topological patterns in Parkinson's disease. *Npj Syst. Biol. Appl.* **2020**, *6*, 38. [CrossRef] [PubMed]
66. Perfeito, R.; Cunha-Oliveira, T.; Rego, A.C. Reprint of: Revisiting oxidative stress and mitochondrial dysfunction in the pathogenesis of Parkinson disease-resemblance to the effect of amphetamine drugs of abuse. *Free Radic. Biol. Med.* **2013**, *62*, 186–201. [CrossRef]

67. Iovino, L.; Tremblay, M.E.; Civiero, L. Glutamate-induced excitotoxicity in Parkinson's disease: The role of glial cells. *J. Pharmacol. Sci.* **2020**, *144*, 151–164. [CrossRef] [PubMed]
68. García-Sanz, P.; Orgaz, L.; Bueno-Gil, G.; Espadas, I.; Rodríguez-Traver, E.; Kuliseyky, J.; Gutierrez, A.; Dávila, J.C.; González-Polo, R.A.; Fuentes, J.M.; et al. N370S-GBA1 mutation causes lysosomal cholesterol accumulation in Parkinson's disease. *Mov. Disord.* **2017**, *32*, 1409–1422. [CrossRef]
69. Hu, L.; Dong, M.-X.; Huang, Y.-L.; Lu, C.-Q.; Qian, Q.; Zhang, C.-C.; Xu, X.-M.; Liu, Y.; Chen, G.-H.; Wei, Y.-D. Integrated Metabolomics and Proteomics Analysis Reveals Plasma Lipid Metabolic Disturbance in Patients With Parkinson's Disease. *Front. Mol. Neurosci.* **2020**, *13*, 80. [CrossRef] [PubMed]
70. Saiki, M.; Baker, A.; Williams-Gray, C.H.; Foltynie, T.; Goodman, R.S.; Taylor, C.J.; Compston, D.A.S.; Barker, R.A.; Sawcer, S.J.; Goris, A. Association of the human leucocyte antigen region with susceptibility to Parkinson's disease. *J. Neurol. Neurosurg. Psychiatry* **2010**, *81*, 890–891. [CrossRef]
71. PLoS ONE Staff. Correction: Parkinson's disease-associated genetic variation is linked to quantitative expression of inflammatory genes. *PLoS ONE* **2019**, *14*, e0210931.
72. Radad, K.; Moldzio, R.; Rausch, W.-D. Rapamycin protects dopaminergic neurons against rotenone-induced cell death in primary mesencephalic cell culture. *Folia Neuropathol.* **2015**, *53*, 250–261. [CrossRef]
73. Li, Y.I.; Wong, G.; Humphrey, J.; Raj, T. Prioritizing Parkinson's disease genes using population-scale transcriptomic data. *Nat. Commun.* **2019**, *10*, 994. [CrossRef] [PubMed]
74. Kia, D.A.; Zhang, D.; Guelfi, S.; Manzoni, C.; Hubbard, L.; Reynolds, R.H.; Botía, J.; Ryten, M.; Ferrari, R.; Lewis, P.A.; et al. Identification of Candidate Parkinson Disease Genes by Integrating Genome-Wide Association Study, Expression, and Epigenetic Data Sets. *JAMA Neurol.* **2021**. [CrossRef]
75. Wickremaratchi, M.M.; Ben-Shlomo, Y.; Morris, H.R. The effect of onset age on the clinical features of Parkinson's disease. *Eur. J. Neurol.* **2009**, *16*, 450–456. [CrossRef]
76. Simuni, T.; Caspell-Garcia, C.; Coffey, C.; Lasch, S.; Tanner, C.; Marek, K.; PPMI Investigators. How stable are Parkinson's disease subtypes in de novo patients: Analysis of the PPMI cohort? *Parkinsonism Relat. Disord.* **2016**, *28*, 62–67. [CrossRef] [PubMed]
77. Mestre, T.A.; Eberly, S.; Tanner, C.; Grimes, D.; Lang, A.E.; Oakes, D.; Marras, C. Reproducibility of data-driven Parkinson's disease subtypes for clinical research. *Parkinsonism Relat. Disord.* **2018**, *56*, 102–106. [CrossRef] [PubMed]
78. Thenganatt, M.A.; Jankovic, J. Parkinson disease subtypes. *JAMA Neurol.* **2014**, *71*, 499–504. [CrossRef]
79. Espay, A.J.; Schwarzschild, M.A.; Tanner, C.M.; Fernandez, H.H.; Simon, D.K.; Leverenz, J.B.; Merola, A.; Chen-Plotkin, A.; Brundin, P.; Kauffman, M.A.; et al. Biomarker-driven phenotyping in Parkinson's disease: A translational missing link in disease-modifying clinical trials. *Mov. Disord.* **2017**, *32*, 319–324. [CrossRef]
80. Fearnley, J.M.; Lees, A.J. Ageing and Parkinson's disease: Substantia nigra regional selectivity. *Brain* **1991**, *114*, 2283–2301. [CrossRef] [PubMed]
81. Kordower, J.H.; Olanow, C.W.; Dodiya, H.B.; Chu, Y.; Beach, T.G.; Adler, C.H.; Halliday, G.M.; Bartus, R.T. Disease duration and the integrity of the nigrostriatal system in Parkinson's disease. *Brain* **2013**, *136*, 2419–2431. [CrossRef] [PubMed]
82. Shoulson, I. DATATOP: A decade of neuroprotective inquiry. Parkinson Study Group. Deprenyl And Tocopherol Antioxidative Therapy Of Parkinsonism. *Ann. Neurol.* **1998**, *44*, S160–S166. [CrossRef] [PubMed]
83. Rascol, O.; Hauser, R.A.; Stocchi, F.; Fitzer-Attas, C.J.; Sidi, Y.; Abler, V.; Olanow, C.W. AFU Investigators Long-term effects of rasagiline and the natural history of treated Parkinson's disease. *Mov. Disord.* **2016**, *31*, 1489–1496. [CrossRef]
84. Berg, D.; Postuma, R.B.; Adler, C.H.; Bloem, B.R.; Chan, P.; Dubois, B.; Gasser, T.; Goetz, C.G.; Halliday, G.; Joseph, L.; et al. MDS research criteria for prodromal Parkinson's disease. *Mov. Disord.* **2015**, *30*, 1600–1611. [CrossRef] [PubMed]
85. Heinzel, S.; Berg, D.; Gasser, T.; Chen, H.; Yao, C.; Postuma, R.B.; MDS Task Force on the Definition of Parkinson's Disease. Update of the MDS research criteria for prodromal Parkinson's disease. *Mov. Disord.* **2019**, *34*, 1464–1470. [CrossRef]
86. Schierding, W.; Farrow, S.; Fadason, T.; Graham, O.E.E.; Pitcher, T.L.; Qubisi, S.; Davidson, A.J.; Perry, J.K.; Anderson, T.J.; Kennedy, M.A.; et al. Common Variants Coregulate Expression of GBA and Modifier Genes to Delay Parkinson's Disease Onset. *Mov. Disord.* **2020**, *35*, 1346–1356. [CrossRef]
87. Leonard, H.; Blauwendraat, C.; Krohn, L.; Faghri, F.; Iwaki, H.; Ferguson, G.; Day-Williams, A.G.; Stone, D.J.; Singleton, A.B.; Nalls, M.A.; et al. Genetic variability and potential effects on clinical trial outcomes: Perspectives in Parkinson's disease. *J. Med. Genet.* **2020**, *57*, 331–338. [CrossRef] [PubMed]
88. ALZFORUM. Available online: https://www.alzforum.org/therapeutics/aducanumab (accessed on 11 February 2021).

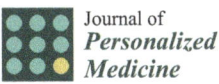

Article

Assessing Lifestyle Behaviours of People Living with Neurological Conditions: A Panoramic View of Community Dwelling Australians from 2007–2018

Nupur Nag [1,*], Xin Lin [1], Maggie Yu [1], Steve Simpson-Yap [1,2], George A. Jelinek [1], Sandra L. Neate [1] and Michele Levin [3]

1 Neuroepidemiology Unit, Centre of Epidemiology and Biostatistics, Melbourne School of Population and Global Health, The University of Melbourne, Parkville, VIC 3010, Australia; xin.lin2@unimelb.edu.au (X.L.); maggie.yu@unimelb.edu.au (M.Y.); steve.simpsonyap@unimelb.edu.au (S.S.-Y.); g.jelinek@unimelb.edu.au (G.A.J.); sandra.neate@unimelb.edu.au (S.L.N.)
2 Menzies Institute for Medical Research, University of Tasmania, Hobart, TAS 7000, Australia
3 Roy Morgan Research Institute, Tonic House, Melbourne, VIC 3000, Australia; michele.levine@roymorgan.com
* Correspondence: nnag@unimelb.edu.au; Tel.: +61-3-8344-7944

Abstract: Neurological disorders pose a substantial health and economic burden to the individual and society, necessitating strategies for effective prevention and disease management. Lifestyle behaviours play a role in risk and management of some neurological disorders; however, overlap between lifestyle behaviours across disorders has not been well explored. We used log-binomial regression to assess associations of selected lifestyle behaviours in community-dwelling Australians (n = 192,091), some of whom self-reported Alzheimer's disease (AD), motor neurone disease (MND), multiple sclerosis (MS), Parkinson's disease (PD) or stroke. Of six lifestyle behaviours, undertaking physical activity was inversely associated with the presence of all neurological disorders except PD. Smoking was positively associated with MND and stroke, and inversely associated with PD. Participants with AD and stroke shared inverse associations with cognitive engagement, face-to-face social interaction and stress-reducing activities, and MS was positively associated with online social interaction and stress-reduction activities. Of eleven food and beverage consumption categories, no associations were seen in MND, ten categories were inversely associated with people with AD or stroke, and six of these with PD. Vegetable and soft drink consumption were associated with MS. Further detailed assessment of commonalities in lifestyle behaviours across neurological disorders may inform potential strategies for risk reduction across disorders.

Keywords: lifestyle behaviours; diet; cross-sectional; population study; neurological disorders

Citation: Nag, N.; Lin, X.; Yu, M.; Simpson-Yap, S.; Jelinek, G.A.; Neate, S.L.; Levin, M. Assessing Lifestyle Behaviours of People Living with Neurological Conditions: A Panoramic View of Community Dwelling Australians from 2007–2018. *J. Pers. Med.* **2021**, *11*, 144. https://doi.org/10.3390/jpm11020144

Academic Editors: K. Ray Chaudhuri and Nataliya Titova

Received: 17 January 2021
Accepted: 16 February 2021
Published: 19 February 2021

Publisher's Note: MDPI stays neutral with regard to jurisdictional claims in published maps and institutional affiliations.

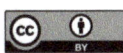

Copyright: © 2021 by the authors. Licensee MDPI, Basel, Switzerland. This article is an open access article distributed under the terms and conditions of the Creative Commons Attribution (CC BY) license (https://creativecommons.org/licenses/by/4.0/).

1. Introduction

The overall burden of neurological disorders continues to increase with an aging population. In 2017, it was estimated that 43% of the Australian population had been diagnosed with a neurological disorder, among these were commonly stroke, Alzheimer's disease (AD) and dementia, and less commonly motor neurone disease (MND), multiple sclerosis (MS) and Parkinson's disease (PD) [1]. These disorders present with a heterogenous array of symptoms including cognitive, psychological and physical impairments, which contribute to reduced quality of life for the individual and pose significant societal and economic burden [2–4]. These current and increasing burdens necessitate the identification of effective and targeted strategies to achieve risk reduction, manage symptoms, and delay progression.

Modifiable lifestyle behaviours, including diet, physical activity, smoking, cognitive reserve and social interaction have been implicated in the onset and progression of some neurological disorders [5–7]. Diets high in saturated fats, including red meat and processed foods, have been associated with increased risk of AD, PD, MS and stroke; while high fruit, vegetable and whole grain intake have been associated with reduced risk [8–11]. Physical activity has been shown to have benefits for healthy aging and neuroplasticity [12,13], with a minimum of 150 min/week of moderate-intense activity being the international recommendation for adults in maintaining a healthy lifestyle [14,15]. Smoking is similarly well-established as a risk factor for dementia, stroke and MS [6,16,17]; its role for PD risk remains debatable with some studies showing a protective effect [5,18]. Cognitive reserve, enhanced by engaging in physical, leisure and intellectually stimulating activities, may be a mechanism for protection against cognitive and functional decline in the presence of brain pathology [6]. Increasing social interaction and reducing stress are also lifestyle recommendations for optimal brain health [19,20].

The evidence for the role of lifestyle behaviours in risk and management of neurological disorders continues to grow, likely acting concurrently for optimal benefits. Indeed, multimodal lifestyle behaviours, combining healthy diet, increased exercise and cognitive training, have shown improved cognitive outcomes in at-risk elderly people and people with MS [21,22] and a reduced risk of secondary stroke and AD [23,24], suggesting a multi-dimensional approach may be beneficial across different disorders.

Despite the evident role of lifestyle in the prevention and management of different neurological disorders, the epidemiological landscape of lifestyle associations across disorders remains under-examined. Herein, we describe and compare the distributions of modifiable lifestyle behaviours in community-dwelling Australians with and without one of five neurological conditions—AD, PD, MND, MS and stroke. In doing so, we aim to identify shared lifestyle profiles of people with these conditions, which may in turn shed new light on targeted risk reduction and effective self-management strategies.

2. Materials and Methods

2.1. Study Design and Participants

Each year, 50,000 randomly selected Australian households in 11 major geographic regions are sampled by Roy Morgan Research Institute [25]. The youngest consenting English-speaking member of the household, aged ≥ 14 years, is interviewed face-to-face by a trained professional. During the interview, the establishment survey including participant demographics is completed and entered into a secure database. Interviewees are then provided with a hard copy of the Single Source Questionnaire (SSQ) for self-completion and asked to return it by post within 30 days to Roy Morgan Research Institutes's Head Office. Completion is incentivised by entry to a monthly monetary draw prize valued at $1000.

The SSQ comprises a 112-page survey, with 10 sections on various consumer behaviours including interests and attitudes, health conditions, lifestyle and purchasing behaviours, and service and technology utilisation. Data from SSQ surveys are scanned and cleaned for analysis on a quarterly cycle.

2.2. Data Collection and Measurement

Participants provided informed consent to Roy Morgan Research Institute for their data to be used for research purposes. The current study was approved by The University of Melbourne, Melbourne School of Population and Global Health Human Ethics Advisory Group, project #1953821.1.

Data extracted includes de-identified adults aged ≥ 18 years that were interviewed from January 2007–September 2018. SSQ non-responder versus responder biases were analysed based on demographics queried in the face-to-face interview. For main analyses, data inclusion was limited to SSQ responders, and data was extracted on demographics, self-reported neurological disorders and researcher-defined lifestyle behaviours using select variables captured in the SSQ (Table 1).

Table 1. Single Source Questionnaire (SSQ) variable inclusions for lifestyle behaviours and food and beverage categories.

Lifestyle	SSQ Variables Queried as Done in the Last 3 Months (Used in Last 4 Weeks, Communication Apps)
Cognitive engagement	Went to a short course/seminar/convention/public lecture; read a novel; read a non-fiction book; used a computer at home; used a computer at work or school; played a musical instrument or sung in a choir; worked on a car; dressmaking
Physical activity	Did some formal exercise; played a sport
Smoker	Current
Social face-to-face	Visited friends/relatives; entertained friends/relatives; held a dinner party
Social online	Facebook Messenger, Skype, Viber, WeChat, WhatsApp, teleconference, telephone
Stress reduction	Hobbies
Food	**SSQ Variables Queried as Consumed in the Last 7 days**
Bakery/cereal	Rolls/bread, porridge, cereals (biscuit, other), toast, bagels
Dairy	Milk (from drinks: white, UHT, flavoured, breakfast), yoghurt (natural, flavoured, drinking), cheese (natural, dip), dairy desserts, ice cream (single, tub)
Fish/seafood	Fish, other seafood
Fruit/vegetables	Fresh, canned, frozen, dried
Meat	Chicken, beef, veal, lamb/mutton, pork, turkey, duck, rabbit, ham/bacon, other cold meats, other meats
Natural grains	Rice, pasta/spaghetti, noodles
Snacks	Pastries, muffins/doughnuts, croissants, biscuits (all), chips, muesli bars, breakfast bars, chocolate (all), lollies/mints/gum, frozen desserts, other snacks
Beverage	**SSQ Variables Queried as Consumed in the Last 7 days**
Alcohol	Beer, wine, cider, spirits
Soft drinks	Cola, lemonade, lemon, orange, other soft drinks (diet and regular), mixers.
Tea/coffee	Tea, coffee (hot and cold)

2.2.1. Classification of Neurological Disorders

Neurological disorders were based on a self-reported tick-box selection of 21 brain and nervous system conditions within 20 condition categories from the section "About your Health". Data were restricted to those reported for 'You', in response to the question "Which of the following illnesses or conditions have you or any other member of your household had in the last 12 months?". Five of 21 listed brain and nervous system conditions were selected as outcome variables: AD, MND, MS, PD and stroke.

Sixteen other SSQ-defined nervous system conditions comprised nine specific neurological conditions (cerebral palsy, chronic fatigue syndrome, epilepsy, nerve damage, neuralgia, neuritis, neuropathy, spinal stenosis, mini stroke) and seven non-specific conditions (face pain, fibromyalgia, frequent headaches, memory problems, meningitis, migraine headaches, tingling sensations).

Participants reporting having more than one of the five conditions of interest ($N = 58$), and those reporting the other nine specific conditions ($N = 722$) were excluded from analysis to allow specificity of the outcome and clarity of signal. The seven non-specific conditions were included in both the comparator population (CP) and neurological disorders of interest populations.

The CP were thus participants who had not self-reported having AD, MND, MS, PD, stroke or any of the nine specific neurological conditions.

2.2.2. Demographics

Demographic variables were categorised as follows: age into tertile year range; BMI according to Word Health Organisation definitions [26]; country of birth from a selection of 13 options: Australia or New Zealand (NZ), Europe, Asia or other (North America, Central and South America, South Pacific, Middle East, Africa, other); religion from a selection of 18 tick-box selection options including 'No religion' dichotomised as No/Yes; education dichotomised to No/Yes for the completion of a university degree; employment status as employed (full and part-time), unemployed, student/home duties, and retired; income aligned with Australian Taxation Office taxable income bracket [27]; remoteness based on postal codes; relationship status dichotomised to partnered (married, de facto, engaged, planning to marry) vs. not partnered (single, separated, divorced, widower); and living status dichotomised to lives with others (partner with/without children, single parent, with parents, boarder, shared household) vs. alone (living alone).

2.2.3. Lifestyle Behaviours

Selected SSQ variables were categorised to lifestyle behaviours identified as being associated with neuronal health in the literature (Table 1). These were then dichotimised (No/Yes) for regression analyses.

2.2.4. Food and Beverage Consumption

Food consumption was based on response to "Which of the following have you eaten in the last 7 days", self-reported tick-box selection on 74 single items within six food categories from the section "Food and Beverages". Selected food items were recategorised into seven groups (Table 1). Reported serves per day of fruit and vegetables were categorised as per Australian recommended daily serves of ≥ 2 and ≥ 5, respectively [28].

Beverage consumption was based on the response to "Consumed in the last 7 days", self-reported tick-box selection on 36 single items, from which soft drinks, tea/coffee, and milk (included with dairy foods) were included for analysis (Table 1).

Alcohol consumption was based on the response to "Brands drunk in the last 7 days", self-reported tick-box selection of brand for beer ($n = 146$), cider ($n = 14$), spirits ($n = 93$), and wine (bottled, cask, fortified, sparkling) and "other"; other were excluded from the analysis.

2.3. Statistical Analysis

SSQ responder bias was assessed using log-binomial regression [29]. Given the large sample size, reliance on statistical significance as a marker of differences resulted in every association being significantly different. We therefore utilised a crude cut-point of a >50% difference as a benchmark for material and meaningful differences, to inform the development of multivariable models for the primary associations of interest.

Characteristics of having one of the five neurological disorders as compared to the CP, were evaluated by log-binomial regression. Multivariable models were adjusted for age, sex and education, these model covariates having been selected on the basis of the literature review and a priori reasoning.

3. Results

3.1. Characteristics of SSQ Non-Responders and Responders

Of participants interviewed from January 2007 to September 2018 ($n = 537{,}327$), 36% ($n = 192{,}091$) returned the SSQ and were aged ≥ 18 years (Table 2).

Compared to non-responders, SSQ responders were more likely to be aged ≥ 40 years ($PR_{40-59} = 1.56$; $PR_{\geq 60} = 1.84$) than 18–39 years. Sex, country of birth, university education, employment status, household income, remoteness, partnered and living status, alcohol consumption and smoking status did not differ more than 50% between the two groups.

3.2. Demographics of Analysis Cohort

Participants with AD, PD or stroke were less likely to be female, and they were more likely to be female for MS ($PR_{AD} = 0.48$; $PR_{MS}= 2.56$; $PR_{PD} = 0.59$; $PR_{stroke} = 0.56$; Table 3). Participants with AD, MND, PD or stroke were more likely to be ≥ 60 years, while participants with MS were more likely to be aged 40–59 years. Participants with stroke were 29% more likely to be obese than the CP. Further, those with AD or stroke were 39% and 36% less likely to be university educated, respectively. Compared to CP, participants with any of the five neurological disorders were more likely to be unemployed or retired. Participants with MND or stroke were less likely to be partnered ($PR_{MND} = 0.50$; $PR_{stroke} = 0.62$) and those with MND or stroke were less likely to live with others (PR_{MND} = 0.43; PR_{stroke} = 0.68). Other characteristics are shown in Table 3.

Table 2. Characteristics of single source survey non-responders and responders.

Characteristic	Non-Responder (N = 345,236)	Responder (N = 192,091)	PR (95% CI)
Sex			
Male	180.2k (68.7%)	82.0k (31.3%)	1.00
Female	165.0k (60.0%)	110.1k (40.0%)	1.28 (1.27, 1.29)
Age, years			
18–39	131.9k (75.8%)	42.2k (24.2%)	1.00
40–59	111.2k (62.2%)	67.5k (37.8%)	**1.56 (1.54, 1.57)**
≥60	102.1k (55.3%)	82.4k (44.7%)	**1.84 (1.83, 1.86)**
Country of birth			
Australia/NZ	251.0k (62.3%)	151.8k (37.7%)	1.00
Europe	40.4k (61.6%)	25.2k (38.4%)	1.02 (1.01, 1.03)
Asia	31.0k (79.5%)	8.0k (20.5%)	0.54 (0.53, 0.55)
Other	22.9k (76.4%)	7.0k (23.6%)	0.63 (0.61, 0.64)
University education			
No	217.3k (63.0%)	127.6k (37.0%)	1.00
Yes	127.9k (66.5%)	64.5k (33.5%)	0.91 (0.90, 0.91)
Employment status			
Employed	205.7k (68.3%)	95.6k (31.7%)	1.00
Unemployed	29.9k (66.8%)	14.8k (33.2%)	1.05 (1.03, 1.06)
Student/Home Duties	29.5k (66.0%)	15.2k (34.1%)	1.07 (1.06, 1.09)
Retired	80.2k (54.7%)	66.5k (45.3%)	1.42 (1.42, 1.44)
Income, AUD			
0–19,999	114.3k (62.2%)	69.5k (37.8%)	1.00
20,000–39,999	86.4k (62.3%)	52.4k (37.7%)	1.00 (0.99, 1.01)
40,000–89,999	103.9k (66.1%)	53.3k (33.9%)	0.90 (0.89, 0.91)
≥90,000	40.4k (70.5%)	16.9k (29.5%)	0.78 (0.77, 0.79)
(Missing)	(202; 80.5%)	(49; 19.5%)	n/a
Remoteness			
Capital city	209.7k (66.2%)	106.9k (33.8%)	1.00
Regional	135.6k (61.4%)	85.2k (38.6%)	1.14 (1.13, 1.15)
Partnered			
No	146.9k (67.3%)	71.4k (32.7%)	1.00
Yes	198.3k (62.2%)	120.7k (37.8%)	1.16 (1.15, 1.17)
Lives with others			
No	69.5k (62.0%)	42.6k (38.0%)	1.00
Yes	272.5k (64.8%)	147.8k (35.2%)	0.93 (0.92, 0.93)
(Missing)	(3.3k; 66.1%)	(1.7k; 34.0%)	n/a
Alcohol consumption, past 7 days			
No	144.7k (64.6%)	79.4k (35.4%)	1.00
Yes	200.6k (64.0%)	112.7k (36.0%)	1.02 (1.01, 1.02)
Current smoker			
No	271.8k (62.6%)	162.2k (37.4%)	1.00
Yes	73.4k (71.1%)	29.9k (28.9%)	0.77 (0.77, 0.78)

Sample sizes were in the unit of thousands (k). Analysis performed using log-binomial regression models. Shown in bold, PR < 0.50 and >1.50 were used as thresholds for material difference between non-responders and responders.

Table 3. Characteristics of neurological disorders referenced to comparator population.

Characteristic	AD (N = 125) PR	95%CI	MND (N = 72) PR	95%CI	MS (N = 441) PR	95%CI	PD (N = 415) PR	95%CI	Stroke (N = 647) PR	95%CI
Sex										
Men	Ref		Ref		Ref		Ref		Ref	
Women	0.48	(0.33,0.69)	1.03	(0.65,1.64)	2.56	(2.04,3.20)	0.59	(0.48,0.71)	0.56	(0.48,0.66)
	P	<0.001	P	=0.91	P	<0.001	P	<0.001	P	<0.001
Age										
18–39	Ref		Ref		Ref		Ref		Ref	
40–59	0.70	(0.30,1.60)	0.70	(0.33,1.51)	2.61	(1.97,3.46)	7.09	(2.55,19.73)	5.54	(3.25,9.43)
≥60	4.58	(2.43,8.62)	1.93	(1.05,3.55)	1.26	(0.93,1.72)	44.79	(16.62,120.68)	14.69	(8.78,24.58)
	PTREND	<0.001	PTREND	=0.034	PTREND	=0.14	PTREND	<0.001	PTREND	<0.001
BMI										
Under/normal	Ref		Ref		Ref		Ref		Ref	
Overweight	1.03	(0.67,1.59)	1.49	(0.84,2.64)	0.97	(0.77,1.23)	1.06	(0.84,1.34)	0.93	(0.76,1.13)
Obese	1.01	(0.63,1.62)	1.07	(0.56,2.02)	1.08	(0.85,1.36)	0.96	(0.74,1.24)	1.29	(1.06,1.57)
	PTREND	=0.97	PTREND	=0.79	PTREND	=0.55	PTREND	=0.77	PTREND	=0.011
Country of birth										
Australia/NZ	Ref		Ref		Ref		Ref		Ref	
Europe	1.04	(0.65,1.67)	1.77	(0.99,3.15)	1.18	(0.90,1.53)	0.81	(0.62,1.06)	0.94	(0.76,1.17)
Asia	3.75	(1.93,7.30)	1.31	(0.37,4.56)	0.18	(0.06,0.55)	0.51	(0.19,1.37)	1.47	(0.91,2.35)
Other	1.61	(0.67,3.91)	2.32	(0.89,6.07)	0.42	(0.20,0.88)	0.75	(0.39,1.46)	1.14	(0.73,1.79)
	PTREND	=0.017	PTREND	=0.031	PTREND	=0.002	PTREND	=0.063	PTREND	=0.47
Religion										
No	Ref		Ref		Ref		Ref		Ref	
Yes	1.34	(0.85,2.11)	0.67	(0.41,1.09)	0.83	(0.67,1.01)	1.13	(0.89,1.42)	1.03	(0.86,1.23)
	P	=0.21	P	=0.11	P	=0.065	P	=0.32	P	=0.77
University education										
No	Ref		Ref		Ref		Ref		Ref	
Yes	0.61	(0.40,0.95)	1.28	(0.80,2.05)	1.19	(0.97,1.45)	0.91	(0.72,1.14)	0.64	(0.52,0.78)
	P	=0.027	P	=0.30	P	=0.088	P	=0.40	P	<0.001
Employment status										
Employed	Ref		Ref		Ref		Ref		Ref	
Unemployed	3.89	(1.82,8.29)	2.70	(1.13,6.44)	2.86	(2.17,3.78)	2.93	(1.83,4.69)	4.46	(3.25,6.12)
Student/home duties	2.30	(0.81,6.48)	2.52	(1.00,6.33)	1.36	(0.95,1.95)	0.66	(0.24,1.85)	3.41	(2.26,5.15)
Retired	3.23	(1.78,5.84)	2.69	(1.19,6.07)	3.18	(2.26,4.48)	3.03	(2.14,4.29)	4.13	(3.09,5.52)
	PTREND	<0.001	PTREND	=0.009	PTREND	<0.001	PTREND	<0.001	PTREND	<0.001
Income, AUD										
0–19,999	Ref		Ref		Ref		Ref		Ref	
20,000–39,999	0.72	(0.48,1.08)	1.32	(0.79,2.22)	0.85	(0.67,1.06)	0.96	(0.77,1.19)	0.67	(0.56,0.80)
40,000–89,999	0.37	(0.21,0.66)	0.58	(0.29,1.16)	0.60	(0.46,0.79)	0.65	(0.48,0.87)	0.34	(0.26,0.43)
>−90,000	0.17	(0.04,0.68)	0.30	(0.07,1.28)	0.57	(0.37,0.87)	0.32	(0.17,0.62)	0.21	(0.12,0.35)
	PTREND	<0.001	PTREND	=0.040	PTREND	<0.001	PTREND	<0.001	PTREND	<0.001
Remoteness										
Capital city	Ref		Ref		Ref		Ref		Ref	
Regional	0.88	(0.62,1.24)	0.83	(0.51,1.33)	1.06	(0.87,1.28)	1.07	(0.88,1.29)	1.03	(0.88,1.20)
	P	=0.46	P	=0.43	P	=0.58	P	=0.52	P	=0.70
Partnered										
No	Ref		Ref		Ref		Ref		Ref	
Yes	0.89	(0.61,1.30)	0.50	(0.31,0.81)	1.00	(0.82,1.22)	0.90	(0.73,1.11)	0.62	(0.53,0.73)
	P	=0.55	P	=0.005	P	=0.98	P	=0.34	P	<0.001
Lives with others										
No	Ref		Ref		Ref		Ref		Ref	
Yes	0.90	(0.60,1.35)	0.43	(0.26,0.71)	0.89	(0.71,1.13)	0.89	(0.71,1.11)	0.68	(0.57,0.81)
	P	=0.62	P	<0.001	P	=0.36	P	=0.32	P	<0.001

Analysis performed using log-binomial regression, adjusted for age, sex and education. Results in boldface denote statistical significance ($p < 0.05$). Abbreviations: AD = Alzheimer's disease; BMI = body mass index; MND = motor neuron disease; MS = multiple sclerosis; PD = Parkinson's disease; Ref: reference category; SES = socioeconomic status.

3.2.1. Lifestyle Associations with Neurological Conditions

Participants with AD or stroke were 52% and 55% less likely to undertake cognitively engaging activities than the CP (Table 4). Participants with either AD, MND, MS or stroke were less likely to undertake physical activity ($PR_{AD} = 0.50$; $PR_{MND} = 0.61$; $PR_{MS} = 0.72$; $PR_{stroke} = 0.69$). Participants with MND or stroke were 2.1 and 1.5 times more likely to be current smokers than the CP, whereas those with PD were 43% less likely. Participants with AD or stroke were 62% and 55% less likely to socialise face-to-face, and those with MS were 68% more likely to socialise online. Participants with AD or stroke were 38% and 24% less likely to engage in stress-reducing activities than the CP, respectively, those with MS were 22% more likely.

Table 4. Associations between lifestyle behaviours and neurological disorders referenced to comparator population.

Lifestyle Behaviour	AD (N = 125)		MND (N = 72)		MS (N = 441)		PD (N = 415)		Stroke (N = 647)	
	PR	(95%CI)	PR	(95%CI)	PR	(95%CI)	PR	(95%CI)	PR	(95%CI)
Cognitive engagement										
No	Ref		Ref		Ref		Ref		Ref	
Yes	0.48	(0.33,0.69)	1.03	(0.59,1.80)	0.99	(0.78,1.26)	0.83	(0.67,1.02)	0.45	(0.38,0.53)
	P	<0.001	P	=0.91	P	=0.94	P	=0.077	P	<0.001
Physical activity										
No	Ref		Ref		Ref		Ref		Ref	
Yes	0.50	(0.33,0.76)	0.61	(0.38,0.96)	0.72	(0.59,0.87)	0.83	(0.68,1.01)	0.69	(0.58,0.81)
	P	=0.001	P	=0.034	P	<0.001	P	=0.064	P	<0.001
Smoker										
No	Ref		Ref		Ref		Ref		Ref	
Yes	1.07	(0.62,1.82)	2.14	(1.21,3.77)	1.13	(0.88,1.46)	0.57	(0.39,0.84)	1.49	(1.22,1.83)
	P	=0.82	P	=0.008	P	=0.34	P	=0.005	P	<0.001
Social face-to-face										
No	Ref		Ref		Ref		Ref		Ref	
Yes	0.38	(0.26,0.57)	1.10	(0.53,2.30)	1.10	(0.79,1.52)	0.93	(0.71,1.21)	0.45	(0.37,0.53)
	P	<0.001	P	=0.80	P	=0.57	P	=0.58	P	<0.001
Social online										
No	Ref		Ref		Ref		Ref		Ref	
Yes	0.36	(0.11,1.16)	1.39	(0.66,2.91)	1.68	(1.29,2.19)	1.07	(0.73,1.58)	0.74	(0.51,1.06)
	P	=0.088	P	=0.39	P	<0.001	P	=0.73	P	=0.10
Stress reduction										
No	Ref		Ref		Ref		Ref		Ref	
Yes	0.62	(0.40,0.99)	1.07	(0.65,1.78)	1.22	(1.00,1.48)	0.88	(0.70,1.10)	0.76	(0.63,0.92)
	P	=0.043	P	=0.78	P	=0.048	P	=0.25	P	=0.004

Analysis performed using log-binomial regression, adjusted for age, sex and education. Results in boldface denote statistical significance ($p < 0.05$). Abbreviations: AD = Alzheimer's disease; MND = motor neuron disease; MS = multiple sclerosis; PD = Parkinson's disease; Ref: reference category.

3.2.2. Food and Beverage Associations with Neurological Disorders

Participants with AD were 55% less likely to consume bakery/cereals, 52% less likely to consume dairy, and 31% less likely to eat fish/seafood. Similar associations were observed among participants with stroke (Table 5).

Participants with AD, PD or stroke were less likely to consume fruit ($PR_{AD} = 0.54$; $PR_{PD} = 0.78$; $PR_{stroke} = 0.61$) or vegetables ($PR_{AD} = 0.41$; $PR_{PD} = 0.71$; $PR_{stroke} = 0.56$). Of participants who consumed fruit in the past 7 days, recommended daily serves were 21% less likely met by participants with stroke. Those with MS were 42% more likely to eat vegetables. Compared to the CP, participants with AD were 61% less likely to consume meat and almost half as likely to eat natural grains and snacks. Participants with PD or stroke were also less likely to consume those foods.

For beverages consumed in the preceding 7 days, participants with AD, PD and stroke were 39%, 33% and 51% less likely to consume alcohol, respectively, than the CP. Soft drinks were 26% less likely to be consumed by participants with MS and tea/coffee were 47% and 33% less likely to be consumed by those with AD or stroke, respectively.

Table 5. Associations between food and beverage consumption and neurological disorders, referenced to the comparator population.

Food & Beverage	AD (N = 125) PR	(95%CI)	MND (N = 72) PR	(95%CI)	MS (N = 441) PR	(95%CI)	PD (N = 415) PR	(95%CI)	Stroke (N = 647) PR	(95%CI)
Food consumed last 7 days										
Bakery/cereals										
No	Ref		Ref		Ref		Ref		Ref	
Yes	0.45	(0.30,0.66)	1.83	(0.79,4.25)	0.96	(0.74,1.25)	0.85	(0.65,1.11)	0.60	(0.49,0.72)
	P **<0.001**		*P* =0.16		*P* =0.75		*P* =0.22		*P* **<0.001**	
Dairy										
No	Ref		Ref		Ref		Ref		Ref	
Yes	0.48	(0.29,0.77)	1.53	(0.55,4.25)	0.97	(0.69,1.37)	0.78	(0.57,1.08)	0.52	(0.42,0.65)
	P **=0.002**		*P* =0.41		*P* =0.86		*P* =0.14		*P* **<0.001**	
Fish/seafood										
No	Ref		Ref		Ref		Ref		Ref	
Yes	0.69	(0.48,0.98)	0.97	(0.60,1.57)	0.87	(0.72,1.06)	1.05	(0.85,1.30)	0.70	(0.60,0.82)
	P **=0.041**		*P* =0.92		*P* =0.17		*P* =0.64		*P* **<0.001**	
Fruit										
No	Ref		Ref		Ref		Ref		Ref	
Yes	0.54	(0.36,0.79)	1.46	(0.72,2.97)	1.13	(0.87,1.47)	0.78	(0.62,0.99)	0.61	(0.51,0.72)
	P **=0.002**		*P* =0.29		*P* =0.36		*P* **=0.044**		*P* **<0.001**	
Fruit ≥ 2 serve/day										
No	Ref		Ref		Ref		Ref		Ref	
Yes	1.04	(0.66,1.62)	1.00	(0.57,1.76)	1.20	(0.96,1.51)	1.21	(0.97,1.52)	0.79	(0.64,0.98)
	P =0.87		*P* =0.99		*P* =0.11		*P* =0.096		*P* **=0.029**	
Vegetables										
No	Ref		Ref		Ref		Ref		Ref	
Yes	0.41	(0.27,0.62)	1.22	(0.56,2.67)	1.42	(1.00,2.02)	0.71	(0.55,0.92)	0.56	(0.46,0.68)
	P **<0.001**		*P* =0.62		*P* **=0.048**		*P* **=0.011**		*P* **<0.001**	
Veg ≥ 5 serve/day										
No	Ref		Ref		Ref		Ref		Ref	
Yes	1.22	(0.59,2.49)	0.94	(0.34,2.57)	1.21	(0.83,1.78)	1.23	(0.84,1.80)	1.29	(0.95,1.75)
	P =0.59		*P* =0.90		*P* =0.32		*P* =0.28		*P* =0.11	
Meat										
No	Ref		Ref		Ref		Ref		Ref	
Yes	0.39	(0.24,0.61)	1.51	(0.55,4.13)	0.90	(0.65,1.25)	0.66	(0.48,0.91)	0.58	(0.46,0.74)
	P **<0.001**		*P* =0.42		*P* =0.53		*P* **=0.010**		*P* **<0.001**	
Natural grains										
No	Ref		Ref		Ref		Ref		Ref	
Yes	0.51	(0.35,0.75)	1.24	(0.69,2.23)	1.08	(0.85,1.36)	0.81	(0.66,1.00)	0.72	(0.61,0.85)
	P **<0.001**		*P* =0.47		*P* =0.53		*P* **=0.047**		*P* **<0.001**	
Snacks										
No	Ref		Ref		Ref		Ref		Ref	
Yes	0.51	(0.33,0.77)	0.98	(0.49,1.95)	0.93	(0.70,1.25)	0.70	(0.55,0.91)	0.53	(0.44,0.64)
	P **=0.002**		*P* =0.95		*P* =0.64		*P* **=0.006**		*P* **<0.001**	
Beverages consumed past 7 days										
Alcohol										
No	Ref		Ref		Ref		Ref		Ref	
Yes	0.61	(0.43,0.89)	1.27	(0.78,2.06)	0.86	(0.71,1.04)	0.67	(0.55,0.82)	0.49	(0.42,0.58)
	P **=0.009**		*P* =0.34		*P* =0.11		*P* **<0.001**		*P* **<0.001**	
Soft drinks										
No	Ref		Ref		Ref		Ref		Ref	
Yes	0.92	(0.62,1.39)	0.99	(0.61,1.62)	0.74	(0.61,0.90)	1.02	(0.83,1.25)	1.10	(0.93,1.31)
	P =0.70		*P* =0.97		*P* **=0.003**		*P* =0.88		*P* =0.26	
Tea/coffee										
No	Ref		Ref		Ref		Ref		Ref	
Yes	0.53	(0.35,0.81)	1.34	(0.68,2.66)	0.82	(0.64,1.04)	0.80	(0.62,1.02)	0.67	(0.55,0.82)
	P **=0.004**		*P* =0.40		*P* =0.10		*P* =0.074		*P* **<0.001**	

Analysis performed using log-binomial regression, adjusted for age, sex and education. Results in boldface denote statistical significance ($p < 0.05$). Abbreviations: AD = Alzheimer's disease; MND = motor neuron disease; MS = multiple sclerosis; PD = Parkinson's disease; Ref: reference category.

4. Discussion

Understanding the overlap in lifestyle behaviours across neurological disorders provides important information on which to potentially base public health interventions and targeted self-management strategies for potential reduced risk as well as improved health. Cross-sectional population data collected annually over 11 years, from community-dwelling Australians, were pooled to assess associations between lifestyle behaviours and five neurological disorders. Undertaking physical activity was inversely associated with all neurological disorders, except PD. Participants with AD and stroke shared inverse associations across four of six lifestyle behaviours and ten of eleven food and beverage consumed categories. Six food and beverage consumed categories were additionally inversely associated with PD. Few associations were found with participants with MS and MND.

Sociodemographic characteristics were generally as expected, with participants with AD, PD and stroke being older males, and with MS more likely to be 40–59-year-old females. Across disorders, similarities were noted in being unemployed or retired, as well as income range, possibly attributable to older age and/or disability common to these disorders. Participants with MND or stroke were less likely to be partnered, and those with AD or stroke less likely to be educated. These and other demographic associations may assist in identifying resources and services required to provide appropriate support and care.

Physical activity was the only lifestyle behaviour shared across all neurological disorders, except PD, being inversely associated. While this aligns with the lack of physical activity undertaken by people with neurological disorders [6,30], it contradicts findings showing a protective impact on PD [31]. Our findings may be attributed to disease-associated disability, or limitations in data collection which queried physical activity broadly as undertaking either formal exercise or sport.

Inverse associations with ten food and beverage consumed categories were observed in participants with AD and stroke, and in participants with PD, with fruit, vegetable, meat, grains, snacks, and alcohol consumed. These findings may reflect the non-specific mode of assessing dietary intake and differential responding between cases and controls. Alternatively, they may reflect the concept of a role of the microbiota-gut-brain-axis in neurodegenerative disorders, whereby the dysregulation of intestinal microbiota through unbalanced nutrition, antibiotics, age, and infection may lead to pathological processes initiating in the gut and then spreading to the brain via the vagus nerve or circulatory system [32,33].

The importance of measuring quantities consumed is evident in associations persisting only between participants with stroke and fruit consumed, when the number of daily serves were assessed. Participants with MS were more and less likely to consume vegetables and soft drinks, respectively, perhaps reflective of a younger demographic's attitudes of a healthy diet. The data captured precludes the ability to determine whether food and beverage consumption and avoidance were adopted after disease diagnosis on the basis of medical recommendations or self-management of symptoms. The shared inverse associations of food and beverages with AD, PD and stroke warrant longitudinal investigations employing a research-focused survey using validated tools for assessing foods consumed that capture serve quantities in addition.

Smoking was positively associated with MND and stroke and inversely associated in PD, aligning with previous studies showing smoking as a strong risk factor for MND and stroke and possibly neuroprotective for PD [34–36]. Although it is an established risk factor [17], we did not find an association between smoking and MS; it may be that the association is weak or dependent on interaction with other risk factors, or due to responders giving up smoking post-diagnosis.

Cognitive engagement, face-to-face social interaction, and undertaking hobbies as a proxy for stress-reducing activities, were inversely associated with AD and stroke. These findings support the concept of cognitive reserve, enhanced by participating in intellectually stimulating activities, in delaying or preventing cognitive decline in the presence of neuropathology [37]. Simultaneously, these activities may be considered stress-reducing, attenuating the impact of psychological stress on the risk of dementia and stroke [38,39]. In participants with MS, positive associations were seen with online social interaction and stress-reduction, likely reflective of the younger and majority female population; both demographics more likely to engage in such activities [40]. People with MS also have high usage of social media for health information and social support [41].

Overall, physical activity was the only shared lifestyle behaviour of AD, MS, MND and stroke. Interventions for regular exercise and sports may therefore effectively impact multiple neurological disorders. Our findings showed inverse associations with all lifestyle behaviours for both AD and stroke, aligning with the latter being an established risk factor for all-cause dementia [42], and the recognized coincidence of cerebrovascular disease and AD [43]. Alternatively, the similarities may be due to the classification of AD in cases of vascular dementia.

The associations between MS and lifestyle factors were different from other neurological disorders. This may be due to differences in demographic characteristics, cause, or symptoms among these disorders, or under-representation of people with MS in the cohort given SSQ responders comprised lower proportions of participants aged 18–39 years, the age range in which MS is usually diagnosed. MND was not associated with most lifestyle factors except physical activity and smoking.

Limitations are acknowledged and include SSQ responders representing only 36% of participants interviewed over 11 years, to contribute to a market research survey. Responder and non-responder characteristics were mostly similar, albeit responders comprising lower proportions of participants aged 18–39 years. Other limitations include measurement errors inherent with self-reported data, potential under-reporting due to the methodology of data collection, incomplete data, unverified clinical diagnosis, temporality of lifestyle behaviours before and after diagnosis and the co-occurrence of conditions which were excluded for clarity of signal. Despite the limitations, our study has important strengths, primarily extensive data variables from a large community-dwelling population that enable the comparison of numerous characteristics, including a range of lifestyle behaviours and food and beverage consumption, across neurological disorders, which may help direct future research in this area.

5. Conclusions and Implementation

The study identified some overlapping associations in lifestyle behaviours and food and beverage consumption in a large community-dwelling population with one of five self-reported neurological disorders. These analyses should be extended to include a comprehensive assessment of the impact of lifestyle behaviours on health outcomes in people with a neurological disorder, to better understand the overlapping role of lifestyle in risk minimisation and disease management.

Cross-sectional studies cannot assess the temporality between modifiable behav-iours and neurological disorders; however, they are important in exploring dis-ease-related characteristics that may inform the planning and allocation of health and research resources. Understanding overlapping relationships across similar disorders may facilitate appropriate and targeted risk reduction and improved self-management through non-invasive and cost-effective methods. Current relationships between life-style factors and neurological disorders need to be further assessed in longitudinal studies to allow the development of effective health interventions in this area.

Author Contributions: Conceptualization, N.N., G.A.J.; methodology, N.N., X.L., S.S.-Y.; validation, X.L.; formal analysis, N.N., X.L.; investigation, M.L.; resources, M.L., G.A.J., S.L.N.; data curation, N.N., S.S.-Y.; writing—original draft preparation, N.N., X.L., M.Y.; writing—review and editing, N.N., X.L., M.Y., S.S.-Y., S.L.N.; visualization, N.N.; supervision, N.N.; project administration, N.N.; funding acquisition, G.A.J., M.L. All authors have read and agreed to the published version of the manuscript.

Funding: Data collection and curation was funded by Roy Morgan Research Institute. The research component was funded by philanthropic gifts to the Neuroepidemiology Unit from Mr Wal Pisciotta and anonymous donors.

Institutional Review Board Statement: This study was approved by The University of Melbourne, Melbourne School of Population and Global Health Human Ethics Advisory Group, project #1953821.1.

Informed Consent Statement: Informed consent was obtained from all subjects involved in the study.

Data Availability Statement: Restrictions apply to the availability of these data. Data was obtained from Roy Morgan Research Institute and may be requested from M.L. with the permission of Roy Morgan Research Institute.

Acknowledgments: The authors gratefully acknowledge survey participants and data collectors and curators at Roy Morgan Research Institute.

Conflicts of Interest: M.L. is the CEO of Roy Morgan Research Institute and data custodian for the Single Source Data. The funders had no role in the study design, data collection, analyses, interpretation, in the writing of the manuscript or in the decision to publish the results.

References

1. Mindgardens Neuroscience Network. Review of the Burden of Disease for Neurological, Mental Health and Substance Use Disorders in Australia. 2019. Available online: https://www.mindgardens.org.au/white-paper/ (accessed on 12 January 2021).
2. Mitchell, A.J.; Kemp, S.; Benito-León, J.; Reuber, M. The influence of cognitive impairment on health-related quality of life in neurological disease. *Acta Neuropsychiatr.* **2010**, *22*, 2–13. [CrossRef]
3. Gandy, M.; Karin, E.; Fogliati, V.J.; Meares, S.; Nielssen, O.; Titov, N.; Dear, B.F. Emotional and cognitive difficulties, help-seeking, and barriers to treatment in neurological disorders. *Rehabil. Psychol.* **2018**, *63*, 563–574. [CrossRef]
4. Prisnie, J.C.; Sajobi, T.T.; Wang, M.; Patten, S.B.; Fiest, K.M.; Bulloch, A.G.; Pringsheim, T.; Wiebe, S.; Jette, N. Effects of depression and anxiety on quality of life in five common neurological disorders. *Gen. Hosp. Psychiatry* **2018**, *52*, 58–63. [CrossRef] [PubMed]
5. Ascherio, A.; Schwarzschild, M.A. The epidemiology of Parkinson's disease: Risk factors and prevention. *Lancet Neurol.* **2016**, *15*, 1257–1272. [CrossRef]
6. Livingston, G.; Sommerlad, A.; Orgeta, V.; Costafreda, S.G.; Huntley, J.; Ames, D.; Ballard, C.; Banerjee, S.; Burns, A.; Cohen-Mansfield, J.; et al. Dementia prevention, intervention, and care. *Lancet* **2017**, *390*, 2673–2734. [CrossRef]
7. Null, G.; Pennesi, L.; Feldman, M. Nutrition and Lifestyle Intervention on Mood and Neurological Disorders. *J. Evid.-Based Integr. Med.* **2017**, *22*, 68–74. [CrossRef]
8. Iacoviello, L.; Bonaccio, M.; Cairella, G.; Catani, M.; Costanzo, S.; D'Elia, L.; Giacco, R.; Rendina, D.; Sabino, P.; Savini, I.; et al. Diet and primary prevention of stroke: Systematic review and dietary recommendations by the ad hoc Working Group of the Italian Society of Human Nutrition. *Nutr. Metab. Cardiovasc. Dis.* **2018**, *28*, 309–334. [CrossRef] [PubMed]
9. Barbaresko, J.; Lellmann, A.W.; Schmidt, A.; Lehmann, A.; Amini, A.M.; Egert, S.; Schlesinger, S.; Nöthlings, U. Dietary Factors and Neurodegenerative Disorders: An Umbrella Review of Meta-Analyses of Prospective Studies. *Adv. Nutr.* **2020**, *11*, 1161–1173. [CrossRef] [PubMed]
10. Black, L.J.; Rowley, C.; Sherriff, J.; Pereira, G.; Ponsonby, A.-L.; Lucas, R.M. A healthy dietary pattern associates with a lower risk of a first clinical diagnosis of central nervous system demyelination. *Mult. Scler. J.* **2019**, *25*, 1514–1525. [CrossRef]
11. Brink, A.C.V.D.; Brouwer-Brolsma, E.M.; Berendsen, A.A.M.; Van De Rest, O. The Mediterranean, Dietary Approaches to Stop Hypertension (DASH), and Mediterranean-DASH Intervention for Neurodegenerative Delay (MIND) Diets Are Associated with Less Cognitive Decline and a Lower Risk of Alzheimer's Disease—A Review. *Adv. Nutr.* **2019**, *10*, 1040–1065. [CrossRef]
12. Physical Exercise for Human Health. In *Advances in Experimental Medicine and Biology*; Springer International Publishing: Berlin/Heidelberg, Germany, 2020; pp. 303–315.
13. Kraft, E. Cognitive function, physical activity, and aging: Possible biological links and implications for multimodal interventions. *Aging Neuropsychol. Cogn.* **2012**, *19*, 248–263. [CrossRef]
14. World Health Organization. Global Recommendations on Physical Activity for Health. Available online: http://www.Who.Int/dietphysicalactivity/publications/9789241599979/en/ (accessed on 24 September 2020).
15. Global Council on Brain Health. *The Brain-Body Connection: GCBH Recommendations on Physical Activity and Brain Health*; Global Council on Brain Health: Washington, DC, USA, 2016.
16. Bailey, R.R. Lifestyle Modification for Secondary Stroke Prevention. *Am. J. Lifestyle Med.* **2016**, *12*, 140–147. [CrossRef]
17. Degelman, M.L.; Herman, K.M. Smoking and multiple sclerosis: A systematic review and meta-analysis using the Bradford Hill criteria for causation. *Mult. Scler. Relat. Disord.* **2017**, *17*, 207–216. [CrossRef] [PubMed]
18. Mappin-Kasirer, B.; Pan, H.; Lewington, S.; Kizza, J.; Gray, R.; Clarke, R.; Peto, R. Tobacco smoking and the risk of Parkinson disease. *Neurology* **2020**, *94*, e2132–e2138. [CrossRef]
19. Global Council on Brain Health. *The Brain and Social Connectedness: GCBH Recommendations on Social Engagement and Brain Health*; Global Council on Brain Health: Washington, DC, USA, 2017.

20. Mitchell, M.B.; Cimino, C.R.; Benitez, A.; Brown, C.L.; Gibbons, L.E.; Kennison, R.F.; Shirk, S.D.; Atri, A.; Robitaille, A.; Macdonald, S.W.S.; et al. Cognitively Stimulating Activities: Effects on Cognition across Four Studies with up to 21 Years of Longitudinal Data. *J. Aging Res.* **2012**, *2012*, 1–12. [CrossRef]
21. Ngandu, T.; Lehtisalo, J.; Solomon, A.; Levälahti, E.; Ahtiluoto, S.; Antikainen, R.; Bäckman, L.; Hänninen, T.; Jula, A.; Laatikainen, T.; et al. A 2 year multidomain intervention of diet, exercise, cognitive training, and vascular risk monitoring versus control to prevent cognitive decline in at-risk elderly people (FINGER): A randomised controlled trial. *Lancet* **2015**, *385*, 2255–2263. [CrossRef]
22. Lee, J.E.; Bisht, B.; Hall, M.J.; Rubenstein, L.M.; Louison, R.; Klein, D.T.; Wahls, T.L. A Multimodal, Nonpharmacologic Intervention Improves Mood and Cognitive Function in People with Multiple Sclerosis. *J. Am. Coll. Nutr.* **2017**, *36*, 150–168. [CrossRef]
23. Lawrence, M.; Pringle, J.; Kerr, S.; Booth, J.; Govan, L.; Roberts, N.J. Multimodal Secondary Prevention Behavioral Interventions for TIA and Stroke: A Systematic Review and Meta-Analysis. *PLoS ONE* **2015**, *10*, e0120902. [CrossRef]
24. Dhana, K.; Evans, D.A.; Rajan, K.B.; Bennett, D.A.; Morris, M.C. Healthy lifestyle and the risk of Alzheimer dementia. *Neurology* **2020**, *95*, e374–e383. [CrossRef] [PubMed]
25. Roy Morgan. How We Collect and Process Single Source Data in Australia. Available online: http://www.Roymorgan.Com/products/single-source/single-source-fact-sheets (accessed on 12 December 2020).
26. WHO Body Mass Index—BMI. Available online: https://www.euro.who.int/en/health-topics/disease-prevention/nutrition/a-healthy-lifestyle/body-mass-index-bmi (accessed on 27 October 2020).
27. Australian Taxation Office. Individual Income Tax Rates. Available online: https://www.ato.gov.au/rates/individual-income-tax-rates/?=top_10_rates (accessed on 1 January 2021).
28. Australian Institute of Health and Welfare. *Australia's Health 2018*; Australia's Health Series no. 16. AUS 221; AIHW: Canberra, Australia, 2018. [CrossRef]
29. Lee, J.; Tan, C.S.; Chia, K.S. A practical guide for multivariate analysis of dichotomous outcomes. *Ann. Acad. Med. Singap.* **2009**, *38*, 714–719.
30. Kinnett-Hopkins, D.; Adamson, B.; Rougeau, K.; Motl, R. People with MS are less physically active than healthy controls but as active as those with other chronic diseases: An updated meta-analysis. *Mult. Scler. Relat. Disord.* **2017**, *13*, 38–43. [CrossRef]
31. Fang, X.; Han, D.; Cheng, Q.; Zhang, P.; Zhao, C.; Min, J.; Wang, F. Association of Levels of Physical Activity With Risk of Parkinson Disease. *JAMA Netw. Open* **2018**, *1*, e182421. [CrossRef] [PubMed]
32. Spielman, L.J.; Gibson, D.L.; Klegeris, A. Unhealthy gut, unhealthy brain: The role of the intestinal microbiota in neurodegenerative diseases. *Neurochem. Int.* **2018**, *120*, 149–163. [CrossRef] [PubMed]
33. Uyar, G.Ö.; Yildiran, H. A nutritional approach to microbiota in Parkinson's disease. *Biosci. Microbiota Food Health* **2019**, *38*, 115–127. [CrossRef]
34. Doyle, P.; Brown, A.; Beral, V.; Reeves, G.; Green, J. Incidence of and risk factors for Motor Neurone Disease in UK women: A prospective study. *BMC Neurol.* **2012**, *12*, 25. [CrossRef]
35. Gallo, V.; Vineis, P.; Cancellieri, M.; Chiodini, P.; Barker, R.A.; Brayne, C.; Pearce, N.; Vermeulen, R.; Panico, S.; Bueno-De-Mesquita, B.; et al. Exploring causality of the association between smoking and Parkinson's disease. *Int. J. Epidemiol.* **2018**, *48*, 912–925. [CrossRef]
36. Pan, B.; Jin, X.; Jun, L.; Qiu, S.; Zheng, Q.; Pan, M. The relationship between smoking and stroke. *Medicine* **2019**, *98*, e14872. [CrossRef]
37. Nelson, M.E.; Jester, D.J.; Petkus, A.J.; Andel, R. Cognitive Reserve, Alzheimer's Neuropathology, and Risk of Dementia: A Systematic Review and Meta-Analysis. *Neuropsychol. Rev.* **2021**, 1–18. [CrossRef]
38. Booth, J.; Connelly, L.; Lawrence, M.; Chalmers, C.; Joice, S.; Becker, C.; Dougall, N. Evidence of perceived psychosocial stress as a risk factor for stroke in adults: A meta-analysis. *BMC Neurol.* **2015**, *15*, 233. [CrossRef]
39. Stuart, K.E.; Padgett, C. A Systematic Review of the Association Between Psychological Stress and Dementia Risk in Humans. *J. Alzheimer's Dis.* **2020**, *78*, 335–352. [CrossRef] [PubMed]
40. Kimbrough, A.M.; Guadagno, R.E.; Muscanell, N.L.; Dill, J. Gender differences in mediated communication: Women connect more than do men. *Comput. Hum. Behav.* **2013**, *29*, 896–900. [CrossRef]
41. Lavorgna, L.; Russo, A.; De Stefano, M.; Lanzillo, R.; Esposito, S.; Moshtari, F.; Rullani, F.; Piscopo, K.; Buonanno, D.; Morra, V.B.; et al. Health-Related Coping and Social Interaction in People with Multiple Sclerosis Supported by a Social Network: Pilot Study With a New Methodological Approach. *Interact. J. Med Res.* **2017**, *6*, e10. [CrossRef]
42. Kuźma, E.; Lourida, I.; Moore, S.F.; Levine, D.A.; Ukoumunne, O.C.; Llewellyn, D.J. Stroke and dementia risk: A systematic review and meta-analysis. *Alzheimer's Dement.* **2018**, *14*, 1416–1426. [CrossRef]
43. Attems, J.; Jellinger, K.A. The overlap between vascular disease and Alzheimer's disease—Lessons from pathology. *BMC Med.* **2014**, *12*, 206. [CrossRef] [PubMed]

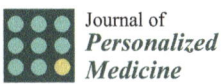

Review

An Innovative Personalised Management Program for Older Adults with Parkinson's Disease: New Concepts and Future Directions

Piyush Varma [1], Lakshanaa Narayan [2], Jane Alty [3,4], Virginia Painter [5,6] and Chandrasekhara Padmakumar [7,*]

1. Faculty of Medicine, Imperial College London, London SW7 2BU, UK; piyush.varma15@imperial.ac.uk
2. Joint Medical Program, University of Newcastle, Callaghan, NSW 2308, Australia; Lakshanaa.Narayan@uon.edu.au
3. Wicking Dementia Research & Education Centre, School of Medicine, Hobart, TAS 7000, Australia; jane.alty@utas.edu.au
4. School of Medicine, University of Tasmania, Hobart, TAS 7000, Australia
5. Department of Geriatric Medicine, Concord Repatriation General Hospital, Concord, NSW 2139, Australia; virginia.painter@health.nsw.gov.au
6. Centre for Education and Research on Ageing, University of Sydney & Concord Repatriation General Hospital, Concord, NSW 2139, Australia
7. Rankin Park Centre, Department of Geriatric Medicine, Parkinson's Disease Service for the Older Person, John Hunter Hospital, HNELHD, Newcastle, NSW 2305, Australia
* Correspondence: Chandrasekhara.Padmakumar@health.nsw.gov.au

Abstract: Introduction: Parkinson's disease is a heterogeneous clinical syndrome. Parkinson's disease in older persons presents with a diverse array of clinical manifestations leading to unique care needs. This raises the need for the healthcare community to proactively address the care needs of older persons with Parkinson's disease. Though it is tempting to categorise different phenotypes of Parkinson's disease, a strong evidence based for the same is lacking. There is considerable literature describing the varying clinical manifestations in old age. This article aims to review the literature looking for strategies in personalising the management of an older person with Parkinson's disease.

Keywords: Parkinson's disease; non-motor symptoms; carer stress; older persons with Parkinson's disease; education

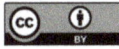

1. Article Highlight

Education, empowerment, and enablement of a person with Parkinson's disease (and carers) is the fundamental cornerstone on which personalised medicine for Parkinson's disease should be based. This article describes a multidisciplinary Parkinson's disease education program, which received wide acceptance from the Parkinson's Disease community.

2. Introduction

Parkinson's disease (PD) has historically been considered a motor disorder with cardinal signs of bradykinesia, tremor, rigidity, and postural instability. However, over the last two decades or so, there has been increased recognition of the importance of non-motor symptoms (NMS), including their typical occurrence prior to the onset of the motor presentation [1]. Current understanding now highlights PD as a multisystem heterogeneous disorder [1,2]. Different patterns of motor and NMS lead to the potential for re-categorisation of PD as a syndrome, or syndromes, rather than a singular disease [1,2].

The mainstay of PD management is dopamine replacement therapy (DRT), such as levodopa, which has been shown to improve PD motor symptoms, function, and quality of life [2]. There is evidence that certain types of NMS may be responsive to dopaminergic therapy whilst others can be more refractory. However, there is increasing recognition that the significant variability of NMS and motor symptoms are likely to require a more nuanced approach to address the overall clinical picture rather than the more traditional "one size fits all" approach [2,3].

This is particularly so in older persons with PD where NMS are common, more severe, and cause substantial impairments in quality of life [3]. Furthermore, management of older persons with PD presents a unique challenge when considering comorbidity, medication, and carer burden. Consequently, there has been emerging interest in advancing the personalisation of PD management for older persons, tailored to the specific needs of the individual [2,4]. In this paper, we present a summary of the literature and discuss the advances made in personalised management in the older adult for the treatment of PD. We will describe a novel model of personalised medicine for older adults with PD that has been very popular in the PD patient community in regional New South Wales (NSW), Australia.

3. What Is Known about the Subtypes of Parkinson's Disease?

A vast array of literature highlights that PD presents with a range of different signs and symptoms between individuals. Distinct PD motor subtypes have been described—such as a tremor-dominant subtype (with a slower rate of progression) and a postural instability gait disorder (PIGD) subtype (with a more rapid rate of progression and higher risk of developing dementia).

NMS, such as rapid-eye movement behavioural disorder, cognitive impairment, mood changes, apathy, and fatigue, vary in frequency and severity between persons with PD [1]. Historically, NMS have been poorly recognised and reported leading to inadequate research into their pathophysiology [3]. A clinical tool designed to assess NMS more objectively was only first introduced in 2005 [3].

Some researchers have hypothesised that separate NMS predominant phenotype exists with non-motor PD subtype clusters, such as cardiovascular, mood changes, perception or hallucination, gastrointestinal, urinary, and sexual function [5,6].

However, despite the advances in our understanding of NMS and the usefulness of subtype classification, this may be premature as considerable overlap is seen. There exists contradictory literature regarding the types of NMS experienced by persons within each subtype. Erro et al. [7] demonstrated that patients within the NMS subtypes were more likely to suffer from urinary incontinence, while motor disease subtype resulted more often in neuropsychiatric and cognitive impairment [7]. However, research elsewhere has demonstrated that the NMS subtype predisposes to significant mood and cognitive impairment, while tremor-dominant disease has a relative sparing of NMS [8,9]. One paper noted that cognitive disturbance helped to distinguish NMS from motor disease later in disease, despite nonspecific features of autonomic disturbance featuring more commonly in NMS [7]. These discrepancies may be in part due to the lack of a standardised classification system of PD subtypes and further reflect its heterogeneity.

4. How Is Parkinson's Disease Different in the Older Person?

Clinical phenotype and progression of PD in older persons is different when compared with their younger disease counterparts with increased severity of motor symptoms and a faster rate of decline despite comparable duration of disease [10]. They demonstrate greater severity of NMS such as pain, sleep, cognition, and apathy [10]. In one paper, where persons with PD were characterised into different clusters according to age of onset, the patients in the older subtype had a faster rate of disease progression and were found to experience greater axial instability, bradykinesia, rigidity, and tremor as compared with their younger counterparts, who experienced milder impairment in both motor and cognitive domains [11].

Older persons with PD have increased risk of cognitive impairment, autonomic dysfunction, and visual hallucinations, when compared with their younger disease counterparts [10]. Often, there is greater caregiver burden due to increased NMS burden and problems with adherence with treatment [10,12]. Since PD-associated cognitive impairment increases with chronological age, older persons are at increased risk of PD dementia [9,10]. They are also more likely to develop hallucinations and deterioration in sleep quality secondary to dopaminergic therapies [10]. Therefore, cognitive impairment should be assessed prior to dopaminergic medication prescription for older persons with PD. Deep brain stimulation surgery is generally not recommended in adults over 70 years old due to the risk of surgical complications and potential cognitive side effects [2].

5. Personalised Medicine for the Older Person with Parkinson's Disease

Management of the older PD patient presents unique challenges with distinct differences in clinical phenotype, progression, and treatment considerations. Optimisation of personalised management within the population of older persons with PD must ensure adequate education, enablement, and empowerment of patients and caregivers, respectively [10,12].

Bloem et al. [12] propose that the modern definition of health has moved from referring to complete absence of illness or accompanying social difficulties, to having the skills required to adjust and take control of one's own condition [12]. Therefore, it is imperative that within a model of patient-centred care, the person with PD (and carers) are given the necessary education regarding their condition and management, so that they can self-manage, and refer to professional advice when required [12].

Educated patients often experience less anxiety associated with their condition [12]. Patients that feel they have greater individual control over their own management, and higher understanding associated with their condition, report increased hope and reduced worry surrounding their illness [13]. This may be especially important in older persons with PD where disease severity, NMS, cognitive impairment, and dopaminergic side effects may adversely affect response to usual pharmacological treatment. Education should extend beyond knowledge of the pathology of the disease, and address the expected lifestyle barriers the patient will experience, as well as how to overcome these [12].

5.1. Parkinson's Disease Multidisciplinary Education Program

Education, enablement, and empowerment of an older person with PD (and their carer) is the fundamental concept behind the Parkinson's Disease Programme, which has been operating at the Rankin Park Centre Day Hospital, John Hunter Hospital, in Newcastle, NSW, Australia over the last two decades (Figure 1).

Ten persons with PD and their main carer are invited to attend an 8-week long PD education program offered by the multidisciplinary team based at the Rankin Park Centre Day Hospital in Newcastle, NSW. During weekly sessions, persons with PD and their carers are provided with information and education sessions, group exercise programs, falls prevention strategies, and a comprehensive geriatric assessment is undertaken by a geriatrician. The goal is to provide improved awareness of the diversity of symptoms, better understanding of the NMS burden, and most importantly enabling the person and carer with optimal non-pharmacological strategies to manage. The major issues addressed amongst the patient cohort include falls, anxiety, depression, and dementia-related issues such as hallucinations and carer stress. This intervention has proved widely acceptable and immensely popular amongst the PD community in the local region. Its success firmly emphasizes the need for similar interventions addressing the individualistic needs of older persons with PD.

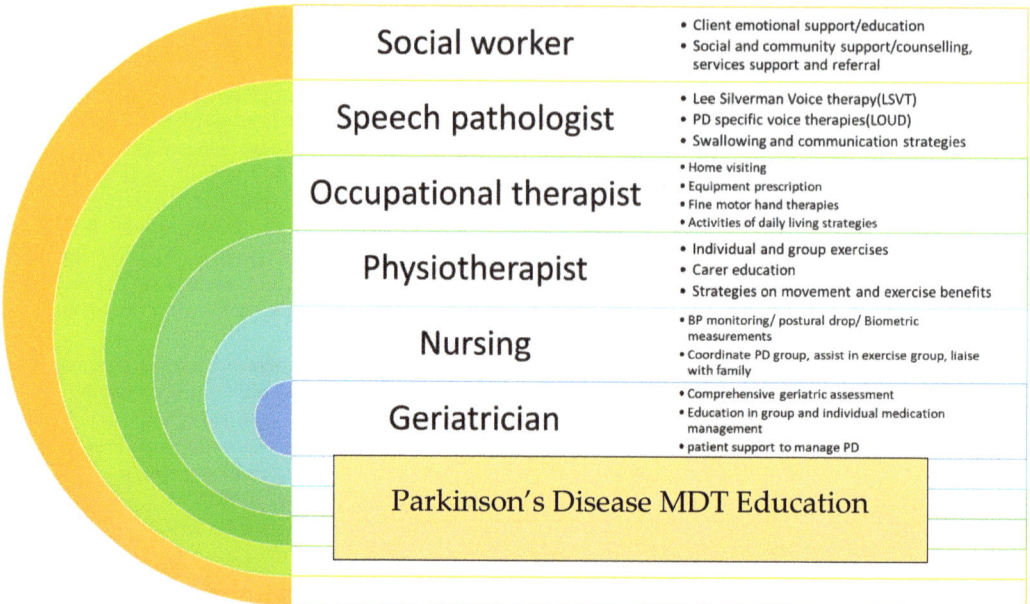

Figure 1. Summary of Parkinson's disease (PD) programme at Rankin Park Centre Day Hospital, John Hunter Hospital, Newcastle, NSW, Australia.

5.2. Comprehensive Geriatric Assessment in the Home

Geriatrician home visit to perform comprehensive geriatric assessment in community-dwelling older persons has been long established in geriatric medicine as a widely accepted and cost-effective means of assessment of the geriatric syndromes. Its benefits on survival and functional outcomes have been demonstrated in the acutely unwell, though evidence is more variable for the community setting. The comprehensive geriatric assessment at home provides a valuable opportunity for first hand assessment of the interaction between the medical and the psychosocial profile of an older person. The carer will feel involved and empowered in delivering the care plans arranged while the service is delivered closer to the person's home. This model has also been utilised at John Hunter Hospital, in Newcastle, NSW, Australia for older persons with PD, with its underlying philosophy demonstrating great potential for extrapolation to a PD service model in the future.

Consideration of additional comorbidities is essential for both the assessment and management of the older person with PD. Firstly, older persons may present with symptoms that mimic the motor and NMS of PD, but are actually secondary to co-existing conditions. For example, slowed walking due to pain or reduced range of arthritic joint movement, or pain, may mimic a bradykinetic gait [10]. Underlying systemic disease can cause fatigue and contribute to autonomic disturbance [10]. Patients with concurrent prostatic enlargement may also complain of urinary retention and/or incontinence [10]. It is essential to recognise these underlying co-existing conditions as many can be alternatively managed, with subsequent impact on improving quality of life [14].

Older persons with PD tend to have a greater number of medications [9]. This polypharmacy poses risks for adverse events, drug-drug interactions, iatrogenic errors, and medication non-adherence, the latter compounded by cognitive impairment. A US study demonstrated that people with PD with poor adherence to treatment were more likely to be hospitalised and require additional care visits at home, compared with those that were adherent [15]. Conversing with the patient to accurately explore any specific barriers to adherence, and using dosette boxes and other aids, may help improve adherence to medication regimens [10]. Patients with a recurrent history of non-adherence may also benefit from pharmacological intervention that is only required once daily, or less [2].

Increased incidence of osteoporosis and higher risk of falls means that older persons with PD are at increased risk of injuries and fractures that significantly hinder daily activities of living [12,16]. Therefore, preventative management against osteoporosis and the loss of bone mass must be emphasised, including with advice on calcium intake, effective vitamin D supplementation, and prompt bisphosphonate therapy when indicated [2]. However, to further enhance patient empowerment, measures must be taken to improve the safety of the patient's daily settings as well. This can be done via use of safety measures within the home, such as handrails and mobility aids, to minimise fall risk [12]. Physiotherapy and careful analysis of the side-effect profile of any coexisting medications are also required to both reduce the risk or extent of osteoporosis, as well as to improve mobility and functionality [12]. Additionally, remote monitoring using sensors and online diaries can be useful in allowing for timely detection of medical problems [12]. Modern technology, such as electronic device typing, also allows clinicians access to information regarding near-falls, so that adaptations can be made to management, before a serious accident occurs [12,17].

5.3. Establishing an Individualised Management Plan for Older Persons with PD through Questionnaire

The challenge of designing a tailor-made treatment regime for an older person will start with identifying and prioritising the key NMS for that individual. This is because, unlike for the motor symptoms, there are no well-established and efficacious treatments for the majority of NMS, including dementia.

One method proposed to help empower patients is through use of patient questionnaires [12]. This enables them to report subjective outcomes of treatment measures to their clinician and streamline the shared decision-making process [12]. Patients and clinicians can more clearly see which interventions are beneficial and which may further contribute to patient issues. This is a vital measure for the future, as recent research demonstrated that persons with PD often feel that they are not adequately included in their own management process [12], which can create a barrier to trust in the patient–physician relationship, as well as failing to sufficiently empower the patient. This empowerment must also extend to carers as well, who are immediately involved and whose well-being can have direct impact on the outcomes for older people with PD. Caring for a person with PD can be emotionally and physically difficult, and the burden placed on carers must be addressed, to avoid increased risk of stress, social withdrawal, and mortality associated with the role [12]. These risks increase the likelihood that older persons with PD, who may be unable to independently care for themselves, are admitted to hospital [12]. In 2008, a unified Non-Motor Symptoms Scale (NMSS) addressed the need for simple identification and comprehensive assessment of NMS in persons with PD based on the NMSQ (Non-motor symptoms questionnaire) [18]. The introduction of NMSQ and NMSS were two fundamental steps in the journey towards proactively addressing the needs of an older person with PD. A deeper understanding of the methodology behind these two tools will be the first steps in designing an individualised, person-specific treatment plan for an older person with PD (Figure 2).

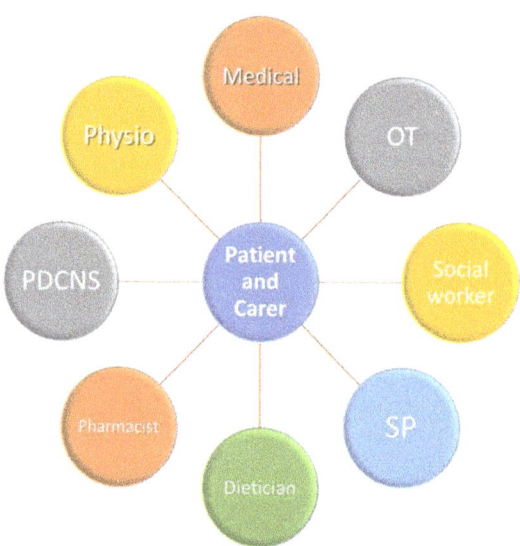

Figure 2. Model of care for the older person with PD. PDCNS: Parkinson's Disease Clinical Nurse Specialist; SP: Speech Pathologist; OT: Occupational Therapist; Physio: Physiotherapist.

6. Conclusions

The heterogeneity of PD is becoming more widely acknowledged. In the future, it is likely that PD will be considered a clinical syndrome, or syndromes, rather than a single disease. This has widespread implications, enabling greater patient awareness around their own condition, and ensuring that symptoms normally attributed to PD are more carefully investigated, in order to ensure that misdiagnosis does not occur. The patient experience of PD is highly variable meaning that generalised treatment approaches fail to address individual patient needs and symptoms. Greater strides need to be taken in clinical practice to maximise education, empowerment, and enablement of PD patients, and to streamline the movement to an era of shared decision-making [12]. Older persons with PD require additional nuances to management approach and these need to be addressed in a timely and proactive manner. This paper aimed to outline several measures that healthcare professionals can take in order to make management as personalised to the older PD patient as possible.

The entire concept of personalised medicine as a template for designing custom made treatment regimens for individual medical conditions is an exciting but at the same time a very early step in medicine.

While it would be the most satisfying step both for the physician and patient alike in the realm of PD, more evidence-based medicine needs to be generated before we can safely design a treatment regime targeting the individual needs of an older person with PD. While it is tempting to generalise the generic principles of managing an older person with a chronic medical condition with emphasis on reducing the polypharmacy and respecting underlying frailty that one expects from an older person with multiple comorbidities, it may not be a rational scientific approach to adopt that approach (Table 1).

Table 1. Take home messages.

Older persons with PD have different care needs compared to a younger person with PD.
We do not have enough evidence-based medicine to identify what those specific care needs are; there is a big scope for future studies in this clinical domain.
There is an increasing amount of evidence advocating the need for monotherapy with L-Dopa in the very frail elderly cohort of people with PD. Whether this is the best approach, we need more studies.
Cognitive impairment plays an important role in deciding which medication should be prescribed in an older person with PD.

The need of the hour is an evidence-based objective approach to answer the question; do we have enough evidence to suggest safe individualised medication regimes to address the medical needs of the older person cohort suffering from Parkinson's disease?

We do hope that our collective thoughts will be the beginning of an evidence-based answer to that question.

Funding: This research received no external funding.

Institutional Review Board Statement: Not applicable.

Informed Consent Statement: Not applicable.

Data Availability Statement: Agree with MDPI research data policies.

Conflicts of Interest: The authors have no relevant or affiliations or financial involvement with any organisation or entity with a financial interest in or conflict with the subject matter.

References

1. Titova, N.; Padmakumar, C.; Lewis, S.J.G.; Chaudhuri, K.R. Parkinson's: A syndrome rather than a disease? *J. Neural Transm.* **2017**, *124*, 907–914. [CrossRef] [PubMed]
2. Titova, N.; Chaudhuri, K.R. Personalized Medicine and Nonmotor Symptoms in Parkinson's Disease. *Int. Rev. Neurobiol.* **2017**, *134*, 1257–1281. [CrossRef] [PubMed]
3. Chaudhuri, K.R.; Healy, D.G.; Schapira, A.H.V. Non-motor symptoms of Parkinson's disease: Diagnosis and management. *Lancet Neurol.* **2006**, *5*, 235–245. [CrossRef]
4. Ginsburg, G.S.; Willard, H.F. Genomic and personalized medicine: Foundations and applications. *Transl. Res.* **2009**, *154*, 277–287. [CrossRef]
5. Mu, J.; Chaudhuri, K.R.; Bielza, C.; De Pedro-Cuesta, J.; Larrañaga, P.; Martinez-Martin, P. Parkinson's Disease Subtypes Identified from Cluster Analysis of Motor and Non-motor Symptoms. *Front. Aging Neurosci.* **2017**, *9*, 301. [CrossRef] [PubMed]
6. Marras, C.; Chaudhuri, K.R. Nonmotor features of Parkinson's disease subtypes. *Mov. Disord.* **2016**, *31*, 1095–1102. [CrossRef] [PubMed]
7. Erro, R.; Vitale, C.; Amboni, M.; Picillo, M.; Moccia, M.; Longo, K.; Santangelo, G.; De Rosa, A.; Allocca, R.; Giordano, F.; et al. The Heterogeneity of Early Parkinson's Disease: A Cluster Analysis on Newly Diagnosed Untreated Patients. *PLoS ONE* **2013**, *8*, e70244. [CrossRef] [PubMed]
8. Lewis, S.J.G.; Foltynie, T.; Blackwell, A.D.; Robbins, T.W.; Owen, A.M.; A Barker, R. Heterogeneity of Parkinson's disease in the early clinical stages using a data driven approach. *J. Neurol. Neurosurg. Psychiatry* **2005**, *76*, 343–348. [CrossRef] [PubMed]
9. Ryden, L.E.; Lewis, S.J.G. Parkinson's Disease in the Era of Personalised Medicine: One Size Does Not Fit All. *Drugs Aging* **2018**, *36*, 103–113. [CrossRef] [PubMed]
10. Lenka, A.; Padmakumar, C.; Pal, P.K. Treatment of Older Parkinson's Disease. *Int. Rev. Neurobiol.* **2017**, *132*, 381–405. [CrossRef] [PubMed]
11. Van Rooden, S.M.; Heiser, W.J.; Kok, J.N.; Verbaan, D.; Van Hilten, J.J.; Marinus, J. The identification of Parkinson's disease subtypes using cluster analysis: A systematic review. *Mov. Disord.* **2010**, *25*, 969–978. [CrossRef] [PubMed]
12. Bloem, B.R.; Henderson, E.J.; Dorsey, E.R.; Okun, M.S.; Okubadejo, N.; Chan, P.; Andrejack, J.; Darweesh, S.K.L.; Munneke, M. Integrated and patient-centred management of Parkinson's disease: A network model for reshaping chronic neurological care. *Lancet Neurol.* **2020**, *19*, 623–634. [CrossRef]
13. Legg, A.M.; Andrews, S.E.; Huynh, H.; Ghane, A.; Tabuenca, A.; Sweeny, K. Patients' anxiety and hope: Predictors and adherence intentions in an acute care context. *Health Expect.* **2014**, *18*, 3034–3043. [CrossRef] [PubMed]
14. Lewis, S.J.G.; Gangadharan, S.; Padmakumar, C.P. Parkinson's disease in the older patient. *Clin. Med.* **2016**, *16*, 376–378. [CrossRef] [PubMed]

15. Fleisher, J.E.; Stern, M.B. Medication nonadherence in Parkinson's disease. *Curr. Neurol. Neurosci. Rep.* **2013**, *13*, 382. [CrossRef] [PubMed]
16. Curtis, J.R.; Safford, M.M. Management of Osteoporosis among the Elderly with Other Chronic Medical Conditions. *Drugs Aging* **2012**, *29*, 549–564. [CrossRef] [PubMed]
17. Espay, A.J.; Hausdorff, J.M.; Sánchez-Ferro, Á.; Klucken, J.; Merola, A.; Bonato, P.; Paul, S.S.; Horak, F.B.; Vizcarra, J.A.; Mestre, T.A.; et al. A roadmap for implementation of patient-centered digital outcome measures in Parkinson's disease obtained using mobile health technologies. *Mov. Disord.* **2019**, *34*, 657–663. [CrossRef] [PubMed]
18. Chaudhuri, K.R.; Martinez-Martin, P. Quantitation of non-motor symptoms in Parkinson's disease. *Eur. J. Neurol.* **2008**, *15*, 2–8. [CrossRef] [PubMed]

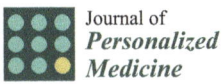

Article

Cerebellar GABA Levels and Cognitive Interference in Parkinson's Disease and Healthy Comparators

Federica Piras [1], Daniela Vecchio [1], Francesca Assogna [1], Clelia Pellicano [1], Valentina Ciullo [1], Nerisa Banaj [1], Richard A. E. Edden [2], Francesco E. Pontieri [3], Fabrizio Piras [1] and Gianfranco Spalletta [1,4,*]

[1] Neuropsychiatry Laboratory, Department of Clinical and Behavioral Neurology, IRCCS Santa Lucia Foundation, Via Ardeatina 306/354, 00179 Rome, Italy; federica.piras@hsantalucia.it (F.P.); d.vecchio@hsantalucia.it (D.V.); f.assogna@hsantalucia.it (F.A.); c.pellicano@hsantalucia.it (C.P.); v.ciullo@hsantalucia.it (V.C.); n.banaj@hsantalucia.it (N.B.); f.piras@hsantalucia.it (F.P.)

[2] Department of Radiology, Kennedy Krieger Institute 707 North Broadway, Johns Hopkins University, Baltimore, MD 21205, USA; richardedden@gmail.com

[3] Department of Neuroscience, Mental Health and Sensory Organs (NESMOS), "Sant'Andrea" University Hospital, via di Grottarossa 1035-1037, 00189 Rome, Italy; fe.pontieri@gmail.com

[4] Menninger Department of Psychiatry and Behavioral Sciences, Baylor College of Medicine, 1977 Butler Blvd., Houston, TX 77030, USA

* Correspondence: g.spalletta@hsantalucia.it; Tel.: +39-06-51501575

Abstract: The neuroanatomical and molecular substrates for cognitive impairment in Parkinson Disease (PD) are far from clear. Evidence suggests a non-dopaminergic basis, and a crucial role for cerebellum in cognitive control in PD. We investigated whether a PD cognitive marker (response inhibition) was differently controlled by g-amino butyric acid (GABA) and/or by glutamate-glutamine (Glx) levels in the cerebellum of idiopathic PD patients, and healthy comparators (HC). Magnetic resonance spectroscopy of GABA/Glx (MEGA-PRESS acquisition sequence) was performed at 3 Tesla, and response inhibition assessed by the Stroop Word-Color Test (SWCT) and the Wisconsin Card Sorting Test (WCST). Linear correlations between cerebellar GABA/Glx levels, SWCT time/error interference effects and WCST perseverative errors were performed to test differences between correlation coefficients in PD and HC. Results showed that higher levels of mean cerebellar GABA were associated to SWCT increased time and error interference effects in PD, and the contrary in HC. Such effect dissociated by hemisphere, while correlation coefficients differences were significant in both right and left cerebellum. We conclude that MRS measured levels of cerebellar GABA are related in PD patients with decreased efficiency in filtering task-irrelevant information. This is crucial for developing pharmacological treatments for PD to potentially preserve cognitive functioning.

Keywords: Parkinson's Disease; cognition; GABAergic signaling; cerebellum; MRS; response inhibition

1. Introduction

Converging evidence indicates that alterations in neurotransmitters beyond the dopamine system are present in Parkinson's Disease (PD), and may disturb fronto-striatal related cognition [1]. Cognitive dysfunction is a well-known precocious non-motor manifestation of PD, and is indicative of risk of developing the disorder in subjects with predictive markers of the illness [2]. Particularly, loss of response inhibition, i.e., the ability to suppress a prepotent behavioral response, is a sensitive measure for diagnosis and progression of PD [3], linked to broader clinical deficits and predictive of later dementia. However, the neuroanatomical and molecular substrates for cognitive impairment in PD are far from clear. Rather than to frank neurodegeneration, cognitive dysfunctions in PD may also be attributable to dysregulation of non-dopaminergic neurotransmitter systems implicated in the disorder, the g-amino butyric acid (GABA) and glutamate (glutamate/glutamine complex: Glx) systems [1,4]. Concurrently, the role of the cerebellum in the pathophysiology of PD has been reconsidered [5], since it participates in compensatory mechanisms to delay symptom onset and to preserve optimal level of performance [6].

Based on the strong cerebellar-cortical interactions during information processing [7], we hypothesized that the cerebellum contributes to response inhibition performance. Therefore, we noninvasively probed, using magnetic resonance spectroscopy (MRS), the relationship between cerebellar GABA/Glx levels and response inhibition performance in a cohort of patients diagnosed with PD and in healthy comparators (HC). We predicted that cerebellar GABAergic signaling would be related in PD to response inhibition measures [1] and that changes in extracellular cerebellar GABA would explain variations in cognitive control efficiency.

2. Materials and Methods

2.1. Participants

In the present case-control correlational study, 25 consecutive subjects diagnosed with PD according to the UK Parkinson's Disease Society Brain Bank diagnostic criteria [8] in the early stages (modified Hoehn and Yahr scale [9] ≤ 2) were initially selected for possible inclusion. All subjects were enrolled at the Movement Disorder Outpatient Services of our Institutions (IRCCS Santa Lucia Foundation; Department of Neuroscience, Mental Health and Sensory Organs, University "Sapienza", Sant'Andrea Hospital) between January 2016 and January 2017. All patients were regularly followed-up in our outpatient clinics and recruited during scheduled visits. Clinical diagnosis of PD was confirmed along a follow-up period of 36-months from symptom onset.

Since there are no published data on the relationship between cerebellar GABA and Glx (Glutamate/Glutamine complex) levels and response inhibition abilities, either in PD or in HC, to determine a sufficient sample size for a two tailed z test on the difference between two independent correlations, a power analysis was conducted using an alpha of 0.05, a power of 0.80, and a very large effect size (Cohen's $q = 1$) in order to detect only effects that would have clinical significance. Based on the aforementioned assumptions, the minimum number of necessary samples to meet the desired statistical constraints is 16 per group.

Dopamine replacement therapy dosages were calculated as daily levodopa equivalents. The following conversion table was applied: 100 mg levodopa = 1 mg pramipexole = 5 mg ropinirole = 5 mg rotigotine [10]. The levodopa equivalent dose of a drug is that which produces the same level of symptomatic control as 100 mg of immediate release L-dopa (taken with carbidopa) and expressed as the amount of levodopa that has a similar effect as the drug taken. The total daily levodopa equivalent dose (mg/day, see Table 1), obtained by adding together the levodopa equivalent dose for each antiparkinsonian drug, provides a summary of the total daily antiparkinsonian medication a patient is receiving. Out of the original group of patients confidently diagnosed with PD, 5 were excluded because were not able to complete the entire magnetic resonance exam, or because of the presence of artefacts or brain abnormalities (see exclusion criteria below). The remaining 20 patients included were age- and gender matched to 20 HC recruited through local advertisement in the same geographical area. HC and PD were screened for a current or lifetime history of DSM-5 mental and personality disorders using the SCID-5 -RV [11] and SCID-5-PD [12].

Table 1. Sociodemographic, clinical, psychopathological-cognitive characteristics, cerebellar GABA, Glx levels and excitation/inhibition balance in the studied samples.

Characteristics (Standard Deviation)	HC (n = 20)	PD (n = 20)	t or χ²	d.f.	p
Age (years/sd)	54.25 (16.62)	58.55 (9.6)	1.09	38	0.27
Males n (%)	12 (60)	10 (50)	0.4	1	0.52
Educational level (years/sd)	14.00 (3.21)	12.65 (3.97)	−1.18	38	0.24
Age at onset (years/sd)	-	55.4 (9.59)	-	-	-
Duration of illness (years/sd)	-	3.51 (1.78)	-	-	-
H&Y score	-	1.47 (0.47)	-	-	-
UPDRS-III score (sd)	-	12.30 (6.01)	-	-	-
Levodopa equivalents (mg/day-sd)	-	335.0 (260.99)	-	-	-
Combined dopamine agonists/levodopa treatment n (%)	-	7 (35)	-	-	-
Dopamine agonists monotherapy n (%)	-	6 (30)	-	-	-
Levodopa monotherapy n (%)	-	3 (15)	-	-	-
non medicated	-	4 (20)	-	-	-
Apathy diagnosis n (%)	-	1 (5)	-	-	-
AS tot. (score/sd)	-	8.75 (5.38)	-	-	-
AS motivation	-	0.60 (0.68)	-	-	-
AS interest	-	1.65 (1.66)	-	-	-
AS effort	-	0.45 (0.75)	-	-	-
AS indifference	-	0.65 (1.22)	-	-	-
HARS tot. (score/sd)	-	7.25 (4.54)	-	-	-
BDI tot. (score/sd)	-	9.10 (6.62)	-	-	-
BDI psychic	-	5.45 (4.51)	-	-	-
BDI somatic	-	3.65 (2.34)	-	-	-
PPRS tot. (score/sd)	-	6.55 (0.82)	-	-	-
PPRS hallucinations	-	1.10 (0.30)	-	-	-
PPRS illusions	-	1.05 (0.22)	-	-	-
PPRS paranoid ideation	-	1.0 (0.0)	-	-	-
PPRS sleep disturbance	-	1.30 (0.57)	-	-	-
PPRS confusion	-	1.0 (0.0)	-	-	-
PPRS sexual preoccupation	-	1.10 (0.45)	-	-	-
MMSE (raw score/sd)	29.50 (1.0)	28.80 (1.05)	2.15	38	**0.04**
M-WCST-sf C	5.95 (0.22)	5.95 (0.22)	0.0	38	1.0
M-WCST-sf P	0.15 (0.36)	1.0 (1.77)	-2.09	38	**0.04**
M-WCST-sf NP	0.60 (0.82)	1.0 (0.97)	−1.40	38	0.38
SWCT-sv IE-T (sec/sd)	31.40 (9.01)	34.55 (10.66)	−1.0	38	0.43
SWCT-sv IE-E	0.20 (0.69)	0.45 (1.05)	−0.88	38	0.09
Mean cerebellar GABA (ppm/sd)	3.48 (0.46)	3.59 (0.61)	−0.60	38	0.55
Cerebellar GABA left	3.53 (0.56)	3.55 (0.76)	−0.11	38	0.91
Cerebellar GABA right	3.44 (0.54)	3.62 (0.82)	−0.82	38	0.41
Mean cerebellar Glx	10.17 (0.99)	10.21 (1.0)	−0.12	38	0.90
Cerebellar Glx left	10.29 (1.31)	10.42 (1.16)	−0.35	38	0.73
Cerebellar Glx right	10.05 (1.29)	9.99 (1.34)	0.14	38	0.89
Mean cerebellar E/I balance (Glx/GABA)	2.97 (0.48)	2.91 (0.56)	0.31	38	0.75
Cerebellar E/I balance (Glx/GABA) left	2.99 (0.60)	3.04 (0.63)	−0.26	38	0.80
Cerebellar E/I balance (Glx/GABA) right	2.99 (0.60)	2.87 (0.70)	0.56	38	0.58

Legend: AS, Apathy Scale; BDI, Beck Depression Inventory; d.f., degree of freedom; E/I excitation/inhibition; GABA, gamma-aminobutyric acid; Glx, Glutamate/Glutamine complex; HC, healthy controls; H&Y, Hoehn and Yahr scale; HARS, Hamilton Anxiety Rating Scale; HC, healthy controls; M-WCST-sf, Modified Wisconsin Card Sorting Test short form; M-WCST-sf C achieved categories; M-WCST-sf NP non-perseverative errors; M-WCST-sf P perseverative errors; MMSE, Minimental State Examination; PD, Parkinson Disease patients; ppm, parts per million; PPRS, Parkinson's Psychosis Rating Scale; SWCT-sv IE-E, Stroop Word-Color Test short form error interference effect; SWCT-sv IE-T, Stroop Word-Color Test short form time interference effect; UPDRS-III scale, Unified Parkinson's Disease Rating Scale Part III motor function. Bold values indicate statistically significant differences.

Inclusion criteria for all subjects were: (1) age between 18 and 65 years, (2) at least eight years of education, and (3) suitability for MRI scanning. Exclusion criteria were: (1) known or suspected history of alcoholism, drug dependence or abuse, other neurological disorders, (2) personality disorder, any present mental disorder (unipolar depressive and anxiety disorders of mild to moderate severity were suitable for recruitment) and past major mental disorders (however, a positive anamnesis for past unipolar mood and/or anxiety disorders of mild to moderate severity was considered acceptable for inclusion), according to DSM-5 criteria, (3) major medical illnesses, i.e., diabetes not stabilized, obstructive pulmonary disease or asthma, hematological/oncological disorders, B12 or folate deficiency as evidenced by blood concentrations below the lower normal limit, pernicious anemia, clinically significant and unstable active gastrointestinal, renal, hepatic, endocrine or cardiovascular system disease, newly treated hypothyroidism, (4) IQ below the normal range according to TIB (Test Intelligenza Breve, Italian analog of the National Adult Reading Test – NART) [13], (5) diagnosis of dementia according to the Movement Disorder Society clinical diagnostic criteria [14], (6) any potential brain abnormalities and vascular lesions as apparent on conventional T2- and FLAIR-scans; in particular, the presence, severity, and location of vascular lesions were rated according to the semi-automated method described elsewhere [15].

Sociodemographic characteristics, clinical features, and dopamine replacement therapy dosages for the PD group are summarized in Table 1.

2.2. Ethics Statement

The study was approved (by a written statement containing a waiver) and undertaken in accordance with the guidelines of the Santa Lucia Foundation Ethics Committee. All participants gave their written informed consent for research after they had received a complete explanation of the study procedures. Information about the potential publication of research results was included in the form, and a signed consent to the processing of personal data obtained from all participants.

2.3. Data Availability Statement

The batch-processing tool for the quantitative analysis of GABA-edited MR spectroscopy spectra used in this study is available for immediate download at https://github.com/richardedden/Gannet3.0/archive/master.zip. Due to a lack of consent of the participants, structural and chemical MRI data cannot be shared publicly, and can only be made available upon reasonable request if data privacy can be guaranteed according to the rules of the European General Data Protection Regulation (EU GDPR). The respective research group has to sign a data use agreement to follow these rules. This statement is in line with our institute's policies and requirements by our funding bodies.

2.4. Neurological and Psychiatric Evaluation

Demographic and neurological features were collected at enrolment by a trained neurologist (CP or FEP) with expertise on parkinsonism. Disease stage was measured by the modified Hoehn and Yahr scale [9], and the severity of motor symptoms by the UPDRS-III scale [16]. Patients diagnosed with PD underwent a detailed neuropsychiatric evaluation. Apathy was diagnosed according to the adapted Marin's criteria [17]. Severity of anxiety symptoms was quantified by the Hamilton Anxiety Rating Scale (HARS) (total score). Severity of depressive symptoms was investigated by the Beck Depression Inventory (BDI) (total score, psychic and somatic sub-scores). Apathy severity was quantified by means of the Apathy Scale (AS) (total score, motivation, interest, effort, indifference/lack of emotion). The Parkinson's Psychosis Rating Scale (PPRS) (total, hallucinations, illusions, paranoid ideation, sleep disturbances, confusion, and sexual preoccupation sub-scores) was used to assess the severity of psychotic symptoms. Clinical interviews and mental disorder diagnoses were made by a senior psychiatrist (GS).

2.5. Cognitive Assessment

After having been screened for global cognitive impairment using the Mini-Mental State Examination (MMSE), all study subjects underwent the Mental Deterioration Battery (MDB) [18]. The latter was performed by two trained neuropsychologists (FeP and FaP) and administered to further exclude, by means of standardized cognitive testing, the presence of major neurocognitive disorder (i.e., scores lower than the tolerance level in at least two MBD tests [14]). Acceptable inter-rater reliability was defined as k > 0.80.

Details on methodology for neuropsychological and psychopathologic evaluations have been published elsewhere [19].

Two traditional set-shifting tests, i.e., the Modified Wisconsin Card Sorting Test short form (M-WCST-sf) [20], and the short version of the Stroop Word-Color Test (SWCT-sv) [21] were administered to explore response inhibition abilities. In these tasks subjects are required to attend to a particular property of a presented visual stimulus, and to select a feature-specific response. In the M-WCST-sf, participants are asked to sort 48 response cards to match either color (red, blue, yellow, or green), form (crosses, circles, triangles, or stars), or number (one, two, three, four) of four stimulus figures. They are expected to accurately sort every response card according to one of three possible sorting criteria, through the feedback (right or wrong) given by the examiner. During the task, the sorting rule changes discreetly from color to form to number of figures, without the participants being informed. Participants have to shift sets accordingly, and to detect the new valid rule by a trial and error procedure. Achieved categories (C), perseverative (P) and non-perseverative (NP) errors were calculated. Set shifting and response inhibition difficulties are indicated by perseverative errors; thus, higher scores represent worse performance. The SWCT-sv comprises three subtests: "word reading" (W), "color naming" (C) and "word-color interference" (I). In the latter, the different stimulus properties interfere with each other since written colored words serve as stimulus displays and participants are instructed to switch between the response rules "color naming" and "word reading." The valid response rule is indicated by an explicit task cue. Response inhibition abilities were evaluated by computing a time interference effect (based on execution time) and an error interference effect (based on number of errors) [21]. Neuropsychological and neuropsychiatric scores are shown in Table 1. Neuropsychological data were collected within 2 days from MRI scanning.

2.6. MRS Acquisition and Processing

Magnetic resonance scanning was conducted on a Philips 3.0 T Achieva system with a 32 channel receiving only head coil (Philips Medical Systems, Best, The Netherlands). Head position was fixed with foam padding to minimize movements.

T1-weighted structural magnetic resonance images were acquired for spectroscopic voxel placement (TR = 300–500 ms, TE = 5.3 msec, matrix = 256 × 228, FOV = 230 × 233, slice thickness = 0.9 mm, flip angle = 8°). T2 and FLAIR sequences were acquired to clinically screen for possible brain pathology. GABA and Glx measurements in the left and right cerebellar hemispheres were obtained using the MEGA-PRESS acquisition sequence (TR = 2.0 s; TE = 68ms; 14 ms editing pulse applied at 1.9 ppm and 7.5 ppm, 256 averages, voxel size 3 × 3 × 3 cm^3), an efficient and reliable sequence for detecting brain level of endogenous GABA [22] and other brain metabolites. Voxel size was sufficient to include each cerebellar hemisphere; all voxels were positioned in the subjects' native space to minimize the signal coming from cerebrovascular fluid (CSF) and skull. Figure 1 shows the location of voxel in the right cerebellum, a typical GABA, Glx MEGA-PRESS spectrum and the fitted GABA, Glx peaks.

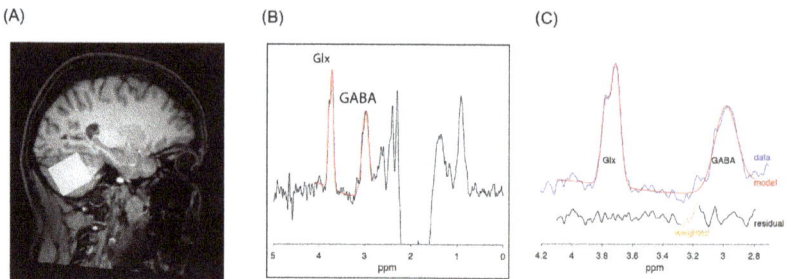

Figure 1. Cerebellar GABA and Glx spectra. Legend: (**A**) Voxel placement in the right hemisphere; (**B**) acquired Magnetic Resonance Spectroscopy (MRS) spectra with gamma-aminobutyric acid (GABA) and Glutamate/Glutamine complex (Glx) peaks in red, and (**C**) zoom on GABA and Glx peaks: acquired data are in blue, fit in red and residual in black.

Quantification was performed using the Gannet 3.0 toolkit (Baltimore, MD, USA), a Matlab-based quantitative batch analysis tool specifically developed for GABA MEGA-PRESS spectra [23]. Gannet contains five modules: GannetLoad, GannetFit, GannetCoRegister, GannetSegment and GannetQuantify. The GannetLoad module is used to parse certain variables from the data headers, apply a line broadening of 3 Hz, and frequency and phase correct the individual spectra using Spectral Registration. GannetFit uses a single-Gaussian model to fit the edited GABA and Glx signals and evaluates both metabolites relative to creatine (Cr). GannetCoRegister takes location and orientation information from the headers of MRI and image data, and generates a binary mask representing the voxel location in the matrix of the image. GannetSegment calls an SPM segmentation of the T1-weighted anatomical image and reports the tissue fractions of the voxel mask generated by GannetCoRegister. GannetQuantify combines modelled peak areas from GannetFit and voxel tissue fractions from GannetSegment with preset values for GABA and Glx and water relaxation and visibility, to deliver concentration values. In order to address differences in GABA and Glx levels of the different tissue compartments that make up the MRS voxel, metabolites concentration was quantified relative to the unsuppressed water signal, corrected for voxel tissue composition (voxel fractions of white, grey matter and cerebrospinal fluid, i.e., alpha-correction).

2.7. Statistical Analysis

PD and HC were first compared in terms of sociodemographic characteristics (age, education level and gender), and cerebellar GABA, Glx (total glutamate+glutamine, as a measure of excitatory function) levels, and Glx/GABA ratios (computed as left, right and mean (left+right/2) cerebellar Glx levels divided by GABA levels to assess the excitation/inhibition balance in the voxel) using chi-square and unpaired t-tests. Paired t-tests were used to compare cerebellar GABA, Glx levels and Glx/GABA ratios between hemispheres within diagnostic groups. In PD, linear correlations (significance was tested by Fisher's r to z transformation) between left, right and mean (left+right/2) GABA, Glx levels and Glx/GABA ratios and dopamine replacement therapy dosages (expressed as daily levodopa equivalents) were computed to verify potential medication effects on GABA and Glx signals measured by MRS [4]. Equally, given the intertwined relationship between dopaminergic replacement therapy and psychiatric symptoms phenomenology in PD, and considering psychosis as a possible medication side effect [24], the correlations between daily levodopa equivalents and AS, HARS, BDI, and PPRS total scores were evaluated. The same psychiatric measures were correlated to M-WCST-sf (perseverative errors, M-WCST-sf P) and SWC-sv (interference effect-time, SWC-sv IE-T, interference effect-errors, SWC-sv IE-E) performance in order to explore the pattern of potential interactions between psychopathology and response inhibition abilities. Whenever significant, correlating factors were used as covariates in partial correlation analyses in order to confirm the strength and direction of the linear relationship between the two random variables, with the effect of a controlling random variable removed.

Linear correlations between cerebellar GABA, Glx levels, Glx/GABA ratios and response inhibition performance, separately for PD and HC, were performed for the M-WCST-sf P, the SWC-sv IE-T and the SWC-sv IE-E. To provide a direct test of a model assuming a different relationship in PD and HC between cerebellar GABA, Glx levels, Glx/GABA ratios and response inhibition performance, the significance of a potential difference between correlation coefficients in the two groups was tested. This was calculated as follows:

$$Z\ observed = (z_1 - z_2) \div (\sqrt{[(1 \div N_1 - 3) + (1 \div N_2 - 3)]}$$

where z_1 and z_2 are the Fisher's transformed values of the two correlations and N_1, N_2 the respective sample size. Significance of the z test was set at $p < 0.01$ (two tailed) after correction for multiple comparisons (0.05/3 response inhibition scores).

3. Results

3.1. Sociodemographic, Neuropsychiatric and Cognitive Features

The two diagnostic groups did not differ for age, gender, and educational attainment. Within the PD patients' cohort, one patient (5%) met diagnostic criteria for apathy [17]. As for mood disorders, two patients (10%) met the DSM 5 criteria for major depressive disorder, while 30% ($n = 6$) was diagnosed with a depressive disorder not otherwise specified. Severity of anxiety and depressive symptoms is reported in Table 1. No PD patient met DSM 5 criteria for psychosis (see Table 1 for PPRS total and sub-scores). Although PD patients significantly differed from HC respect to MMSE total score, no study subject met a formal diagnosis of major neurocognitive disorder [14]. The two groups significantly differed respect to number of perseverative errors in the M-WCST-sf, with a borderline significant trend for the SWC-sv error interference effect (see Table 1).

A significant negative correlation in the patients' group was observed between HARS total score and daily levodopa equivalents (see Table 2). No other significant correlation was observable in PD patients between any neuropsychiatric tests scores and response inhibition abilities as indexed by the M-WCST-sf P, the SWC-sv IE-T and the SWC-sv IE-E scores.

Table 2. Correlations in Parkinson's Disease patients, between neuropsychiatric tests scores, dopamine replacement therapy and response inhibition tests scores.

	Levodopa eq. r to z (p level)	M-WCST-sf P r to z (p level)	SWCT-sv IE-T r to z (p level)	SWCT-sv IE-E r to z (p level)
AS tot	−0.06 (0.81)	0.14 (0.55)	0.10 (0.68)	0.16 (0.50)
HARS tot	**−0.52 (0.02)**	−0.11 (0.64)	−0.16 (0.49)	0.06 (0.79)
BDI tot	−0.13 (0.58)	0.03 (0.90)	−0.04 (0.85)	−0.11(0.64)
PPRS tot	0.37 (0.10)	0.04 (0.88)	−0.06 (0.80)	0.25 (0.30)

Legend: AS, Apathy Scale; BDI, Beck Depression Inventory; HARS, Hamilton Anxiety Rating Scale; M-WCST-sf, P Modified Wisconsin Card Sorting Test short form perseverative errors; PPRS, Parkinson's Psychosis Rating Scale; r to z, Fisher's r to z transformation; SWCT-sv IE-E, Stroop Word-Color Test short form, error interference effect; SWCT-sv IE-T, Stroop Word-Color Test short form, time interference effect. Daily levodopa equivalent doses are expressed as mg/day. Bold values indicate statistically significant differences.

3.2. Cerebellar GABA, Glx Levels and Excitation/Inhibition Balance

The cerebellar metabolite levels and their excitation/inhibition balance did not differ between PD and HC (sees Table 1). Concentrations of GABA, Glx and excitation/inhibition balance did not differ between right and left cerebellar hemispheres in either diagnostic group.

In PD, mean cerebellar Glx concentration was correlated with daily levodopa dosages, with a tendency toward significance for the correlation between the latter and Glx level in the right cerebellar hemisphere (see Table 3). No other significant correlation between daily levodopa dosages and cerebellar metabolite concentrations was observed.

In HC, mean cerebellar GABA level positively correlated with the SWCT-sv IE-T score (see Table 3 and Figure 2). In PD, a positive correlation was observed between mean GABA level and the SWCT-sv IE-E score. Focusing on hemispheres, a positive significant correlation was detected between left cerebellar GABA level and the SWCT-sv IE-E score in the PD cohort, while right cerebellar GABA level negatively correlated with the SWCT-sv IE-T score in HC, and positively in PD (see Table 3 and Figure 2).

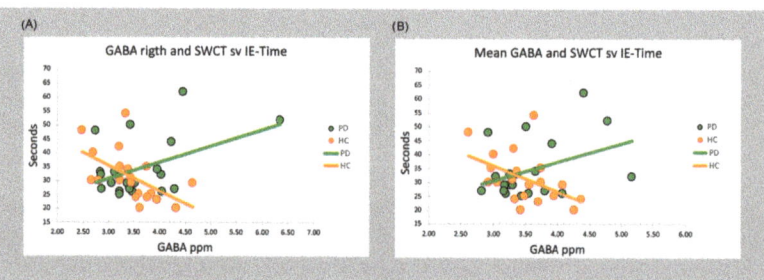

Figure 2. Bivariate scattergrams of the differential relationship in experimental groups between cerebellar gamma-aminobutyric acid (GABA) and cognitive interference. Legend: (**A**) right and (**B**) left and right mean values of GABA cerebellar concentration and response inhibition performance in patients diagnosed with Parkinson Disease (PD) and Healthy Comparators (HC), as measured through the time (in seconds) Interference Effect of the Stroop Word-Color Test short version (SWCT sv IE-Time). ppm: parts per million.

No significant correlations were observed between mean, left and right Glx levels and neuropsychological measures indexing response inhibition abilities. However, given the significant correlation between daily levodopa dosage and mean cerebellar Glx level, and in an attempt to correct for this effect, partial correlations were calculated between the latter and WSCT-sf P, SWCT-sv IE-T and SWCT-sv IE-E scores in PD. Again, no significant correlation emerged when the effect of dopamine replacement treatment was removed, apart from a tendency toward significance for the relationship between the WSCT-sf P score and mean cerebellar Glx levels ($r = 0.40$; $p = 0.08$). A positive significant correlation was observed in HC between the SWCT-sv IE-T score and the excitation/inhibition balance in the right cerebellar hemisphere. No other significant correlation was present in both groups between the measured cerebellar metabolites, the excitation/inhibition balance within the cerebellar voxel and scores indexing response inhibition abilities.

3.3. Comparisons between PD and HC Correlation Coefficients

After FDR correction for multiple comparisons, the difference between HC and PD correlation coefficients was significant for the interdependence between mean cerebellar GABA level and the SWCT-sv IE-T and IE-E scores (negative in HC and positive in PD) and between the SWCT-sv IE-E score and left cerebellar GABA levels (negative in HC and positive in PD). A significant difference in correlation coefficients was also observed for the relationship between right GABA levels and the SWCT-sv IE-T score (negative in HC and positive in PD) (see Table 3).

Table 3. Correlations between cerebellar GABA, Glx levels, excitation/inhibition balance and dopamine replacement therapy (daily levodopa equivalents), response inhibition measures in the studied samples and results from the test of difference between correlation.

	Mean GABA r to z (p level)			GABA left r to z (p level)			GABA right r to z (p level)		
	HC = 20	PD = 20	Z-test z (p level)	HC = 20	PD = 20	Z-test z (p level)	HC=20	PD = 20	Z-test z (p level)
levodopa eq. (mg/day)	-	0.007 (.98)	-	-	0.06 (0.80)	-	-	−0.05 (0.85)	-
M-WCST-sf P	0.05 (0.82)	0.31 (0.19)	−0.79 (ns)	0.11 (0.64)	0.11 (0.63)	0 (ns)	−0.03 (0.91)	0.35 (0.12)	−1.15 (ns)
SWCT-sv IE-T	−0.47 (0.03)	0.39 (0.09)	−2.69 (0.007) *	−0.25 (0.29)	0.13 (0.59)	−1.13 (ns)	−0.55 (0.01)	0.45 (0.04)	−3.22 (0.001) *
SWCT-sv IE-E	−0.42 (0.06)	0.48 (0.03)	−2.83 (0.005) *	−0.30 (0.20)	0.53 (0.01)	−2.62 (0.009) *	−0.40 (0.08)	0.21 (0.36)	−1.86 (ns)

	Mean Glx r to z (p level)			Glx left r to z (p level)			Glx right r to z (p level)		
	HC = 20	PD = 20	Z-test z (p level)	HC = 20	PD = 20	Z-test z (p level)	HC = 20	PD = 20	Z-test z (p level)
levodopa eq. (mg/day)	-	−0.50 (0.02)	-	-	−0.36 (0.11)	-	-	−0.43 (0.06)	-
M-WCST-sf P	0.06 (0.80)	0.31 (0.18)	−0.76 (ns)	−0.28 (0.24)	0.21 (0.36)	−1.46 (ns)	0.37 (0.10)	0.28 (0.24)	0.29 (ns)
SWCT-sv IE-T	0.07 (0.78)	0.09 (0.71)	−0.06 (ns)	−0.002 (0.1)	−0.01 (0.96)	0.02 (ns)	0.10 (0.67)	0.14 (0.54)	−0.12 (ns)
SWCT-sv IE-E	−0.18 (0.44)	0.30 (0.19)	−1.43 (ns)	−0.25 (0.28)	0.06 (0.79)	−0.92 (ns)	−0.02 (0.94)	0.40 (0.08)	−1.29 (ns)

	Mean E/I (Glx/GABA) r to z (p level)			E/I (Glx/GABA) left r to z (p level)			E/I (Glx/GABA) right r to z (p level)		
	HC = 20	PD = 20	Z-test z (p level)	HC = 20	PD = 20	Z-test z (p level)	HC = 20	PD = 20	Z-test z (p level)
levodopa eq. (mg/day)	-	−0.29 (0.21)	-	-	−0.32 (0.17)	-	-	−0.21 (0.37)	-
M-WCST-sf P	−0.03 (0.89)	−0.12 (0.61)	0.26 (ns)	−0.28 (0.23)	−0.06 (0.79)	−0.66 (ns)	0.25 (0.29)	−0.13 (0.58)	1.13 (ns)
SWCT-sv IE-T	0.40 (0.07)	−0.28 (0.23)	2.07 (0.03)	0.13 (0.59)	−0.19 (0.42)	0.94 (ns)	0.51 (0.02)	−0.22 (0.35)	2.29 (0.02)
SWCT-sv IE-E	0.27 (0.25)	−0.22 (.36)	1.46 (ns)	0.06 (0.81)	−0.35 (0.13)	1.24 (ns)	0.37 (0.10)	−0.03 (0.90)	1.22 (ns)

Legend: HC, healthy controls; E/I excitation/inhibition; GABA, gamma-aminobutyric acid; Glx, Glutamate/Glutamine complex; M-WCST-sf P, Modified Wisconsin Card Sorting Test short form perseverative errors; ns, non-significant; PD, Parkinson disease patients; r to z, Fisher's r to z transformation; SWCT-sv IE-E, Stroop Word-Color Test short form, error interference effect; SWCT-sv IE-T, Stroop Word-Color Test short form, time interference effect. *Significant after correction for multiple comparisons (i.e., $p < 0.01$ see text for reference). Bold values indicate statistical significance.

4. Discussion

Here the role of cerebellar tonic inhibition in cognitive functioning was investigated under a pathological clinical condition and compared to what observed under normal physiological condition. Specifically, the correlation between GABA and Glx cerebellar levels (as measured by MRS) [25] and proper response inhibition (as typically assessed through time and error interference effects in the Stroop test) [20] was tested in a cohort of non-demented patients with PD and in HC. We found that while in PD patients increased GABAergic tonic inhibition in the cerebellum was associated with decreased efficiency in filtering task-irrelevant information, the reverse correlation was observable in HC.

Such results crucially demonstrate, in the first place, that the GABAergic neurochemical profile in the cerebellum is linked to response inhibition in both HC and patients diagnosed with PD. Since response inhibition is one of the most sensitive measures for characterizing the cognitive phenotype in PD [3], our results critically confirm the non-dopaminergic basis of this key cognitive deficit [26]. This extends to PD patients previous findings demonstrating that aberrant GABAergic inhibitory regulation of prefronto-cerebellar circuits underlies impairments in executive control [27].

Our results also substantiate that the cerebellum is a critical node in the distributed neural circuits subserving cognition [7] in PD also [28], and that this region should be increasingly recognized as being involved in the pathophysiology of the disorder [5]. They finally suggest that MR spectroscopic assessment of cerebellar GABA in PD may be a potential biomarker [29] in those patients showing changed performance in executive functioning tests [30].

Although the role of persistent cerebellar GABAergic inhibition in shaping brain function has been intensively studied, evidence is limited to animal studies and the motor and learning domains. Mediated through an activation of extrasynaptic $GABA_A$ receptors by the tonically released GABA, tonic inhibition exerts a powerful action in cognitive functions by controlling neuronal excitability. Since it enforces a dynamic control of motor coordination [31] regulating the rate, rhythm and accuracy of movements, so it may also regulate the speed, capacity and appropriateness of mental and cognitive processes.

Indeed, the cerebellum is thought to mediate cortical information processing via closed cortico-cerebellar loops [32]. The unique connections to different areas of the cortex suggest that it may be involved in the executive control processes performed by the lateral prefrontal cortex (PFC) [33]. While the PFC sends signals to posterior portions of the brain to bias relevant over irrelevant information, cerebellar GABA-dependent tonic inhibition regulates sensory information transmission across the cerebellar cortex [34]. Thus, this mechanism may participate to the PFC-based enhancement of task-relevant information processing [35]. The here reported correlation between cerebellar GABA levels and response inhibition both in PD patients and HC, strongly supports this hypothesis suggesting that a balance of neurotransmitter activity in the cerebellum [34] regulates the gating of sensory information in the PFC. The observed hemispheric dissociation further supports this assumption. Indeed, GABA-dependent inhibition in the left cerebellar hemisphere correlated with the error interference effect in PD. Concurrently, tonic inhibition in the right cerebellar hemisphere was related to the time interference effect in both PD patients and HC. Contralateral cerebellar-cerebral connections with the PFC possibly exploited the reported correlations, as the left PFC is responsible for resolving semantic conflict, and the right PFC for response conflict [36].

However, we found that the relationship between cerebellar GABA-dependent tonic inhibition and response inhibition was reversed in PD patients. Actually, potential changes in cerebellar output in PD are still largely unknown. Indirect evidence suggests some functional changes in the cerebellar-cerebral circuitry, which may support compensatory mechanisms to the basal ganglia dysfunction [5,37]. Indeed, the here observed reversed association between cerebellar GABA-dependent tonic inhibition and preserved response inhibition in PD patients suggests the potential enactment of some kind of compensation to support optimal levels of performance [6]. For example, executive dysfunction in PD revolves around prefrontal dopamine systems [38]. Response inhibition in particular, evokes dopamine release in the PFC of HC [39], and dopamine pharmacological manipulation improves response inhibitory behavior [40] in PD patients also [41]. Animal studies demonstrate that cerebellar Purkinje cells output can modulate dopamine efflux in the PFC [42]. Thus, changes in cerebellar GABAergic transmission may be compensatory mechanisms for counteracting cognitive impairment associated with prefrontal dopaminergic dysfunction in PD. Alternatively, variations in cerebellar GABA-dependent tonic inhibition may compensate for the down-regulation of inhibitory neurotransmission in the frontal cortex observed in PD, as also suggested by molecular studies [43,44]. Since the level of inhibition is critically important for creating the attentional set that facilitates the selection of task-relevant representations in the Stroop task, it is clear that efficient inhibitory neurotransmission in the PFC is crucial for optimal performance [45]. Additionally, although the cerebellum receives mainly noradrenergic and serotonergic projections, there is also evidence for dopamine. The cerebellar cortex contains a high density of dopamine receptors, thus implying that cerebellar output may be affected by dopamine depletion in PD, but also by dopamine replacement therapy. Indeed, levodopa increases cerebellar activity restoring it to that observed in healthy controls in PD patients on medication after overnight withdrawal of dopaminergic replacement therapy [46]. Therefore, the here observed correlation between cerebellar GABA levels and normal response inhibition in PD might be indirectly related to medication status, and to the levodopa-related boost in activity in the basal ganglia (and the cerebellum) owing to the direct connections and enhanced connectivity after medication [47], between these structures. However, although preliminary given the case-control cross-sectional nature of the present finding, the observation that cerebellar metabolite levels and their excitation/inhibition balance were not correlated to dopamine replacement therapy dosages would suggest that both a potential dopamine depletion effect on cerebellar output and a possible indirect effect of medication status on cerebellar metabolite levels are unlikely.

Nevertheless, the reported inverted association (respect to what observed in HC) in PD patients may also be a disease-related change. It is, indeed, possible that GABA concentrations in the cerebellum are increased in the early stages of the disorder. This change would be a consequence of dopamine depletion in the basal ganglia, and related to the executive dysfunctions observed in early PD [1]. The evidence of cerebellar microstructural changes and GABA-related neuronal dysfunctions in the tremor-dominant subtype of PD [48–50] further suggests that such abnormalities may lead to pathologic activity along the cerebellar-cortical pathways. Yet, in our sample of medicated patients, both cerebellar GABA levels and response inhibition performance were not different from that of HC. Although dopamine replacement medication may have "normalized" cerebellar tonic inhibition and cognitive performance [41] in PD patients, no relationship was observed between daily levodopa-equivalent dosages and cerebellar GABA levels. Moreover, although within a very limited sub-sample (only four patients), cerebellar GABA levels in unmedicated PD subjects were always within the range (+/- 2 standard deviations from mean) of those measured in medicated PD patients. In contrast, a significant negative association was found in PD patients between mean cerebellar Glx levels and levodopa-equivalent dosages suggesting that glutamate levels were modulated by dopamine replacement therapy. However, Glx levels in the small sub-sample of unmedicated PD patients were comparable to Glx concentrations in the medicated sample. Future studies comparing groups of medicated and unmedicated patients or with a longitudinal approach, either within the same patients, or with patients at different levels of disease duration/progression will further clarify this issue.

Actually, a first limitation of the present study is that the investigation of the relationship between GABA/Glx levels in the cerebellum and cognition in a sample of medicated PD patients may be influenced by the treatment itself. However, while dopamine replacement therapy was negatively correlated to mean cerebellar Glx levels, Glx did not affect response inhibition performance. Thus, the intervening effect of treatment on our main result is unlikely, also considering the null difference in cerebellar metabolite levels and their excitation/inhibition balance between medicated patients and the small sub-sample of unmedicated PD patients. Second, it might be argued that MRS cannot distinguish between synaptic and intracellular stores of GABA, thus impeding a detailed and definitive interpretation of the neurophysiological significance of our findings. Nevertheless, according to recent consensus, MRS is most sensitive to extracellular unbound GABA, which is involved in tonic inhibition [25]. Since such local tonic inhibition was related to cognitive efficiency in counteracting interference in both samples, we assumed that extracellular cerebellar GABA, which MRS can measure, participated to response inhibition. We therefore interpreted our findings at the macro-circuit system level postulating that a change in GABAergic neurotransmission within cerebellar-cerebral networks, served to maintain an optimal level of performance in PD patients [5]. Future studies measuring extracellular GABA in more than one cortical region within the executive control network (cerebellum included) will contribute to clarify the dynamic of cerebellar-cerebral networks and their relation with cognition. Additionally, the potentiality for MR spectroscopic assessment of cerebellar GABA in PD as a diagnostic biomarker should be further investigated [29]. Given the putative role of the cerebellum in the pathophysiology of the disorder, and he here reported relationship between cerebellar GABAergic signaling and measures for diagnosis and progression of PD [3], the neurochemical profile in the cerebellum might constitute an additional diagnostic marker [29] of the disorder.

A further potential limitation of the present study is the relatively small sample size, which might have increased the risk for type I error. However, a very large effect (Cohen's $q > 0.90$) was observed for the difference in HC and PD correlation coefficients between mean cerebellar GABA levels and response inhibition performance, thus suggesting that the analyses were not underpowered (post-hoc computed beta = 0.80). Nevertheless, a further study including a larger sample is warranted also considering the significant (although not surviving to multiple comparisons) test of difference between HC and PD correlation coefficients between the excitation/inhibition balance in the cerebellum and measures of response inhibition.

5. Conclusions

Here we demonstrate for the first time, that cognitive efficiency in counteracting interference is related to GABA-dependent tonic inhibition in the cerebellum both under physiological and pathological conditions. We also underline that increased tonic inhibition in the cerebellum, relative to response inhibition, is associated to normal levels of performance in PD patients. Given the cross-sectional nature of the present study we could not establish the potential longitudinal "cost" of the observed change in the relationship between GABAergic neurotransmission and cognition in PD. However, our finding provides strong evidence that the cerebellum should be considered as a primary site for systems-level compensation in the disorder [5]. Considering the neuroprotective role of GABAergic inhibition [51], future intervention studies are necessary to test how the modulation of GABAergic mechanisms changes PD cognitive symptoms, and to establish whether GABA plays a compensatory or pathophysiological role in Parkinson's disease. This is of clinical relevance since pharmacologically boosting GABAergic neurotransmission in PD patients modulates aberrant neuronal network oscillations at beta frequency [52], which seems to restore cognitive functions, at least in stroke patients.

Author Contributions: Conceptualization, F.P. (Federica Piras), F.P. (Fabrizio Piras) and G.S.; data curation, F.A., V.C. and N.B.; formal analysis, F.P. (Federica Piras) and D.V.; investigation, D.V., V.C. and N.B.; methodology, F.P. (Federica Piras), F.A., C.P., R.A.E.E., F.E.P., F.P. (Fabrizio Piras) and G.S.; project administration, F.A., N.B. and G.S.; resources, F.A., C.P., F.E.P., F.P. (Fabrizio Piras) and G.S.; software, D.V. and R.A.E.E.; supervision, R.A.E.E. and G.S.; validation, D.V.; writing—original draft, F.P. (Federica Piras); writing–review and editing, F.E.P., F.P. (Fabrizio Piras) and G.S. All authors have read and agreed to the published version of the manuscript.

Funding: Italian Ministry of Health RC17, RC18, RC19 and RC20. The funding source had no involvement in study design, conduct.

Conflicts of Interest: The authors declare no conflict of interest.

References

1. Murueta-Goyena, A.; Andikoetxea, A.; Gómez-Esteban, J.C.; Gabilondo, I. Contribution of the GABAergic system to non-motor manifestations in premotor and early stages of Parkinson's disease. *Front. Pharmacol.* **2019**, *10*, 1294. [CrossRef] [PubMed]
2. Youn, S.; Kim, T.; Yoon, I.Y.; Jeong, J.; Kim, H.Y.; Han, J.W.; Kim, J.M.; Kim, K.W. Progression of cognitive impairments in idiopathic REM sleep behaviour disorder. *J. Neurol. Neurosurg. Psychiatry* **2016**, *87*, 890–896. [CrossRef] [PubMed]
3. MacDonald, H.J.; Byblow, W.D. Does response inhibition have pre- and postdiagnostic utility in Parkinson's disease? *J. Mot. Behav.* **2015**, *47*, 29–45. [CrossRef] [PubMed]
4. O'Gorman Tuura, R.L.; Baumann, C.R.; Baumann-Vogel, H. Beyond dopamine: GABA, glutamate, and the axial symptoms of Parkinson disease. *Front. Neurol.* **2018**, *9*, 806. [CrossRef] [PubMed]
5. Lewis, M.M.; Galley, S.; Johnson, S.; Stevenson, J.; Huang, X.; McKeown, M.J. The role of the cerebellum in the pathophysiology of Parkinson's disease. *Can. J. Neurol. Sci.* **2013**, *40*, 299–306. [CrossRef] [PubMed]
6. Palmer, S.J.; Li, J.; Wang, Z.J.; McKeown, M.J. Joint amplitude and connectivity compensatory mechanisms in Parkinson's disease. *Neuroscience* **2010**, *166*, 1110–1118. [CrossRef]
7. Schmahmann, J.D.; Guell, X.; Stoodley, C.J.; Halko, M.A. The Theory and Neuroscience of Cerebellar Cognition. *Annu. Rev. Neurosci.* **2019**, *42*, 337–364. [CrossRef]
8. Daniel, S.E.; Lees, A.J. Parkinson's Disease Society Brain Bank, London: Overview and research. *J. Neural Transm. Suppl.* **1993**, *39*, 165–172.
9. Goetz, C.G.; Poewe, W.; Rascol, O.; Sampaio, C.; Stebbins, G.T.; Counsell, C.; Giladi, N.; Holloway, R.G.; Moore, C.G.; Wenning, G.K.; et al. Movement Disorder Society Task Force report on the Hoehn and Yahr staging scale: Status and recommendations. *Mov. Disord.* **2004**, *19*, 1020–1028. [CrossRef]
10. Tomlinson, C.L.; Stowe, R.; Patel, S.; Rick, C.; Gray, R.; Clarke, C.E. Systematic review of levodopa dose equivalency reporting in Parkinson's disease. *Mov. Disord.* **2010**, *25*, 2649–2653. [CrossRef]
11. First, M.; Williams, J.; Karg, R.; Spitzer, R. *Structured Clinical Interview for DSM-5—Research Version (SCID-5 for DSM-5, Research Version; SCID-5-RV)*; American Psychiatric Association: Arlington, VA, USA, 2015.
12. First, M.B. *SCID-5-PD: Structured Clinical Interview for DSM-5 Personality Disorders: Includes the Self-Report Screener Structured Clinical Interview for DSM-5 Screening Personality Questionnaire (SCID-5-SPQ)*; American Psychiatric Association: Arlington, VA, USA, 2016; ISBN 9781585624744.
13. Sartori, G.; Colombo, L.; Vallar, G.; Rusconi, M.L.; Pinarello, A. TIB. Test di intelligenza breve per la valutazione del quoziente intellettivo attuale e pre-morboso. *Prof. Psicol.* **1997**, *1*, 2–24.
14. Emre, M.; Aarsland, D.; Brown, R.; Burn, D.J.; Duyckaerts, C.; Mizuno, Y.; Broe, G.A.; Cummings, J.; Dickson, D.W.; Gauthier, S.; et al. Clinical diagnostic criteria for dementia associated with Parkinson's disease. *Mov. Disord.* **2007**, *22*, 1689–1707. [CrossRef] [PubMed]
15. Iorio, M.; Spalletta, G.; Chiapponi, C.; Luccichenti, G.; Cacciari, C.; Orfei, M.D.; Caltagirone, C.; Piras, F. White matter hyperintensities segmentation: A new semi-automated method. *Front. Aging Neurosci.* **2013**, *5*, 76. [CrossRef] [PubMed]
16. Goetz, C.G.; Tilley, B.C.; Shaftman, S.R.; Stebbins, G.T.; Fahn, S.; Martinez-Martin, P.; Poewe, W.; Sampaio, C.; Stern, M.B.; Dodel, R.; et al. Movement Disorder Society-Sponsored Revision of the Unified Parkinson's Disease Rating Scale (MDS-UPDRS): Scale presentation and clinimetric testing results. *Mov. Disord.* **2008**, *23*, 2129–2170. [CrossRef] [PubMed]
17. Starkstein, S.E. Apathy and Withdrawal. *Int. Psychogeriatr.* **2000**, *12*, 135–137. [CrossRef]
18. Carlesimo, G.A.; Caltagirone, C.; Gainotti, G. The Mental Deterioration Battery: normative data, diagnostic reliability and qualitative analyses of cognitive impairment. *Eur. Neurol.* **1996**, *36*, 378–384. [CrossRef]
19. Spalletta, G.; Robinson, R.G.; Cravello, L.; Pontieri, F.E.; Pierantozzi, M.; Stefani, A.; Long, J.D.; Caltagirone, C.; Assogna, F. The early course of affective and cognitive symptoms in de novo patients with Parkinson's disease. *J. Neurol.* **2014**, *261*, 1126–1132. [CrossRef]
20. Nelson, H.E. A Modified Card Sorting Test Sensitive to Frontal Lobe Defects. *Cortex* **1976**, *12*, 313–324. [CrossRef]
21. Caffarra, P.; Vezzadini, G.; Dieci, F.; Zonato, F.; Venneri, A. A short version of the Stroop test: Normative data in an Italian population sample. *Nuova Riv. Neurol.* **2002**, *12*, 111–115.
22. Mullins, P.G.; McGonigle, D.J.; O'Gorman, R.L.; Puts, N.A.J.; Vidyasagar, R.; Evans, C.J.; Edden, R.A.E. Current practice in the use of MEGA-PRESS spectroscopy for the detection of GABA. *Neuroimage* **2014**, *86*, 43–52. [CrossRef]
23. Edden, R.A.E.; Puts, N.A.J.; Harris, A.D.; Barker, P.B.; Evans, C.J. Gannet: A batch-processing tool for the quantitative analysis of gamma-aminobutyric acid–edited MR spectroscopy spectra. *J. Magn. Reson. Imaging* **2014**, *40*, 1445–1452. [CrossRef] [PubMed]
24. Rondot, P.; de Recondo, J.; Coignet, A.; Ziegler, M. Mental disorders in Parkinson's disease after treatment with L-DOPA. *Adv. Neurol.* **1984**, *40*, 259–269. [PubMed]
25. Dyke, K.; Pépés, S.E.; Chen, C.; Kim, S.; Sigurdsson, H.P.; Draper, A.; Husain, M.; Nachev, P.; Gowland, P.A.; Morris, P.G.; et al. Comparing GABA-dependent physiological measures of inhibition with proton magnetic resonance spectroscopy measurement of GABA using ultra-high-field MRI. *Neuroimage* **2017**, *152*, 360–370. [CrossRef] [PubMed]

26. Ye, Z.; Altena, E.; Nombela, C.; Housden, C.R.; Maxwell, H.; Rittman, T.; Huddleston, C.; Rae, C.L.; Regenthal, R.; Sahakian, B.J.; et al. Selective serotonin reuptake inhibition modulates response inhibition in Parkinson's disease. *Brain* **2014**, *137*, 1145–1155. [CrossRef] [PubMed]
27. Piras, F.; Piras, F.; Banaj, N.; Ciullo, V.; Vecchio, D.; Edden, R.A.E.; Spalletta, G. Cerebellar GABAergic correlates of cognition-mediated verbal fluency in physiology and schizophrenia. *Acta Psychiatr. Scand.* **2019**, *139*, 582–594. [CrossRef] [PubMed]
28. Nishio, Y.; Hirayama, K.; Takeda, A.; Hosokai, Y.; Ishioka, T.; Suzuki, K.; Itoyama, Y.; Takahashi, S.; Mori, E. Corticolimbic gray matter loss in Parkinson's disease without dementia. *Eur. J. Neurol.* **2010**, *17*, 1090–1097. [CrossRef] [PubMed]
29. Mazuel, L.; Chassain, C.; Jean, B.; Pereira, B.; Cladière, A.; Speziale, C.; Durif, F. Proton MR spectroscopy for diagnosis and evaluation of treatment efficacy in Parkinson disease. *Radiology* **2016**, *278*, 505–513. [CrossRef]
30. Dujardin, K.; Leentjens, A.F.G.; Langlois, C.; Moonen, A.J.H.; Duits, A.A.; Carette, A.S.; Duhamel, A. The spectrum of cognitive disorders in Parkinson's disease: A data-driven approach. *Mov. Disord.* **2013**, *28*, 183–189. [CrossRef]
31. Woo, J.; Min, J.O.; Kang, D.S.; Kim, Y.S.; Jung, G.H.; Park, H.J.; Kim, S.; An, H.; Known, J.; Kim, J.; et al. Control of motor coordination by astrocytic tonic GABA release through modulation of excitation/inhibition balance in cerebellum. *Proc. Natl. Acad. Sci. USA* **2018**, *115*, 5004–5009. [CrossRef]
32. Schmahmann, J.D. The cerebrocerebellar system. In *Essentials of Cerebellum and Cerebellar Disorders: A Primer for Graduate Students*; Springer International Publishing: Cham, Switzerland, 2016; pp. 101–115. ISBN 9783319245515.
33. Bellebaum, C.; Daum, I. Cerebellar involvement in executive control. *Cerebellum* **2007**, *6*, 184–192. [CrossRef]
34. Duguid, I.; Branco, T.; London, M.; Chadderton, P.; Häusser, M. Tonic inhibition enhances fidelity of sensory information transmission in the cerebellar cortex. *J. Neurosci.* **2012**, *32*, 11132–11143. [CrossRef] [PubMed]
35. Purmann, S.; Pollmann, S. Adaptation to recent conflict in the classical color-word Stroop-task mainly involves facilitation of processing of task-relevant information. *Front. Hum. Neurosci.* **2015**, *9*, 88. [CrossRef] [PubMed]
36. Milham, M.P.; Banich, M.T.; Webb, A.; Barad, V.; Cohen, N.J.; Wszalek, T.; Kramer, A.F. The relative involvement of anterior cingulate and prefrontal cortex in attentional control depends on nature of conflict. *Cogn. Brain Res.* **2001**, *12*, 467–473. [CrossRef]
37. Appel-Cresswell, S.; De La Fuente-Fernandez, R.; Galley, S.; McKeown, M.J. Imaging of compensatory mechanisms in Parkinson's disease. *Curr. Opin. Neurol.* **2010**, *23*, 407–412. [CrossRef]
38. Narayanan, N.S.; Rodnitzky, R.L.; Uc, E.Y. Prefrontal dopamine signaling and cognitive symptoms of Parkinson's disease. *Rev. Neurosci.* **2013**, *24*, 267–278. [CrossRef]
39. Albrecht, D.S.; Kareken, D.A.; Christian, B.T.; Dzemidzic, M.; Yoder, K.K. Cortical dopamine release during a behavioral response inhibition task. *Synapse* **2014**, *68*, 266–274. [CrossRef]
40. Nandam, L.S.; Hester, R.; Wagner, J.; Cummins, T.D.R.; Garner, K.; Dean, A.J.; Kim, B.N.; Nathan, P.J.; Mattingley, J.B.; Bellgrove, M.A. Methylphenidate but not atomoxetine or citalopram modulates inhibitory control and response time variability. *Biol. Psychiatry* **2011**, *69*, 902–904. [CrossRef]
41. Manza, P.; Amandola, M.; Tatineni, V.; Li, C.R.; Leung, H.-C. Response inhibition in Parkinson's disease: A meta-analysis of dopaminergic medication and disease duration effects. *NPJ Park. Dis.* **2017**, *3*, 1–10. [CrossRef]
42. Mittleman, G.; Goldowitz, D.; Heck, D.H.; Blaha, C.D. Cerebellar modulation of frontal cortex dopamine efflux in mice: Relevance to autism and schizophrenia. *Synapse* **2008**, *62*, 544–550. [CrossRef]
43. Lanoue, A.C.; Blatt, G.J.; Soghomonian, J.J. Decreased parvalbumin mRNA expression in dorsolateral prefrontal cortex in Parkinson's disease. *Brain Res.* **2013**, *1531*, 37–47. [CrossRef]
44. Lanoue, A.C.; Dumitriu, A.; Myers, R.H.; Soghomonian, J.J. Decreased glutamic acid decarboxylase mRNA expression in prefrontal cortex in Parkinson's disease. *Exp. Neurol.* **2010**, *226*, 207–217. [CrossRef] [PubMed]
45. Kühn, S.; Schubert, F.; Mekle, R.; Wenger, E.; Ittermann, B.; Lindenberger, U.; Gallinat, J. Neurotransmitter changes during interference task in anterior cingulate cortex: Evidence from fMRI-guided functional MRS at 3 T. *Brain Struct. Funct.* **2016**, *221*, 2541–2551. [CrossRef] [PubMed]
46. Martinu, K.; Degroot, C.; Madjar, C.; Strafella, A.P.; Monchi, O. Levodopa influences striatal activity but does not affect cortical hyper-activity in Parkinson's disease. *Eur. J. Neurosci.* **2012**, *35*, 572–583. [CrossRef] [PubMed]
47. Mueller, K.; Jech, R.; Ballarini, T.; Holiga, Š.; Růžička, F.; Piecha, F.A.; Möller, H.E.; Vymazal, J.; Růžička, E.; Schroeter, M.L. Modulatory Effects of Levodopa on Cerebellar Connectivity in Parkinson's Disease. *Cerebellum* **2019**, *18*, 212–224. [CrossRef] [PubMed]
48. Boecker, H.; Weindl, A.; Brooks, D.J.; Ceballos-Baumann, A.O.; Liedtke, C.; Miederer, M.; Sprenger, T.; Wagner, K.J.; Miederer, I. GABAergic dysfunction in essential tremor: An11C-flumazenil PET study. *J. Nucl. Med.* **2010**, *51*, 1030–1035. [CrossRef] [PubMed]
49. Gironell, A.; Figueiras, F.P.; Pagonabarraga, J.; Herance, J.R.; Pascual-Sedano, B.; Trampal, C.; Gispert, J.D. Gaba and serotonin molecular neuroimaging in essential tremor: A clinical correlation study. *Park. Relat. Disord.* **2012**, *18*, 876–880. [CrossRef] [PubMed]
50. Zhang, X.; Santaniello, S. Role of cerebellar GABAergic dysfunctions in the origins of essential tremor. *Proc. Natl. Acad. Sci. USA* **2019**, *116*, 13592–13601. [CrossRef]

51. Van Nuland, A.J.M.; den Ouden, H.E.M.; Zach, H.; Dirkx, M.F.M.; van Asten, J.J.A.; Scheenen, T.W.J.; Toni, I.; Cools, R.; Helmich, R.C. GABAergic changes in the thalamocortical circuit in Parkinson's disease. *Hum. Brain Mapp.* **2020**, *41*, 1017–1029. [CrossRef]
52. Hall, S.D.; Prokic, E.J.; McAllister, C.J.; Ronnqvist, K.C.; Williams, A.C.; Yamawaki, N.; Witton, C.; Woodhall, G.L.; Stanford, I.M. GABA-mediated changes in inter-hemispheric beta frequency activity in early-stage Parkinson's disease. *Neuroscience* **2014**, *281*, 68–76. [CrossRef]

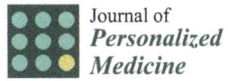

Article

Relationship between Blood and Standard Biochemistry Levels with Periodontitis in Parkinson's Disease Patients: Data from the NHANES 2011–2012

João Botelho [1,2,*], Patrícia Lyra [1], Luís Proença [3], Catarina Godinho [1], José João Mendes [1] and Vanessa Machado [1,2]

1. Clinical Research Unit (CRU), Centro de Investigação Interdisciplinar Egas Moniz (CiiEM), Instituto Universitário Egas Moniz, 2829-511 Almada, Portugal; patricialyra10@gmail.com (P.L.); cgodinho@egasmoniz.edu.pt (C.G.); jmendes@egasmoniz.edu.pt (J.J.M.); vmachado@egasmoniz.edu.pt (V.M.)
2. Periodontology Department, Clinical Research Unit (CRU), CiiEM, Egas Moniz, CRL, 2829-511 Almada, Portugal
3. Quantitative Methods for Health Research Unit (MQIS), CiiEM, Egas Moniz, CRL, 2829-511 Almada, Portugal; lproenca@egasmoniz.edu.pt
* Correspondence: jbotelho@egasmoniz.edu.pt; Tel.: +351-969848394

Received: 29 June 2020; Accepted: 23 July 2020; Published: 25 July 2020

Abstract: People with Parkinson's Disease (PD) are associated with the presence of periodontitis. We aimed to compare blood and standard biochemical surrogates of PD patients diagnosed with periodontitis with PD individuals without periodontitis. This retrospective cohort study used a sample from the National Health and Nutrition Examination Survey (NHANES) 2011–2012 that underwent periodontal diagnosis ($n = 3669$). PD participants were identified through specific PD reported medications. Periodontitis was defined according to the 2012 case definition, using periodontal examination data provided. Then, we compared blood levels and standard chemical laboratory profiles of PD patients according to the presence of periodontitis. Multivariable regression was used to explore this dataset and identify relevant variables towards the presence of periodontitis. According to the medication report, 37 participants were eligible, 29 were secure and 8 were unsecure PD medications regimens. Overall, PD cases with periodontitis presented increased levels of White Blood Cells (WBC) ($p = 0.002$), Basophils ($p = 0.045$) and Segmented neutrophils ($p = 0.009$), and also, lower levels of Total Bilirubin ($p = 0.018$). In the PD secure medication group, a significant difference was found for WBC ($p = 0.002$) and Segmented neutrophils ($p = 0.002$) for the periodontitis group. Further, WBC might be a discriminating factor towards periodontitis in the global sample. In the secure PD medication, we found gender, segmented neutrophils and Vitamin D2 to be potential discriminative variables towards periodontitis. Thus, periodontitis showed association with leukocyte levels alterations in PD patients, and therefore with potential systemic changes and predictive value. Furthermore, Vitamin D2 and gender showed to be associated with periodontitis in with secure medication for PD. Future studies should assess in more detail the potential systemic repercussion of the presence of periodontitis in PD patients.

Keywords: Parkinson's disease; movement disorders; periodontitis; periodontal disease; hematologic tests; Vitamin D; oral health

1. Introduction

Periodontitis is a chronic inflammatory condition that targets the supporting structures of the teeth [1]. Dental plaque build-up, periodontopathic microbial specificity and the host immune response can collectively be considered as periodontitis etiology factors [2]. The presence of periodontal pockets, inflamed gingiva and alveolar bone loss in certain teeth or tooth sites clinically characterizes periodontitis, which can ultimately result in tooth loss [3]. Apart from its effects in the oral cavity, periodontitis repercussions also instigate slight systemic inflammation, which end up setting off or aggravating known chronic inflammatory diseases, such as cardiovascular diseases including high blood pressure [4], diabetes mellitus [5], rheumatoid arthritis [6] Furthermore and Alzheimer's Disease [7–9]. Being one of the most prevalent conditions of the adult population worldwide, periodontitis frequency seems to be higher in the male gender while also increasing with age [10].

Parkinson's disease (PD) is the second most frequent slowly progressive neurodegenerative condition that mostly affects the central nervous system [11]. Still with elusive causal factors to date, sporadic PD appears to be the conjugation of both genetic and environmental risk factors [12,13]. Being a heterogeneous disorder, PD clinical phenotype is characterized by a broad range of motor and non-motor symptoms, differing in onset age (which is most common at 65–70 years of age) and disease progression rates (faster in late-onset forms) [11,14]. PD classical motor features include resting tremor, muscular rigidity and bradykinesia, while a wide number of other motor and non-motor features contribute to PD disability and the deterioration of PD patients' overall quality of life [15]. Dopaminergic drugs like levodopa and functional neurosurgery are still standard treatments, although tending to be a universal solution to a non-uniform disease [16,17]. PD increases with age and tends to affect more men than women [18–20]. In an overall aging population, PD cases are expected to duplicate in the next couple decades [17,21].

To date, the relationship between PD and periodontitis stands with PD associated motor impairments and cognitive decline that compromises oral hygiene habits and causes the deterioration of patient's oral status [22]. Consequently, PD individuals seem to be at high risk of developing periodontitis [23–27]. Furthermore, it has been proposed that chronic neuroinflammation secondary to periodontitis systemic outcomes may lead to PD pathogenesis, initiation and progression [8,22,28]. However, to the best of our knowledge, the systemic repercussion of the presence of periodontitis on blood and biochemical surrogates on PD has never been investigated. Our hypothesis is that, as an infection, periodontitis in PD subjects might result in an increase of the leukocyte levels, though for the remaining levels this is still undetermined.

Therefore, our primary aim was to compare blood and standard biochemical levels between periodontitis and non-periodontitis cases among Parkinson's disease patients. Additionally, we aimed to evaluate if such changed biomarkers might contribute to predict the presence of periodontitis in PD patients.

2. Material and Methods

2.1. Population

The National Health and Nutrition Examination Survey (NHANES) 2011–2012 data is a representative multistage probability sample of non-institutionalized U.S. civilians survey to assess the health status through the Centers for Disease Control and Prevention (CDC) and Prevention National Center for Health Statistics (NCHS) website at https://www.cdc.gov/nchs/nhanes/index.htm. In this retrospective cohort study, periodontal examination data from the NHANES 2011–2012 was extracted. Our analysis deemed the following exclusion criteria: younger than 18 years of age; participants with medical exclusion from periodontal exam; non-complete periodontal status and edentulous patients.

Oral health data collection protocols were approved by the CDC, NCHS Research Ethics Review Board, Atlanta (USA), and all participants gave written informed consent. All the examinations were conducted in a mobile examination center (see in detail in [29]).

2.2. PD Definition

PD cases were confirmed through specific PD reported medications according to the NHANES database. In this way, patients reporting the use of Benztropine, Carbidopa, Levodopa, Ropinirole, Methyldopa, Entacapone, Cabergoline, Orphenadrine and Pramipexole were categorized as PD cases [30,31]. Then, we divided participants as PD cases according to secure PD medication (Benztropine, Carbidopa, Levodopa, Ropinirole, Methyldopa and Entacapone) [30,31] and unsecure PD medication (Cabergoline, Orphenadrine and Pramipexole) [30–34]. The unsecure PD group was defined because Cabergoline is used to treat high levels of prolactin hormone [32], Orphenadrine is used to treat muscle spasms in musculoskeletal conditions [33] and Pramipexole is also used to treat restless legs syndrome (RLS) [34].

2.3. Periodontal Clinical Examination

Periodontitis was defined as a minimum of 2 or more sites with clinical attachment loss (CAL) ≥ 3 mm and a periodontal pocket depth (PPD) ≥ 4 mm or one site with PPD ≥ 5 mm, as described by Eke et al. (2012). Data from the Periodontal Examination of NHANES 11–12 were treated through appropriate algorithms in Microsoft Office (MO) Excel to render the respective periodontal diagnosis. From this, we were able to render the number of missing teeth.

2.4. Demographics Characteristics

The demographic variables included were age, gender, smoking status and number of teeth. From the self-reported questionnaire, we categorized smoking status as current smoker (smoked more than 100 cigarettes and currently smoking), former smoker (smoked more than 100 cigarettes and currently not smoking) and non-smoker (never smoked). Diabetes mellitus was categorized as "yes" or "no" according to the self-reported questionnaire. High blood pressure was categorized according to previous medical confirmation of high blood pressure and if taking prescription for hypertension.

2.5. Blood and Standard Biochemical Profile Levels

Blood levels data included White Blood Cell (WBC) count (10^9/L), percentage of Lymphocyte (%), percentage of Monocyte (%), percentage of Segmented Neutrophils (%), percentage of Eosinophils (%), percentage of Basophils (%), Lymphocyte (10^9/L), Monocyte (10^9/L), Segmented neutrophils (10^9/L), Eosinophils (10^9/L), Basophils (10^9/L), Red Blood Cell (RBC) count (million cells/uL), Hemoglobin (g/dL), Hematocrit (%), Mean Cell Volume (MCV) (fL), Mean Cell Hemoglobin (MCH) (pg), Mean Cell Hemoglobin Concentration (MCHC) (g/dL), Red Cell Distribution (RCD) width (%), Platelet count (10^9/L), Mean Platelet Volume (MPV) (fL).

For the Standard Biochemical Profile levels we included Albumin (g/dL), Alanine aminotransferase (ALT) (U/L), Aspartate aminotransferase (AST) (U/L), Alkaline phosphatase (AP) (U/L), Blood Urea Nitrogen (mg/dL), Total Calcium (mg/dL), Creatine Phosphokinase (CPK) (IU/L), Cholesterol (mg/dL), Bicarbonate (mmol/L), Creatinine (mg/dL), Gamma Glutamyl Transferase (GGT) (U/L), Glucose, Serum (mg/dL), Iron (refrigerated) (ug/dL), Lactate Dehydrogenase (LDH) (U/L), Phosphorus (mg/dL), Total Bilirubin (mg/dL), Total Protein (g/dL), Uric Acid (mg/dL), Sodium (mmol/L), Potassium (mmol/L), Chloride (mmol/L), Osmolality (mmol/Kg), Globulin (g/dL), Triglycerides (mg/dL), 25-hydroxyvitamin D2 (25OHD2) (nmol/L), 25-hydroxyvitamin D3 (25OHD3) (nmol/L).

2.6. Data Management and Analysis

Data were uploaded through SAS Universal Viewer for Windows and handled with MS Excel. For each periodontal case definition, specific MS Excel datasets were derived in order to formulate appropriate algorithms to define the periodontal status according to the case definition. Data analysis was performed using IBM SPSS Statistics version 25.0 for Windows (IBM CORP: ARMONK, NY, USA). Descriptive measures are reported through mean ± standard deviation (SD) for continuous variables, and number of cases (n), percentage (%) for categorical variables. The main outcome variable was the presence of periodontitis (P+ vs. P−). We compared baseline variables between periodontitis and non-periodontitis groups. Explicit comparison of mean values was performed by t-Student test when data assumptions for the application of this test were met (normality and homoscedasticity). Mann–Whitney test was used, as an alternative comparison technique, when those assumptions were not verified. To compare significant variables between the subgroups P(−) and P(+) we graphically computed the tendency of WBC, segmented neutrophils and basophils counts according to age using scatterplots from ggplot2 package for R version 4.0, and tendency was computed and fitted via 'geom_smooth'. Then, we made regression analyses in the overall and only in secure PD cases. Preliminary analyses were performed using univariate models. Next, a multivariable model was constructed for the presence of periodontitis. Only variables showing a significance $p \leq 0.25$ in the univariate model were included in the multivariable stepwise procedure. Predictor variables considered in this procedure were: gender (female as reference), WBC count (10^9/L), Segmented neutrophils (10^9/L) and 25-hydroxyvitamin D2 (25OHD2) (nmol/L). The contribution of each variable to the model was evaluated by Wald statistics. A multivariable stepwise adjusted logistic regression procedure was used to model the influence of the investigated factors towards the presence of periodontitis in PD patients. A significance level of 5% was set in all inferential analyses.

3. Results

3.1. Population

From a total of 9756 participants, 3669 individuals had completed periodontal examination. From these, 37 (32 to 80 years old, 57.6 ± 14.6) participants were identified as taking PD medications, 29 secure (32 to 80 years old, 59.6 ± 14.7) and 8 unsecure PD (36 to 73 years old, 50.5 ± 12.5) medications regimens (Table 1). There were no age differences between PD cases with periodontitis (P+) and without periodontitis (P−). Males comprised 40.5% of the sample. The majority of subjects were non-smokers (55.9%). Diabetes and high blood pressure cases were evenly distributed. The number of missing teeth did not differ between PD cases with periodontitis and without periodontitis.

Table 1. Participants characteristics.

Variable	Global (n = 37)			Secure PD Medication (n = 29)		
	P(−)	P(+)	p-value †	P(−)	P(+)	p-Value †
Age, mean (SD) (years)	53.1 (14.6)	61.6 (13.8)	0.069	55.9 (15.4)	62.6 (13.8)	0.215
Gender, n (%)						
Female	12 (44.4)	10 (27.0)	0.204	10 (34.5)	7 (24.1)	0.071
Male	5 (13.5)	10 (27.0)		3 (10.3)	9 (31.0)	
Smoking habits, n (%)						
Never	11 (29.7)	12 (44.4)		7 (24.1)	9 (31.0)	
Former	5 (13.5)	5 (13.5)	0.668	5 (17.2)	4 (13.8)	0.588
Active	1 (2.7)	3 (8.1)		1 (3.4)	3 (10.3)	
Diabetes Mellitus, n (%)	3 (8.1)	2 (5.4)	0.498	3 (10.3)	2 (6.9)	0.453
High Blood Pressure, mean (SD)	10 (27.0)	10 (27.0)	0.591	9 (31.0)	9 (31.0)	0.474
Missing Teeth, mean (SD)	3.9 (5.8)	4.5 (4.3)	0.302	5.1 (6.2)	4.6 (4.6)	0.362

† Chi-square test for categorical variables and Mann–Whitney test for continuous variables, $p < 0.05$. P(−)—No Periodontitis, P(+)—Periodontitis.

3.2. Blood and Standard Biochemical Levels

Complete blood count with 5-part differential was used to compare blood levels of the periodontitis group defined by NHANES measures with the subset of subjects considered periodontally healthy (Table 2). Overall, periodontitis group presented increased levels of WBC ($p = 0.002$), Basophils ($p = 0.045$) and Segmented Neutrophils ($p = 0.009$), also displayed graphically (Figure 1). In the PD secure medication group, the same difference was found for WBC ($p = 0.002$) and Segmented Neutrophils ($p = 0.002$) for the periodontitis group (Figure 1).

Then, we investigated the standard biochemistry profile levels to investigate the systemic status of these participants according to the presence of periodontitis (Table 3). The only meaningful result was found in the global sample, where the periodontitis group presented lower levels of Total Bilirubin ($p = 0.018$).

Table 2. Hematologic levels of PD patients with periodontitis and without periodontitis.

Variable	Global (n = 37)			Secure PD Medication (n = 29)		
	P(−)	P(+)	p-Value [†]	P(−)	P(+)	p-Value [†]
WBC count (10^9/L)	5.57 (1.28)	7.28 (2.19)	0.002	5.25 (1.02)	7.26 (2.36)	0.002
Lymphocyte (%)	28.75 (6.19)	26.38 (6.91)	0.284	28.84 (6.47)	25.35 (5.87)	0.144
Monocyte (%)	7.36 (3)	7.01 (2.09)	0.988	7.65 (3.36)	6.89 (2.07)	0.812
Segmented neutrophils (%)	60.25 (7.48)	62.85 (8.34)	0.330	59.37 (7.53)	63.88 (6.82)	0.103
Eosinophils (%)	3.16 (2.2)	3.1 (1.5)	0.752	3.66 (2.27)	3.22 (1.56)	0.682
Basophils (%)	0.51 (0.36)	0.75 (0.95)	0.537	0.52 (0.38)	0.73 (1.05)	0.846
Lymphocyte (10^9/L)	1.59 (0.49)	1.89 (0.66)	0.137	1.52 (0.5)	1.81 (0.63)	0.179
Monocyte (10^9/L)	0.39 (0.17)	0.5 (0.19)	0.104	0.38 (0.19)	0.49 (0.19)	0.121
Segmented neutrophils (10^9/L)	3.38 (0.98)	4.61 (1.66)	0.009	3.12 (0.72)	4.68 (1.73)	0.002
Eosinophils (10^9/L)	0.18 (0.13)	0.23 (0.13)	0.297	0.21 (0.14)	0.23 (0.14)	0.682
Basophils (10^9/L)	0.01 (0.03)	0.06 (0.08)	0.045	0.01 (0.03)	0.06 (0.08)	0.101
RBC count (million cells/uL)	4.37 (0.36)	4.45 (0.4)	0.528	4.28 (0.31)	4.48 (0.44)	0.186
Hemoglobin (g/dL)	13.64 (1.35)	13.92 (1.2)	0.519	13.35 (1.22)	14.02 (1.22)	0.155
Hematocrit (%)	39.85 (3.42)	40.48 (3.98)	0.614	39.13 (3.08)	40.9 (4.15)	0.213
MCV (fL)	91.34 (4.56)	91 (3.18)	0.794	91.48 (5.24)	91.33 (2.91)	0.922
MCH (pg)	31.23 (1.89)	31.29 (1.4)	0.919	31.17 (2.16)	31.32 (1.36)	0.822
MCHC (g/dL)	34.18 (0.84)	34.39 (1.01)	0.516	34.05 (0.89)	34.29 (1.1)	0.532
RCD width (%)	12.94 (1.05)	12.78 (0.69)	0.940	13.02 (1.2)	12.93 (0.5)	0.650
Platelet count (10^9/L)	213.82 (41.73)	243.3 (86.16)	0.598	205.62 (38.2)	246.44 (91.76)	0.329
MPV (fL)	8.21 (1.19)	8.17 (0.8)	0.752	8.14 (1.27)	8.13 (0.79)	0.714

[†] Mann-Whitney for continuous variables without normal distribution and t-test for continuous data with normal distribution, $p < 0.05$. Lymphocytes (%), Segmented neutrophils (%), RBC, Hemoglobin, Hematocrit, MCV and MCH were compared with t-test, and remaining with Mann-Whitney test. P(−)—No Periodontitis, P(+)—Periodontitis; WBC—White Blood Cells; RBC—Red Blood Cells; MCV—Mean Cell Volume; MCH—Mean Cell Hemoglobin; MCHC—Mean Cell Hemoglobin Concentration; RCD—Red Cell Distribution; MPV—Mean Platelet Volume.

Table 3. Standard biochemical levels of PD patients with periodontitis and without periodontitis.

Variable	Global (n = 37)			Secure PD Medication (n = 29)		
	P(−)	P(+)	p-Value [†]	P(−)	P(+)	p-Value [†]
Albumin (g/dL)	4.19 (0.31)	4.02 (0.97)	0.775	4.15 (0.32)	3.99 (1.09)	0.714
ALT (U/L)	21.53 (11.12)	20.6 (15.54)	0.517	21.77 (12.45)	21.25 (17.32)	0.682
AST (U/L)	24.53 (8.22)	22.95 (10.68)	0.821	25.38 (9.26)	23 (11.87)	0.650
AP (U/L)	76.41 (26.04)	75.45 (28.62)	0.916	81.92 (27.02)	75.19 (30.63)	0.540
Blood urea nitrogen (mg/dL)	14.12 (6.71)	14.00 (7.83)	0.916	14.92 (7.39)	14.06 (8.68)	0.812
Total calcium (mg/dL)	9.25 (0.39)	8.94 (2.13)	0.209	9.28 (0.42)	8.81 (2.37)	0.449
CPK (IU/L)	117.71 (69.34)	114.4 (71.15)	0.798	113.92 (67.13)	118.5 (73.93)	0.619
Cholesterol (mg/dL)	179.41 (39)	175.15 (48.95)	0.869	176.08 (42.41)	174.94 (54.9)	0.619
Bicarbonate (mmol/L)	25.06 (2.11)	23.1 (5.96)	0.232	25.38 (2.06)	22.69 (6.55)	0.092
Creatinine (mg/dL)	0.92 (0.29)	0.87 (0.3)	0.869	0.95 (0.31)	0.88 (0.33)	0.880
GGT (U/L)	20.76 (14.06)	26.9 (30.47)	0.684	21.92 (15.47)	29.19 (33.77)	0.812
Glucose, serum (mg/dL)	107.82 (51.97)	91.45 (27.09)	0.892	113.54 (58.4)	93.31 (29.78)	0.914
Iron, refrigerated (ug/dL)	89.12 (30.64)	74.65 (38.59)	0.080	85.15 (31.26)	72.88 (42.46)	0.170
LDH (U/L)	131.06 (24.8)	122.25 (36.4)	0.557	138.85 (21.86)	122.81 (39.98)	0.268
Phosphorus (mg/dL)	3.51 (0.51)	3.59 (0.9)	0.232	3.48 (0.57)	3.52 (0.99)	0.398
Total bilirubin (mg/dL)	0.68 (0.22)	0.5 (0.21)	0.016	0.64 (0.19)	0.51 (0.23)	0.110
Total Protein (g/dL)	6.92 (0.6)	6.63 (1.66)	0.940	6.82 (0.59)	6.61 (1.86)	0.475
Uric acid (mg/dL)	4.81 (1.39)	4.95 (1.65)	0.794	4.73 (1.31)	5.14 (1.74)	0.487
Sodium (mmol/L)	139.06 (1.92)	132.3 (31.19)	0.869	139.15 (1.68)	130.44 (34.83)	0.880
Potassium (mmol/L)	4.01 (0.27)	3.84 (0.98)	0.752	4.04 (0.25)	3.84 (1.1)	1.000
Chloride (mmol/L)	104.76 (2.61)	98.85 (23.45)	0.270	104.31 (2.56)	97.38 (26.16)	0.398
Osmolality (mmol/Kg)	278.65 (5.74)	264.75 (62.47)	0.619	279.38 (5.69)	261.31 (69.84)	0.779
Globulin (g/dL)	2.73 (0.45)	2.62 (0.77)	0.916	2.67 (0.45)	2.61 (0.86)	0.779
Triglycerides (mg/dL)	119.82 (86.92)	161.5 (109.11)	0.149	109.31 (68.72)	178.63 (115.18)	0.068
25OHD2+25OHD3 (nmol/L)	75.56 (21.29)	77.11 (34.24)	0.873	71.14 (18.69)	68.59 (30.07)	0.792
25OHD2 (nmol/L)	4.27 (8.53)	11.12 (33.31)	0.478	4.93 (9.73)	4.52 (12.07)	0.423
25OHD3 (nmol/L)	71.28 (23.24)	65.97 (32.46)	0.578	66.18 (21.07)	64.03 (29.9)	0.829
epi-25OHD3 (nmol/L)	3.47 (2.11)	3.68 (2.19)	0.557[†]	2.89 (1.28)	3.7 (2.36)	0.351

[†] Mann-Whitney for continuous variables without normal distribution and t-test for continuous data with normal distribution, $p < 0.05$. Uric Acid and epi-25OHD3 were compared with Mann-Whitney test, and the remaining with t-test. P(−)—No Periodontitis, P(+)—Periodontitis; ALT—Alanine aminotransferase; AST—Aspartate aminotransferase; AP—Alkaline phosphatase; CPK—Creatine Phosphokinase; GGT—Gamma glutamyl transferase; LDH—Lactate dehydrogenase; 25OHD2—25-hydroxyvitamin D2; 25OHD3— 25-hydroxyvitamin D3.

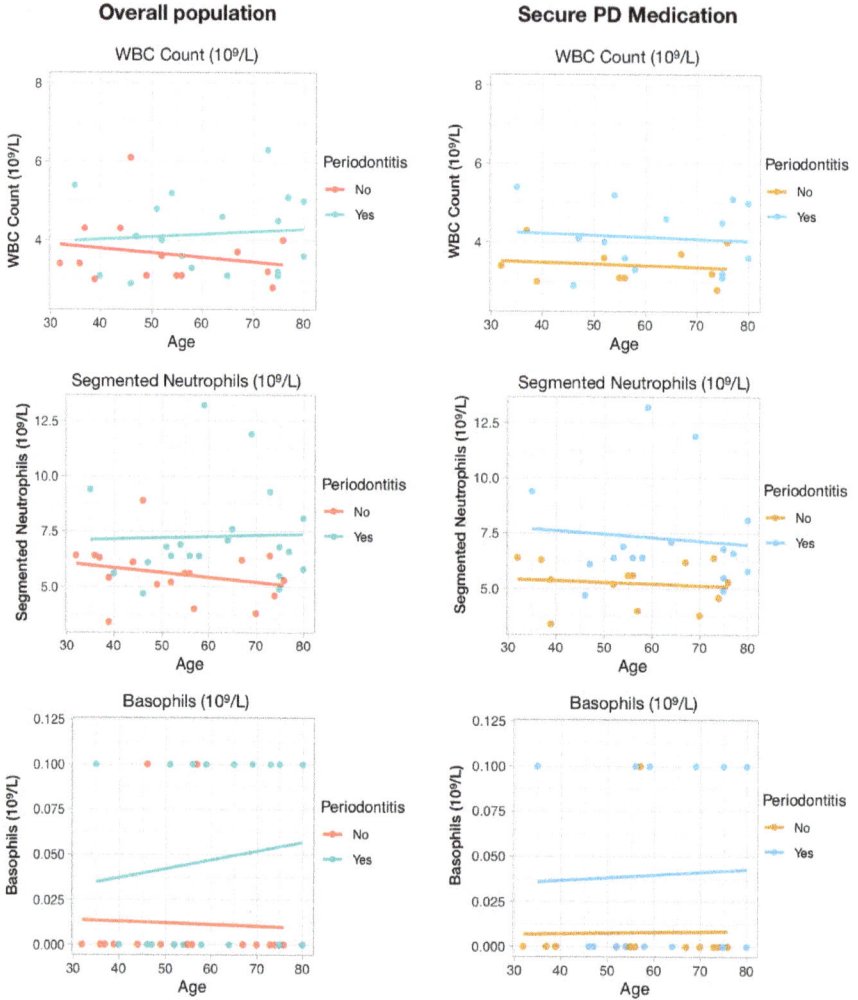

Figure 1. Comparison of WBC Count, Segmented neutrophils and Basophils serum levels between Periodontitis and no Periodontitis PD participants both in the overall sample and Secure PD medications. Lines represent graphically the tendency.

3.3. Predictive Models of Periodontitis on PD Patients

In order to analyze which factors would discriminate the periodontitis presence, we performed multivariable stepwise regression analyses considering each factor. In the overall sample, blood WBC levels were consistently identified as a discriminative factor towards periodontitis (B = 0.773, p =0.025) (Table 4). Among the participants with secure PD medication, we found discriminative factors to be gender (male) (B = 5.126, p = 0.026), Segmented Neutrophils (B = 4.232, p = 0.027) and 25OHD2 (B = −0.127, p = 0.060). The second model evidenced an improved score for correct classification (89.7%).

Table 4. Final reduced logistic regression models for the overall population ($n = 37$) and patients with secure PD medication ($n = 29$).

	Crude Model				Adjusted Model			
	B	p-Value	Exp(B)	95% CI for Exp(B)	B	p-Value	Exp(B)	95% CI for Exp(B)
Model 1—Overall population ($n = 37$) [1]								
WBC count (10^9/L)	0.773	0.025	2.1	1.1–4.2	0.773	0.025	2.2	1.1–4.3
Model 2—Secure PD medication ($n = 29$) [2]								
Gender (male)	5.064	0.024	158.3	2.0–12760.6	5.126	0.026	19.2	1.2–297.1
Segmented neutrophils (10^9/L)	3.727	0.090	41.6	0.6–3069.7	4.232	0.027	14.2	1.57–128.8
25OHD2 (nmol/L)	−0.130	0.058	0.9	0.8–1.0	−0.127	0.060	0.9	0.8–1.0

[1] $R^2(n) = 0.291$, % correct classification = 75.0%. [2] $R^2(n) = 0.730$, % correct classification = 89.7%. B—unstandardized regression coefficient; WBC—White Blood Cells.

4. Discussion

In the present representative study from the NHANES 2011–2012, periodontitis was associated with increased serum levels in PD patients. Therefore, our hypothesis was confirmed, in which leukocyte levels (WBC count, segmented neutrophils and basophils) and bilirubin were increased in periodontitis cases in this particular population. Furthermore, for the overall population WBC count showed potential predictive value towards periodontitis, while for secure PD medications gender, segmented neutrophils and 25OHD2 were the meaningful elements.

The link between periodontitis and leukocytosis is well documented [35–40]. This result is expected given the infectious nature of periodontitis where bacteria invade the periodontal tissues via the ulcerated epithelium, and leukocytes, in particular neutrophils, are triggered towards the periodontal injury [40–42]. Neutrophils had been associated with periodontitis pathogenesis [40,43,44] and were established as key players involved in many inflammatory chronic and aging-related diseases [44]. Neutrophils represent the vast majority (≥95%) of leukocytes recruited to the periodontal pocket [45]. Despite the homeostasis role of neutrophils in the healthy periodontium [3], they are impaired in periodontitis [1]. The chronic recruitment of excessive neutrophil, and therefore the increase of its serum counts, is learned as a consequence of the persisting microbial dysbiotic challenge [44]. The newness of this study is the likelihood of such parameters presenting predictive value towards periodontitis in PD cases, and future research is warranted to confirm this possibility.

Furthermore, male gender presented a higher risk to have periodontitis, this result being in line with previous reports that show males have a higher prevalence of periodontitis both in representative [10,46,47] and PD populations [23–26]. This result is of particular relevance because, in the same fashion as periodontitis, PD is more prevalent in men [18–20]. Additionally, the prevalence of periodontitis in this age-group is in line with previous studies developed in this region, where this age groups have high levels of periodontal disease [46–48].

Additionally, the presence of 25OHD2 in the predictive models is also in accordance with previous studies, where individuals with periodontitis were associated with lower levels of Vitamin D, compared to non-periodontitis [49–53]. Further, Vitamin D concentrations were associated with higher periodontal destruction, severe periodontitis stages and higher tooth loss [54–58]. Vitamin D also influences the immune response through the regulation of cathelicidin [59]. Interestingly, cathelicidin is an antimicrobial peptide produced by neutrophils and has been shown that dysregulated neutrophils in periodontitis lead to a low secretion of cathelicidin [60], though this should be further investigated. Therefore, Vitamin D levels may be an interesting clinical surrogate to consider in this link of periodontitis with PD, though it demands more studies to allow strong conclusions. However, we should carefully interpret these findings because of the lack of significance according to the periodontal status but its predictive value to infer periodontitis.

The present report has limitations important to mention and discuss. Despite this sample deriving from a large representative U.S. population survey, the final number of included patients was small.

However, this small number can be explained by the fact that PD affects 1% of individuals over 60 [11]. In our study, the overall prevalence of PD patients confirmed by medication represented 0.4% of the entire population and 1.0% of the sample that was examined for periodontitis. Thus, the sample size of this study limits the validity of these results and warrants future confirmation with prospective studies, since there are inherent biases in cross-sectional studies, such as selection bias. Notwithstanding, the identification of PD patients was also a limitation, since was based on the medication consumption present in the NHANES database with inherent selection bias. While for some medications this is somehow secure (Benztropine, Carbidopa, Levodopa, Ropinirole, Methyldopa and Entacapone) for others this is not the case (Cabergoline, Orphenadrine and Pramipexole) [30–34]. Yet, PD clinical diagnosis is even now considered to be speculative, since a definitive diagnosis always implies a post-mortem examination [13,61]. Another shortcoming is the medication itself since this survey was carried out in 2011–2012, and a large variation of medication gained therapeutic relevance in recent years. Furthermore, therapeutic adherence in PD is sub-optimal in a significant proportion of patients with PD [62], and we may have had a sample shortage due to this reason. Further, this approach does not deliver any causality rather an associative conclusion, and future studies should investigate in more depth how PD and periodontitis relate systemically, and if treating periodontitis might alleviate these elevated surrogates. Moreover, white blood cells and neutrophils were used as proxy of systemic inflammation and PISA as proxy to oral inflammation, though more evidence, such as immunohistochemistry staining of the periodontal tissues, indicating the infiltration level of neutrophils, monocytes and related white blood cells are warranted to further confirm our results to expand this matter. Lastly, the number of analyzed markers may be considered excessive, as future studies will narrow analysis to the most relevant measures.

In spite of these limitations, this article has important strengths. Our report is the first to depict the potential effect of the presence of periodontitis on the systemic status of PD. Further, NHANES is prospectively a reliable source of data to determine associations as previously demonstrated [63], and public data bank analysis (such as NHANES) are key towards more comprehensive oral health studies. Furthermore, we were able to produce predictive estimates using serum surrogates, which may be clinically relevant for the multidisciplinary team of PD. These results underline the importance of oral health care and how it can become unbalanced with the progression of this neurodegenerative disease, and the importance of more studies to investigate the systemic influence of periodontitis on PD.

5. Conclusions

Periodontitis was associated with an increase of white blood cells count, segmented neutrophils and basophils in PD patients. Furthermore, white blood cells count, segmented neutrophils, Vitamin D2 and gender showed discriminatory value to predict the existence of periodontitis in PD cases. Future studies should assess in more detail the potential systemic repercussion of the presence of periodontitis in PD patients.

Author Contributions: Conceptualization, J.B., V.M.; methodology, J.B.; validation, V.M., L.P. and J.B.; formal analysis, J.B.; investigation, J.B., V.M., P.L., C.G. and J.J.M.; resources, J.B., V.M.; data curation, J.B.; writing—original draft preparation, all authors.; writing—review and editing, all authors; supervision, V.M. All authors have read and agreed to the published version of the manuscript.

Funding: This research received no external funding.

Conflicts of Interest: The authors declare no conflict of interest

References

1. Hajishengallis, G. Periodontitis: From microbial immune subversion to systemic inflammation. *Nat. Rev. Immunol.* **2014**, *15*, 30–44. [CrossRef] [PubMed]
2. Slots, J. Periodontitis: Facts, fallacies and the future. *Periodontol. 2000* **2017**, *75*, 7–23. [CrossRef] [PubMed]

3. Darveau, R.P. Periodontitis: A polymicrobial disruption of host homeostasis. *Nat. Rev. Genet.* **2010**, *8*, 481–490. [CrossRef] [PubMed]
4. Aguilera, E.M.; Suvan, J.; Buti, J.; Czesnikiewicz-Guzik, M.; Ribeiro, A.; Orlandi, M.; Guzik, T.J.; Hingorani, A.D.; Nart, J.; D'Aiuto, F. Periodontitis is associated with hypertension: A systematic review and meta-analysis. *Cardiovasc. Res.* **2019**, *116*, 28–39. [CrossRef]
5. Preshaw, P.M.; Alba, A.L.; Herrera, D.; Jepsen, S.; Konstantinidis, A.; Makrilakis, K.; Taylor, R. Periodontitis and diabetes: A two-way relationship. *Diabetologia* **2012**, *55*, 21–31. [CrossRef] [PubMed]
6. Hussain, S.B.; Botelho, J.; Machado, V.; Zehra, S.A.; Mendes, J.J.; Ciurtin, C.; Orlandi, M.; Aiuto, F.D. Is there a bidirectional association between rheumatoid arthritis and periodontitis? A systematic review and meta-analysis. *Semin. Arthritis Rheum.* **2020**, *50*, 414–422. [CrossRef]
7. Dominy, S.S.; Lynch, C.; Ermini, F.; Benedyk, M.; Marczyk, A.; Konradi, A.; Nguyen, M.; Haditsch, U.; Raha, D.; Griffin, C.; et al. Porphyromonas gingivalisin Alzheimer's disease brains: Evidence for disease causation and treatment with small-molecule inhibitors. *Sci. Adv.* **2019**, *5*, eaau3333. [CrossRef]
8. Hashioka, S.; Inoue, K.; Miyaoka, T.; Hayashida, M.; Wake, R.; Oh-Nishi, A.; Inagaki, M. The Possible Causal Link of Periodontitis to Neuropsychiatric Disorders: More Than Psychosocial Mechanisms. *Int. J. Mol. Sci.* **2019**, *20*, 3723. [CrossRef]
9. Dioguardi, M.; Crincoli, V.; Laino, L.; Alovisi, M.; Sovereto, D.; Mastrangelo, F.; Russo, L.L.; Muzio, L.L. The Role of Periodontitis and Periodontal Bacteria in the Onset and Progression of Alzheimer's Disease: A Systematic Review. *J. Clin. Med.* **2020**, *9*, 495. [CrossRef]
10. Ebersole, J.L.; Al-Sabbagh, M.; Gonzalez, O.A.; Dawson, D.R. Ageing effects on humoral immune responses in chronic periodontitis. *J. Clin. Periodontol.* **2018**, *45*, 680–692. [CrossRef]
11. Tysnes, O.-B.; Storstein, A. Epidemiology of Parkinson's disease. *J. Neural Transm.* **2017**, *124*, 901–905. [CrossRef]
12. De Lau, L.M.; Breteler, M.M. Epidemiology of Parkinson's disease. *Lancet Neurol.* **2006**, *5*, 525–535. [CrossRef]
13. Kalia, L.V.; Lang, A.E. Parkinson's disease. *Lancet* **2015**, *386*, 896–912. [CrossRef]
14. Foltynie, T.; Brayne, C.; Barker, R.A. The heterogeneity of idiopathic Parkinson's disease. *J. Neurol.* **2002**, *249*, 138–145. [CrossRef]
15. Poewe, W.; Seppi, K.; Tanner, C.M.; Halliday, G.M.; Brundin, P.; Volkmann, J.; Schrag, A.E.; Lang, A.E. Parkinson disease. *Nat. Rev. Dis. Prim.* **2017**, *3*, 1–21. [CrossRef] [PubMed]
16. Obeso, J.A.; Rodríguez-Oroz, M.C.; Goetz, C.G.; Marín, C.; Kordower, J.H.; Rodriguez, M.; Hirsch, E.C.; Farrer, M.J.; Schapira, A.H.V.; Halliday, G.M. Missing pieces in the Parkinson's disease puzzle. *Nat. Med.* **2010**, *16*, 653–661. [CrossRef] [PubMed]
17. Johnson, M.E.; Stecher, B.; Labrie, V.; Brundin, L.; Brundin, P. Triggers, Facilitators, and Aggravators: Redefining Parkinson's Disease Pathogenesis. *Trends Neurosci.* **2018**, *42*, 4–13. [CrossRef]
18. Schrag, A.; Quinn, N.P.; Irving, R.J.; Oram, S.H.; Boyd, J.; Rutledge, P.; Mcrae, F.; Bloomfield, P. Cross sectional prevalence survey of idiopathic Parkinson's disease and parkinsonism in London Ten year audit of secondary prevention in coronary bypass patients. *BMJ* **2000**, *321*, 21–22. [CrossRef]
19. Alves, G.; Müller, B.; Herlofson, K.; HogenEsch, I.; Telstad, W.; Aarsland, D.; Tysnes, O.-B.; Larsen, J.P. Incidence of Parkinson's disease in Norway: The Norwegian ParkWest study. *J. Neurol. Neurosurg. Psychiatry* **2009**, *80*, 851–857. [CrossRef]
20. Ferreira, J.J.; Gonçalves, N.; Valadas, A.; Januário, C.; Silva, M.R.; Nogueira, L.; Vieira, J.L.M.; Lima, A.B. Prevalence of Parkinson's disease: A population-based study in Portugal. *Eur. J. Neurol.* **2017**, *24*, 748–750. [CrossRef]
21. Ray Dorsey, E.; Elbaz, A.; Nichols, E.; Abd-Allah, F.; Abdelalim, A.; Adsuar, J.C.; Ansha, M.G.; Brayne, C.; Choi, J.Y.J.; Collado-Mateo, D.; et al. Global, regional, and national burden of Parkinson's disease, 1990–2016: A systematic analysis for the Global Burden of Disease Study 2016. *Lancet Neurol.* **2018**, *17*, 939–953. [CrossRef]
22. Kaur, T.; Uppoor, A.; Naik, D. Parkinson's disease and periodontitis—The missing link? A review. *Gerodontology* **2015**, *33*, 434–438. [CrossRef] [PubMed]
23. Einarsdóttir, E.R.; Gunnsteinsdóttir, H.; Hallsdóttir, M.H.; Sveinsson, S.; Jónsdóttir, S.R.; Olafsson, V.G.; Bragason, T.H.; Saemundsson, S.R.; Holbrook, W.P.; Sæmundsson, S.R. Dental health of patients with Parkinson's disease in Iceland. *Spec. Care Dent.* **2009**, *29*, 123–127. [CrossRef] [PubMed]

24. Hanaoka, A.; Kashihara, K. Increased frequencies of caries, periodontal disease and tooth loss in patients with Parkinson's disease. *J. Clin. Neurosci.* **2009**, *16*, 1279–1282. [CrossRef]
25. Nakayama, Y.; Washio, M.; Mori, M. Oral health conditions in patients with Parkinson's disease. *J. Epidemiol.* **2004**, *14*, 143–150. [CrossRef]
26. Van Stiphout, M.A.E.; Marinus, J.; van Hilten, J.J.; Lobbezoo, F.; de Baat, C. Oral Health of Parkinson's Disease Patients: A Case-Control Study. *Parkinsons. Dis.* **2018**, *2018*, e13. [CrossRef]
27. Schwarz, J.; Heimhilger, E.; Storch, A. Increased periodontal pathology in Parkinson's disease. *J. Neurol.* **2006**, *253*, 608–611. [CrossRef]
28. Chen, C.-K.; Wu, Y.-T.; Chang, Y.-C. Periodontal inflammatory disease is associated with the risk of Parkinson's disease: A population-based retrospective matched-cohort study. *PeerJ* **2017**, *5*, e3647. [CrossRef]
29. Eke, P.I.; Dye, B.A.; Wei, L.; Thornton-Evans, G.O.; Genco, R.J. Prevalence of Periodontitis in Adults in the United States: 2009 and 2010. *J. Dent. Res.* **2012**, *91*, 914–920. [CrossRef]
30. Fox, S.H.; Katzenschlager, R.; Lim, S.Y.; Ravina, B.; Seppi, K.; Coelho, M.; Poewe, W.; Rascol, O.; Goetz, C.G.; Sampaio, C. The movement disorder society evidence-based medicine review update: Treatments for the motor symptoms of Parkinson's disease. *Mov. Disord.* **2011**, *26*, 2–41. [CrossRef]
31. Seppi, K.; Weintraub, D.; Coelho, M.; Perez-Lloret, S.; Fox, S.H.; Katzenschlager, R.; Hametner, E.-M.; Poewe, W.; Rascol, O.; Goetz, C.G.; et al. The Movement Disorder Society Evidence-Based Medicine Review Update: Treatments for the non-motor symptoms of Parkinson's disease. *Mov. Disord.* **2011**, *26*, S42–S80. [CrossRef] [PubMed]
32. Anna, B.G.S.; Musolino, N.R.C.; Gadelha, M.R.; Marques, C.; Castro, M.; Elias, P.C.L.; Vilar, L.; Lyra, R.; Martins, M.R.A.; Quidute, A.R.P.; et al. A Brazilian multicentre study evaluating pregnancies induced by cabergoline in patients harboring prolactinomas. *Pituitary* **2019**, *23*, 120–128. [CrossRef] [PubMed]
33. Abd-Elsalam, S.; Ebrahim, S.; Soliman, S.; Alkhalawany, W.; Elfert, A.; Hawash, N.; Elkadeem, M.; Badawi, R. Orphenadrine in treatment of muscle cramps in cirrhotic patients. *Eur. J. Gastroenterol. Hepatol.* **2019**, 1. [CrossRef] [PubMed]
34. De Biase, S.; Pellitteri, G.; Gigli, G.L.; Valente, M. Advancing synthetic therapies for the treatment of restless legs syndrome. *Expert Opin. Pharmacother.* **2019**, *20*, 1971–1980. [CrossRef]
35. Nibali, L.; Darbar, U.; Rakmanee, T.; Donos, N.; Nibali, L. Anemia of inflammation associated with periodontitis: Analysis of two clinical studies. *J. Periodontol.* **2019**, *90*, 1252–1259. [CrossRef]
36. Temelli, B.; Ay, Z.Y.; Aksoy, F.; Büyükbayram, H.I.; Doguc, D.K.; Uskun, E.; Varol, E. Platelet indices (mean platelet volume and platelet distribution width) have correlations with periodontal inflamed surface area in coronary artery disease patients: A pilot study. *J. Periodontol.* **2018**, *89*, 1203–1212. [CrossRef]
37. Kumar, B.P.; Khaitan, T.; Ramaswamy, P.; Sreenivasulu, P.; Uday, G.; Velugubantla, R.G. Association of chronic periodontitis with white blood cell and platelet count—A Case Control Study. *J. Clin. Exp. Dent.* **2014**, *6*, e214–e217. [CrossRef]
38. Wang, X.; Meng, H.; Xu, L.; Chen, Z.; Shi, D.; Lv, D. Mean platelet volume as an inflammatory marker in patients with severe periodontitis. *Platelets* **2014**, *26*, 67–71. [CrossRef]
39. Papapanagiotou, D.; Nicu, E.A.; Bizzarro, S.; Gerdes, V.E.; Meijers, J.C.; Nieuwland, R.; Van Der Velden, U.; Loos, B.G. Periodontitis is associated with platelet activation. *Atherosclerosis* **2009**, *202*, 605–611. [CrossRef]
40. Hirschfeld, J. Dynamic interactions of neutrophils and biofilms. *J. Oral Microbiol.* **2014**, *6*, 135. [CrossRef]
41. Ryder, M.I. Comparison of neutrophil functions in aggressive and chronic periodontitis. *Periodontol. 2000* **2010**, *53*, 124–137. [CrossRef]
42. Aboodi, G.M.; Goldberg, M.B.; Glogauer, M. Refractory Periodontitis Population Characterized by a Hyperactive Oral Neutrophil Phenotype. *J. Periodontol.* **2011**, *82*, 726–733. [CrossRef] [PubMed]
43. Loesche, W.J.; Robinson, J.P.; Flynn, M.; Hudson, J.L.; Duque, R.A. Reduced oxidative function in gingival crevicular neutrophils in periodontal disease. *Infect. Immun.* **1988**, *56*, 156–160. [CrossRef] [PubMed]
44. Hajishengallis, G. New developments in neutrophil biology and periodontitis. *Periodontol. 2000* **2019**, *82*, 78–92. [CrossRef] [PubMed]
45. DeLima, A.J.; Van Dyke, T.E. Origin and function of the cellular components in gingival crevice fluid. *Periodontol. 2000* **2003**, *31*, 55–76. [CrossRef] [PubMed]
46. Machado, V.; Botelho, J.; Amaral, A.; Proença, L.; Alves, R.; Rua, J.; Cavacas, M.A.; Delgado, A.S.; Mendes, J.J. Prevalence and extent of chronic periodontitis and its risk factors in a Portuguese subpopulation: A retrospective cross-sectional study and analysis of Clinical Attachment Loss. *PeerJ* **2018**, *6*, e5258. [CrossRef]

47. Botelho, J.; Machado, V.; Proença, L.; Alves, R.; Cavacas, M.A.; Amaro, L.; Mendes, J.J. Study of Periodontal Health in Almada-Seixal (SoPHiAS): A cross-sectional study in the Lisbon Metropolitan Area. *Sci. Rep.* **2019**, *9*. [CrossRef]
48. Botelho, J.; Machado, V.; Proença, L.; Oliveira, M.J.; Cavacas, M.A.; Amaro, L.; Águas, A.; Mendes, J.J. Perceived xerostomia, stress and periodontal status impact on elderly oral health-related quality of life: Findings from a cross-sectional survey. *BMC Oral Health* **2020**, *20*, 1–9. [CrossRef]
49. Anbarcioglu, E.; Kirtiloglu, T.; Ozturk, A.; Kolbakir, F.; Acıkgoz, G.; Colak, R. Vitamin D deficiency in patients with aggressive periodontitis. *Oral Dis.* **2018**, *25*, 242–249. [CrossRef]
50. Agrawal, A.A.; Kolte, A.P.; Kolte, R.A.; Chari, S.; Gupta, M.; Pakhmode, R. Evaluation and comparison of serum vitamin D and calcium levels in periodontally healthy, chronic gingivitis and chronic periodontitis in patients with and without diabetes mellitus—A cross-sectional study. *Acta Odontol. Scand.* **2019**, *77*, 592–599. [CrossRef]
51. Ebersole, J.L.; Lambert, J.; Bush, H.M.; Emecen-Huja, P.; Basu, A. Serum Nutrient Levels and Aging Effects on Periodontitis. *Nutrients* **2018**, *10*, 1986. [CrossRef] [PubMed]
52. Isola, G.; Alibrandi, A.; Rapisarda, E.; Matarese, G.; Williams, R.C.; Leonardi, R. Association of vitamin D in patients with periodontitis: A cross-sectional study. *J. Periodontal Res.* **2020**, 1–11. [CrossRef] [PubMed]
53. Ketharanathan, V.; Torgersen, G.R.; Petrovski, B. Éva; Preus, H.R. Radiographic alveolar bone level and levels of serum 25-OH-Vitamin D3 in ethnic Norwegian and Tamil periodontitis patients and their periodontally healthy controls. *BMC Oral Health* **2019**, *19*, 83. [CrossRef] [PubMed]
54. Millen, A.E.; Hovey, K.M.; LaMonte, M.J.; Swanson, M.; Andrews, C.A.; Kluczynski, M.A.; Genco, R.J.; Wactawski-Wende, J. Plasma 25-hydroxyvitamin D concentrations and periodontal disease in postmenopausal women. *J. Periodontol.* **2012**, *84*, 1243–1256. [CrossRef] [PubMed]
55. Antonoglou, G.N.; Knuuttila, M.; Niemela, O.; Raunio, T.; Karttunen, R.; Vainio, O.; Hedberg, P.; Ylöstalo, P.; Tervonen, T. Low serum level of 1,25(OH)2D is associated with chronic periodontitis. *J. Periodontal Res.* **2014**, *50*, 274–280. [CrossRef] [PubMed]
56. Dietrich, T.; Joshipura, K.; Dawson-Hughes, B.; Bischoff-Ferrari, H.A. Association between serum concentrations of 25-hydroxyvitamin D3 and periodontal disease in the US population. *Am. J. Clin. Nutr.* **2004**, *80*, 108–113.
57. Zhan, Y.; Samietz, S.; Holtfreter, B.; Hannemann, A.; Meisel, P.; Nauck, M.; Völzke, H.; Wallaschofski, H.; Dietrich, T.; Kocher, T. Prospective Study of Serum 25-hydroxy Vitamin D and Tooth Loss. *J. Dent. Res.* **2014**, *93*, 639–644. [CrossRef]
58. Botelho, J.; Machado, V.; Proença, L.; Delgado, A.S.; Mendes, J.J. Vitamin D Deficiency and Oral Health: A Comprehensive Review. *Nutrients* **2020**, *12*, 1471. [CrossRef]
59. Chung, C.; Silwal, P.; Kim, I.; Modlin, R.L.; Jo, E.-K. Vitamin D-Cathelicidin Axis: At the Crossroads between Protective Immunity and Pathological Inflammation during Infection. *Immune Netw.* **2020**, *20*, 1–26. [CrossRef]
60. Marinho, M.C.; Pacheco, A.B.F.; Costa, G.C.V.; Ortiz, N.D.; Zajdenverg, L.; Sansone, C. Quantitative gingival crevicular fluid proteome in type 2 diabetes mellitus and chronic periodontitis. *Oral Dis.* **2018**, *25*, 588–595. [CrossRef]
61. Lebouvier, T.; Neunlist, M.; Varannes, S.B.D.; Coron, E.; Drouard, A.; N'Guyen, J.-M.; Chaumette, T.; Tasselli, M.; Paillusson, S.; Flamand, M.; et al. Colonic Biopsies to Assess the Neuropathology of Parkinson's Disease and Its Relationship with Symptoms. *PLoS ONE* **2010**, *5*, e12728. [CrossRef] [PubMed]
62. Sisodiya, S.M.; Grosset, D. Medication Adherence in Patients with Parkinson's Disease. *CNS Drugs* **2014**, *29*, 47–53. [CrossRef]
63. Montero, E.; Herrera, D.; Sanz, M.; Dhir, S.; Van Dyke, T.; Sima, C. Development and validation of a predictive model for periodontitis using NHANES 2011–2012 data. *J. Clin. Periodontol.* **2019**, *46*, 420–429. [CrossRef] [PubMed]

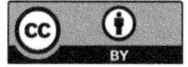

© 2020 by the authors. Licensee MDPI, Basel, Switzerland. This article is an open access article distributed under the terms and conditions of the Creative Commons Attribution (CC BY) license (http://creativecommons.org/licenses/by/4.0/).

MDPI
St. Alban-Anlage 66
4052 Basel
Switzerland
Tel. +41 61 683 77 34
Fax +41 61 302 89 18
www.mdpi.com

Journal of Personalized Medicine Editorial Office
E-mail: jpm@mdpi.com
www.mdpi.com/journal/jpm

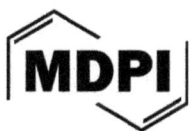